Performing Brains on Screen

Performing Brains on Screen

Fernando Vidal

Routledge
Taylor & Francis Group
LONDON AND NEW YORK

First published in 2022 by Amsterdam University Press Ltd.

Published 2025 by Routledge
4 Park Square, Milton Park, Abingdon, Oxon OX14 4RN
605 Third Avenue, New York, NY 10158

Routledge is an imprint of the Taylor & Francis Group, an informa business

ISBN: 9789462989146 (hbk)
ISBN: 9781041184027 (pbk)
ISBN: 9781003701217 (ebk)
NUR 670

Cover illustration: Martín Malamud.

Cover design: Coördesign, Leiden

DOI: 10.5117/9789462989146

For Product Safety Concerns and Information please contact our EU representative:
GPSR@taylorandfrancis.com
Taylor & Francis Verlag GmbH, Kaufingerstraße 24, 80331 München, Germany

For Cayetana, my filmmaker sister,
this souvenir of our time with Hieronymus Bosch

Table of Contents

Acknowledgments

Numerous film specialists seem to have chosen their field of studies out of their love for the cinema, as a spontaneous way to turn recreational fun into scholarly endeavor. This strikes me as being especially the case of those who write about the categories to which many of the movies discussed here belong: low-budget B-to-Z productions, many critically demolished at the time of their first screening, but later attaining "cult" status (the same applies to the pulp magazines we also discuss). The pleasure in which their vocation originates often manifests in their texts; their enjoyment shines through in their sense of humor and their frequently immense erudition, and in the best instances, they lead their readers to partake in their fun and to open up, both critically and aesthetically, to worlds they (the readers) had perhaps snubbed or simply ignored. I arrived at these movies in a different way, starting from a thoroughly filmless intellectual history of the human viewed as a "cerebral subject." The remarks on film in an article by the medievalist Caroline Bynum (1995), a mentor and friend, helped me realize the potential of cinema for this topic. As I studied the history of modern subjectivities and the contemporary "neuroscientific turn," my attention was directed to performances of the brain on screen, and to the large-scale exploration whose results are offered here. With time, I've come to feel like a member of the community of academics whose interest in "bad movies" began as a pleasant pastime; and if I learned to enjoy them (and, frankly, to prefer them over most multimillion-dollar productions), it is in no small measure thanks to their insights and their enthusiastic and expert scholarship.

Over the years, too, a number of cinephiles, hardly any of them film or media studies professionals, provided me with information, titles, suggestions, commentaries, and even copies of pictures that were desperately unavailable (unfortunately, a few remained unobtainable, and the same must be said of some books, mainly in languages other than English). To all of them, as well as to the two demanding reviewers of this book's manuscript, I give my heartfelt thanks. Mention should be also made of the pseudonymous persons who share rare pearls on YouTube and other platforms. Although many more of the films I discuss are found there now than at the beginning of my inquiry, it is always gratifying to see friends and colleagues puzzle or grin over the bizarre DVDs, and even VHS cassettes, that sit on my shelves.

I owe a special debt to Hansun Hsiung and Martín Malamud.

Typescripts of the plays by Peggy Webling and John Balderston on which James Whale's 1931 *Frankenstein* is based were deposited in the Library of

Congress, Washington, DC, in 1928 and 1931. The Library, however, is not allowed to deliver copies. The quotations that appear in Chapter 5 come from the extensive notes Dr. Hsiung took down for me during a visit to Washington while he was a postdoctoral fellow at the Max Planck Institute for the History of Science, Berlin. It is a pleasure to acknowledge his extremely generous help. (It turned out that Balderston's play had been published in 2010; the volume, however, provides no sources and misleadingly suggests that the text is that of the film script.)

Martín Malamud – a draftsman of fantastic skill and brilliant imagination, and a dear friend from the years at the Colegio Nacional de Buenos Aires – graciously agreed to do the cover of this book. We hope readers will like it as much as we enjoyed our collaboration. ¡Gracias, Martín!

Finally, thanks are due to institutions that variously provided support, collegiality, and scholarly context, in particular: the Max Planck Institute for the History of Science (Berlin), the Pontifical Catholic University of Rio de Janeiro, the Centre Alexandre Koyré and the École des Hautes Études en Sciences Sociales (Paris), ICREA (Catalan Institution for Research and Advanced Studies), the Center (now Institute) for the History of Science at the Autonomous University of Barcelona, and the Medical Anthropology Research Center at the Department of Anthropology, Philosophy and Social Work (Rovira i Virgili University, Tarragona).

Note on References and Images

No page numbers are provided for quotations from e-books or online articles.

For technical reasons, this book does not include the images referred to in the text. They are referenced in the text as "Brainfilms," followed by the illustration number, and can be downloaded here: https://www.academia.edu/49648716/Brainfilms.

1. Brainhood and the Cinema

Abstract
This chapter outlines the main themes of *Performing Brains on Screen*. It explains the emphasis on *performance* (rather than mere representation), and critically examines the "deficit model" in the public understanding of science, the relevance of filmic genres, the interpretive strategy of "symptomatic reading," and ways of approaching philosophy in film or film as philosophy. It discusses varieties of "brainfilms" and the universe of B movies, which form an important part of the filmic material examined in the rest of the book. It also sketches the history of the emergence of the view of the human as "cerebral subject," as well as the "neuroscientific turn" in contemporary culture, both of which are central frameworks for the filmic performance of brains.

Keywords: brainfilm, cerebral subject, deficit model, neuroscientific turn, symptomatic reading, performance

Performing Brains on Screen explores how fiction film has enacted the belief that human beings are essentially their brains. It is a chapter in the history of two interrelated phenomena: on the one hand, a medium, the cinema; and on the other, the making of subjectivities as sustained by the view that humans are basically "cerebral subjects." The statement *You are your brain* embodies one of the most widespread and influential ways of understanding the human in contemporary culture. The ideology of the "neuro" it encapsulates began to acquire prominence in the nineteenth century. However, it has become truly global only since the "Decade of the Brain" in the 1990s, largely thanks to the increase in the range of application of brain-imaging technologies, which in turn gave impulse to a protean "neuroscientific turn" across many disciplines and social and intellectual spaces (Littlefield and Johnson 2012; Vidal and Ortega 2017). The cinema, though, has been using brains as a MacGuffin, as well as more substantially rehearsing avatars of the cerebral subject, before the rise of the "neuro" as a major global creed. It has done so by turning physical brains into the

Vidal, F., *Performing Brains on Screen*. Taylor & Francis Group, 2022
DOI 10.5117/9789462989146_CH01

protagonists of filmic action (as in the 1950s movies that show terrestrial or extraterrestrial "disembodied brains" pursuing generally evil intentions), or by giving brains (gruesomely displayed or invisible inside someone's head) an explicitly major role, as in brain transplantation films or their less carnal successors since the 1980s, in which brainmind contents are transferred and manipulated by means of information technologies.

Brains function in those movies as "characters," as fictional beings to which we ascribe the ability to think and act, and whose motivation is largely responsible for setting the action in motion (Eder 2010; Eder, Jannidis, and Schneider 2010). Their quality of character is nevertheless synecdochic: the isolated organ can play its role because it contains the mind and the personal identity of the individual to which it belonged. Thus, a significant number of the movies considered here enact personality or identity transfers, a popular theme since the earliest days of science fiction. On screen as on paper, brain transplantations and brains detached from bodies (with or without heads) have had the most "melodramatic potential" (Stableford 2006, 329). Nevertheless, as we shall see, all the existing ways of representing the brain and its activity, from the phrenological chart to contemporary neuroimaging, as well as developments ranging from the cerebral localization of sensory functions to the modern cognitive neurosciences, have made it into both film and literature. The result across media, genres, and styles has always been an aestheticizing and fetishizing of the brain, and alongside this, a reinforcement of its position as a modern cultural icon.

The most relevant filmic productions for a history of how brains have been performed can be characterized as *brain movies* or *brain-and-memory movies*. The former category has been defined so as to include productions involving wicked brains or malevolent brain-like entities (Senn and Johnson 1992, 99–109). It can nevertheless be enlarged to encompass all pictures, mostly from the 1940s to 1970s, where the brain visually appears as a main character. I will sometimes call them *brainfilms*, using Jeffrey Sconce's term for designating cinematic "narratives organized around the icon of the human brain" (Sconce 1995a, 281). Surgery, usually brain transplantation, is in these pictures a key visual and narrative ingredient, and functions as a primary device for unfolding main or secondary plots centered on what happens when an individual's brain (and therefore, so go the stories, the person) ends up located in someone else's body.

As for *brain-and-memory movies*, countless pictures assume that one's personal identity is defined fundamentally by one's memories. That assumption has long been a prime filmic resource, and the corpus of films where it is enacted as a basis for narrative and visual development is extremely large. Here I shall consider only the intersection between brain and memory – in other words, pictures that, while not always turning the brain itself into a protagonist, explicitly locate memories in the cerebral substance, and have plots and visuals that involve handling the brain as physical organ. In these productions, which date mostly from the 1980s onward, the computational approach tends to supersede the surgical, which prevailed in earlier films. Their manipulation of brain matter and contents usually entails micro-electronic procedures or computer-like operations for inserting, copying, transferring, selling, buying, controlling, grafting, deleting, downloading, or uploading "embrained" information. These procedures often require implanting microchips, and are conveyed through visuals reminiscent of neuroimagery. In this way, brainmind contents, consisting primarily of memories, can be engineered so that experiences, beliefs, information, and eventually an individual's entire identity are recorded and visualized, modified and programmed.

In spite of considerable differences – in their scripts, plots, visuals and special effects, in their representations of science and technology, in their characters and narrative types, in their styles and ambitions – both brain and brain-and-memory movies explore the relationships between having a body and being a brain, and assume that personhood and personal identity consist primarily of cerebral contents. Memory transfers turn out to be functional equivalents of brain transplantations: if A has B's brain, then A must have B's memories; and giving A's memories to B generally implies grafting or otherwise removing, altering, or displacing brain substance. Films that perform brains assume that the cerebral self is basically memorial, and that the memorial self is naturally cerebral. That is their intellectual core.

These features can be examined for their ideological and potentially philosophical meanings and related to long-standing debates about definitions of personhood and criteria of personal identity (Korfmacher 2006; Olson 2008. On brain identity as criterion, see Northoff and Wagner 2017). We should, however, keep in mind that motion pictures seek above all to make money and to entertain. Some elements or contents to which we could be tempted to attribute profound or revealing meanings respond to more mundane needs, as well as to goals and constraints internal to the cinema and its production. At the same time, most movies make things clear and (even if superficially) evoke deeper messages. They do so by means of didactic moments that provide scientific-sounding explanations, or cogitate on the ethical, philosophical, or societal implications of the action. These conspicuous, often clichéd and frustratingly distracting sequences (known in science-fiction narrative as "expository lumps") are heavy on dialogue, and often provide the "information" by means of voice-over.

Performing Brains on Screen documents this little-charted territory, describing how the cinema has functioned as a space where a core notion of the contemporary world has been assumed and conveyed, and at the very same time problematized and challenged. Indeed, while the motion pictures examined here invariably start out by asserting that we are our brains, most question their own initial claim or undermine its most reductionistic implications. The "neuronovels" that appeared in the early and mid-2000s share this strategy of ambivalence: they give the impression of adhering to the ideology of the cerebral subject, but tend to use *neuro* idioms and materials less as ideological assertions than as figurative possibilities with the potential to frame narratives about individual and social experience.

As a result of such strategies, the ways brains are performed on screen suggest that definitive solutions to the challenges they raise are unlikely to be forthcoming. Murray Smith notes that Carl Reiner's *All of Me* (1984) – a comedy in which a rich woman's soul is accidentally transferred to her lawyer's body, where it must coexist with the lawyer's own soul – seems simultaneously committed to dualism and monistic physicalism. Rather than interpreting the film's handling of identity as a symptom of philosophical inconsistency, he proposes seeing such paradoxical treatment "as a compact dramatization of our conflicting intuitions about the place of body in personal identity" (Smith 2006, 40). Undeniably, movies enact in numerous ways issues and questions that, whether individual, relational, collective, or global, are independent of them. In addition, however, *Performing Brains on Screen* assumes that motion pictures do not merely dramatize the offscreen world. Rather, it posits that, to the extent that movies are embedded in culture and are themselves part of the contexts where those issues and questions take root and are mobilized, they contribute to producing them, shaping them and transforming them.

The "Deficit Model" and the Agency of Film

This may seem obvious, but it is common to approach motion pictures as if they were factually truthful reflections of the world. Such a tendency, apparently spontaneous and in any case widespread, is particularly clear in commentary about movies that are perceived as conveying verifiable information, such as biopics, and pictures that involve historical actors and events, or science and scientists. The inclination to judge fiction films with regard to informative accuracy neglects the fact that, in most cases, their main goal is not to inform, but to entertain and make money, and that, by their very nature, they are obliged neither to instruct nor to follow what some experts and audiences regard as established fact. Even scientists who understand the constraints of the movie industry, the limits of what film can achieve when it comes to communicating "real science," and the "active feedback between real science and Hollywood science" insist that "society and the movie industry could benefit by better presentations of science on screen" (Perkowitz 2007, 215, 227). In contrast to such a turn of mind, I shall seldom discuss scientific information. It is clear that "science drives fiction and fiction drives sciences" in ways that have historically engaged both fantasies and research about the brain (Brake and Hook 2008). Nevertheless, even when a movie conveys science-inspired visuals and scientific-sounding idioms, I will not try to assess the extent to which it respects, reflects, represents, or distorts established hypotheses, ongoing investigations, or accepted knowledge. The trap I thereby wish to avoid goes by the name of the "deficit model."

The "deficit model" designates a way of approaching the public understanding of science and science communication that emphasizes scientific illiteracy and the need to educate the public. The label emerged in the 1990s to describe an established mode of analysis and practice characterized by the assumption "that *public understanding of science* coincides with *scientific literacy*," the belief that the ability to understand science as divulged by experts "guarantees favorable attitudes toward science and technological innovation," and the tendency to make the public answerable for the shortcomings of its relationship to science (Bucchi and Neresini 2007, 450). Since then, the deficit model has been the object of much empirical research and critical analysis in media studies, education, science studies, and the sociology of science and technology. Scholars and institutions engaged in science communication policy have developed alternative approaches aimed at taking account of contexts, giving room to lay expertise, or furthering public engagement (Brossard and Lewenstein 2010). In 2002, British scientists proposed replacing the label "Public Understanding of Science" with "Public Engagement in Science and Technology" (Holden 2002). This shift "from PUS to PEST" then became the narrative officially adopted "across continents and by governments, scientific societies, intergovernmental bodies, civil society organizations and many more interests" (Trench 2008, 120). By 2007, the journal *Public Understanding of Science* could proclaim, "We have clearly moved from the old days of the deficit frame" (Einsiedel 2007, 5). Yet less than a decade later, it launched an essay competition on the question, "Why does the 'deficit model' not go away?" (Bauer 2016, 398).

Scientists, too, have nervously asked the same question. Noting that the deficit model is "wrong" and nonetheless endures, a 2017 report of the US National Academies of Sciences, Engineering, and Medicine called for the use of systemic and contextual approaches to achieve more effective communication, which it considered especially necessary "when science related to contentious issues is involved in public controversy" (NAS 2017). Motion pictures are seen as a major means of attaining that goal. Public and private initiatives worldwide encourage filmmakers to tackle science and technology topics with the goal of informing audiences adequately about them and encouraging an appreciation for science. In spite of putatively democratizing aims, these initiatives uphold scientists' claims to absolute epistemic authority. Their outlook was captured in a 2009 *Nature Physics* editorial celebrating the globalization of science film festivals, which characterized "a good science film" as "a good film in which good (correct) science is central to the plot, or at least has a strong supporting part" (Anon. 2009).

Beyond science communication, the endurance of the deficit model is part of a broader and longer-lasting phenomenon: the persistence of realism as a criterion for judging figurative artworks. Resemblance and representation can be assessed according to a variety of criteria; the terms associated with the realist outlook, such as *accuracy*, *authenticity*, *fidelity*, *truthfulness*, or *verisimilitude*, are neither univocal nor self-contained (Vidal 2018). As linguist Roman Jakobson (1921) remarked a century ago, the concept and phenomenon of realism are extremely elastic. A range of artistic movements have adopted faithfulness to reality as their guiding maxim, and realism can be brought about in many different, even incompatible ways, from following accepted representational norms to violating them systematically in order to make viewers confront "the real" that lies beyond representation. More than a "period style," therefore, realism is a "recurrent effect" (McHale 2008, 7) – and one that has been prominent in the history of film aesthetics.

Insofar as the cinema is able to use all modes of representation and narration, and thus to "engender a unique event of sight and sound that *need* be perceived neither as a real event nor as an illusion of such an event" (Seel 2008, 166), it is as indifferent to realism as it is to anti-realism. Film, however, has long been understood as entertaining an ontological or indexical relation with reality. The "evidential force" Roland Barthes (1980, 89) found in photography seems potentiated by movies' capacity to combine time and movement, as well as by the resulting reality effects and their physical, emotional, and intellectual impact. This realist stance prevailed until the 1960s (Aitken 2001,

Chaps. 7–8; Aitken 2006, 2016; Thomson-Jones 2008, Chap. 2). The analytic focus later shifted from an interest in the phenomenal depiction of reality to the analysis of semiological means and conventions (Stam, Burgoyne and Flitterman-Lewis 1992, Part V). Since the mid-1990s, however, realist perspectives have re-emerged in world cinema and television, supported by a "cognitivist" perspective (Nagib and Mello 2009) according to which "perceptual recognition of something in the [filmic] image is on the whole neither arbitrary nor culturally variable" (Bordwell 2015).

Without going further into the problem of realism or the conditions of perceptual recognition, let us repeat the obvious: motion pictures are always documents bearing traces of contents, structures, and events that exist before, beneath, above, and beyond the screen. One way or another, they articulate values, beliefs, and concerns that subsist without them. They can therefore be approached as the expression and elaboration of issues that circulate in the "outside world." Nevertheless, since the cinema belongs in that world and movies are integral to the contexts they supposedly reflect, they must be considered as active agents in structuring them. That is why not every film is best analyzed by the methodical application of the interpretive strategy known as "symptomatic reading," which sees each and every feature as an expression of latent or concealed meanings (Best and Marcus 2009). This is another form of realism, one focused not on the most manifest appearance, but on unconscious, hidden signification. Distancing oneself from realist modes implies a caveat about film and philosophy: exploring philosophical issues through film and discussing movies as if they were philosophical thought experiments can be fun and illuminating; they should not, however, abolish film as film, nor neglect the contextual conditions, from the technical and the commercial to the aesthetic and the political, in which pictures are produced. Furthermore, dealing with "film as film" means paying attention not only to the textual and narrative dimensions of plots and dialogues, which are the focus of most philosophical commentary, but also to specifically cinematographic features, techniques and operations.

As explained above, *Performing Brains on Screen* considers movies as important pieces in the history of the cerebral subject. This view of what humans are belongs in the history of debates about personhood and personal identity. These are venerable and interrelated philosophical problems. It is therefore by no means surprising that the cinema has dealt with them and that it has in turn attracted philosophical attention. Yet, in spite of the popularity and variety of the film-as-philosophy outlook and of the conviction that the cinema can "do philosophy" (including ethics), there is no universal consensus concerning the viability of motion pictures as a medium for philosophical ideas. The matter of principle is complicated by the existence of competing currents – from the now less-favored psychoanalytic and semiotic to the trendier outlooks of post-colonialism, gender studies or queer theory, and especially "film-philosophy" as "an aesthetic, self-reflective, interpretative approach that puts philosophy in dialogue with film as an alternative way of thinking" (Sinnerbrink 2011, 7). These currents blend with a range of modes claimed for the philosophical relevance of moving pictures: they can illustrate theories; they can offer counterexamples to philosophical claims; they can themselves make such claims; sometimes their very form conveys philosophical content (for example, about time); or they can participate in philosophically-informed social criticism (Wartenberg 2009; see also Herzogenrath 2017; and Carroll, Di Summa and Loht 2019, Part IV).

In much larger numbers and in more languages than are referenced here, the spectrum of analytic styles is also huge, from Julio Cabrera's (1999) unpretentious introduction to philosophy through film to Slavoj Žižek's idiosyncratic and characteristically histrionic performance in *The Pervert's Guide to Cinema* (itself a motion picture) or, with regard to the less-trodden field of ethics, from those resolutely anchored in theory to others who wish to address ordinary spectators' experience (examples include, respectively, Sinnerbrink 2016 and Clémot 2018; see the overview by Sinnerbrink and Trahair 2016, and Choi and Frey 2016 for the broader range of "cine-ethics"). Finally, objections to film-as-philosophy include the charge that movies are incapable of pursuing general truths, which is the goal of most academic philosophy; that they rarely make their philosophically relevant claims explicit; that philosophically-inclined scholars read into movies their interests and preferences, and therefore overinterpret the film they examine; or that movies' philosophical content is for the most part banal or trivial (Wartenberg 2009, 2016).

With regard to these discussions, *Performing Brains on Screen* recognizes that filmmakers can assert a position, or formulate and explore philosophical issues. Yet it does not expect them to provide systematic arguments, defend a cause, or even overtly pose and answer questions – only (as Beatriz Sarlo [1993] said of Borges's stories) to generate them by way of the mise-en-scène. This book also distances itself from a certain kind of focus on the *image*. As Gilles Deleuze postulated, filmmakers (in their movies) think not so much in concepts as in *images-mouvement* and *images-temps*. Numerous film-philosophers before and after Deleuze have made related claims or assumed a similar standpoint, or extended the Deleuzian outlook in complex neuro-cognitive directions (Pisters 2012). Through its many incarnations, the basic idea is that, in contrast to discourse, which analyzes and rationalizes, the filmic image denotes and shows without naming or explaining; it is autonomous from language; it conveys presence. In short, while the cinema renounces "abstract thinking," it is, as Jean-Luc Godard put it, *une forme qui pense* (Cerf 2009, 20; Morgan 2013, Chap. 4).

Such a position, however, emphasizes the image at the expense of the fact that, in the vast majority of cases, what we see on screen is not just an image, albeit moving, but a performance, albeit in images. It may well be that film does not enable access to characters' subjective states and restricts spectators to a third-person viewpoint (Knight 2009, 619). Yet, while it surely cannot solve the "problem of other minds" (Avramides 2019), it can exhibit circumstances and conditions of possibility of subjective and intersubjective experience. More generally, motion pictures can set up philosophically significant thought experiments, but instead of "arguing" their premises, empirical consequences and logical corollaries, they *perform* them (on whether and how films can function as thought experiments, see Dadlez 2019). This has a distinct advantage over argumentation. While it is in the nature of thought experiments to be simplified models (and that is why they can be criticized as implausible, vague, or blind to real-world alternatives), cinematic performances tend to redirect thinking toward "real life." This often happens in absurd ways and in the absence of any profound intention. Pictures can *enact* thought experiments even when, in doing so, they typify filmic clichés. In those cases, their hackneyed character does not diminish their interest, since the fact that they recur and become commonplace is in itself telling.

Bs to Zs

Sa place, nulle dans l'histoire de l'Art, est immense dans l'histoire sentimentale des sociétés.
Marcel Proust, "Éloge de la mauvaise musique,"
Les Plaisirs et les Jours (1896)

Marcel Proust observed that it is "bad music," far more than the good, which has gradually "been filled with the dreams and the tears of mankind." Even if we do not enjoy it (and he did), we should respect it, he said, not out of "the charity of good taste" but because we understand its social role. For the place of bad music, "insignificant in the history of art, is huge in the sentimental history of societies" (Proust 1896, 149). Crucial to that effect, as Proust noted, is the repetition of themes and melodies that, though "worthless in the eyes of an artist," cut across social classes and touch the hearts of multitudes. Something similar must be recognized of "bad movies."

As the indologist Wendy Doniger (2005, 5–6) noted, "What we call mythemes when they occur in myths, we call clichés when they occur in B movies." Claude Lévi-Strauss (1963, 211) coined *mythème* to name the "gross constituent units" of myth; he defined them as "bundles" of relations that "can be put to use and combined so as to produce a meaning." It follows that a myth consists of the totality of its variants, that its analysis should consider all of them, and that there is no such a thing as the "true" or "authentic" version of a myth. Thus, for example, in interpreting the Oedipus myth, one should include Sigmund Freud's use of it, which adds to the myth itself (ib., 216–217). With less structuralist rigor, these observations apply to our movies: they offer significant differences, while sharing a constituent unit made up of a character (the protagonist whose brain is somehow disturbed by an external force), an event (the alteration of the brain), and a theme (living with a transformed brain or as a brain that has been placed in particular circumstances). That unit recurs across media, genres, and styles. Its clichéd nature, however, is especially apparent in B movies (on them in general, see Memba 2006; Mérigeau and Bourgoin 1983; and Davis 2012 for the period most relevant for our discussion; and Cross 1982 and Tesson 1997 for richly illustrated books).

Indeed, B movies thrive on cliché, whose success largely depends on being formulaic and combining commonplaces. As Umberto Eco (2019, 21) noted, "Two clichés are laughable. A hundred clichés are affecting." Writing about the pictures he called "schlock/kitsch/hack movies" (s/k/h), some of which are technically Bs, Charles Flynn (1975, 8) remarked that audiences like them because they see in them "the myth in its purest form." Many of the films to be discussed here belong in that simultaneously clichéd and mythic universe, whose main features are largely determined by the circumstances of their production. B movies originated in the United States in the 1930s. Their main motivation was economic: depression-era exhibitors hoped to attract audiences by featuring two films; cheap and quickly made, the lower-quality B was the second feature in those double bills (Flynn and McCarthy 1975). Production took place in Hollywood's "Poverty Road," as small B movie studios came to be known from the late 1920s to the mid-1950s. The category overlaps with genres: Westerns were common in early Bs, while a combination of horror and science fiction became popular in the 1950s.

From the point of view of style, B movies shared several features (not all present at the same time, and none by itself enough to define them), such as illogical, inconsistent, or outlandish plots, outrageous imagery, careless production (continuity flaws are legion), simplistic action, or stereotypical characters. As time went by, they featured increasingly repellent freaks and allowed ever greater and more explicit levels of (often combined) violence, nudity, and gruesomeness. B, and the even "lower" C and Z movies, as well as "exploitation" film, which since the 1960s has flourished thanks to gore, splatter, and the sensationalistic treatment of lurid and prurient themes, have in the meantime gained academic respectability (Perkins and Verevis 2014 includes discussions on this point).

The "negative" vocabulary just employed is actually meant to be descriptive, and highlights the very traits that have turned a good number of B or s/k/h into "cult" (on the notion, see Mathijs and Mendik 2008, Introduction, and Mathijs and Sexton 2011). "Imperfection," as Eco perceptively explained, is indeed intrinsic to such pictures:

> To give rise to a cult, a film must already be inherently ramshackle, shaky and disconnected in itself. A perfect film ... remains imprinted in our memory as a whole, in the form of an idea or a principal emotion; but only a ramshackle film survives in a disjointed series of images and visual high points. It should show not one central idea, but many. It should not reveal a coherent "philosophy of composition," but it should live on, and by virtue of, its magnificent instability. (Eco 2019, 215)

The cult status that movies in these categories have achieved often partakes in the aesthetic of camp, and implies parodic or ironic pleasures: fans routinely proclaim they relish them precisely because they find them so awful. Placing a production in the *so bad it's good* category is not easy, beginning with the fact that "badness" itself has become canonical and is not always as transgressive as it may seem (MacDowell and McCulloch, 2019; Sconce, 2019). Be that as it may, most brainfilms possess features and an enjoyable bizarreness that situate them among the disparate subgenres that constitute the universe of "paracinema." As Jeffrey Sconce (1995b, 372) insightfully noted, paracinema is

> less a distinct group of films than a particular reading protocol, a counter-aesthetic turned subcultural sensibility devoted to all manner of cultural detritus. In short, the explicit manifesto of paracinematic culture is to

> valorize all forms of cinematic "trash," whether such films have been either explicitly rejected or simply ignored by legitimate film culture.

Sconce's characterization of paracinema applies to many of the earlier movies discussed here, and sheds light on the filmic background of later performances of brains on screen.

Although sometimes obsessively labeled, paracinematic productions tend to highlight the capacity that genres have to combine and recombine, the fluidity of their boundaries, the relative nature and impurity of judgments of taste, and the interpenetration of filmic sources, references, and traditions. That is why I shall refrain from giving weight to classifications, which, though sometimes helpful, may also slant analysis and interpretation. An instance of this phenomenon can be found in science fiction. Many productions to which the sci-fi label has been attached can be considered "a species of horror, substituting futuristic technologies for supernatural forces" (Carroll 1990, 13–14). Transplantation pictures, discussed here in Chapter 3, illustrate this well. They fictionalize a future where the potentialities of science are actualized, but they tend to do so in a horror mode. The connection has something intrinsic to it. As Emily Russell (2019, 195–196, and more generally Chap. 6) points out in her history of organ exchange, the genre of horror "is appropriate to the expression of lingering fears about organ transplant not simply because it is the genre of fear, but because so many shared foundational concerns underpin both horror and transplantation," including the transgression of boundaries and an emphasis on physicality.

The most basic use of generic concepts consists of establishing taxonomies. Genre, however, also exists as a process in which concepts are created, redefined, subdivided, combined, and used for different purposes (Altman 2000). Moreover, a central theme or premise, such as the claim that "we are cerebral subjects," does not play the same narrative or conceptual role in philosophical, political or science fiction movies, and these may in turn differ from comedy, romance, or satire in several respects, including the degree of "seriousness" with which they take that theme or premise. From the viewpoint of reception, clues to a film's genre influence viewers' expectations, attitudes toward verisimilitude, and emotional and intellectual responses. As for internal film analysis, understanding single productions as a whole, even auteur movies, requires placing them within larger patterns that include genre. In short, since genres transcend individual motion pictures, they facilitate navigating large masses of material, tracking relations, and identifying intertextual figures. Moreover, insofar as genre choices participate in the construction of a picture as much as in its reception, identifying genre dynamics helps connect the various dimensions of a film's existence, from the commercial to the critical. Nevertheless, because (as illustrated above with science fiction and horror), genres interpenetrate and cross over, and because I here study a theme that has been enacted in virtually all narrative and stylistic modes, I shall not usually go beyond mentioning a movie's genre as a practical way of situating one of its aspects, rather than using *genre* as an analytic category.

The brain motif not only cuts across genres but also, as mentioned, across media. Variations in the plots, characters, and settings we see on screen can be encountered in literature of diverse kinds, long and short, high and low – from novels and short stories to comics, manga, the pulps, and at least one bubblegum trading card series of 1962, *Mars Attacks!* Especially important in connection with the filmic universe of the Bs to the Zs is the science fiction published, mainly in the United States between the late nineteenth and the mid-twentieth century, in the cheap magazines known as "pulp" because of the kind of paper on which they were printed. Chapter 2 is devoted to that context.

Filmic Brains in the Neurobiological Age

Brain movies act out the brain as the somatic limit of the self. The replacement of other inner organs, such as lung, heart or kidney, may affect our sense of self, but not radically alter our personal identity. Replace the brain, however, and you replace the person; as philosopher Roland Puccetti (1969, 70) put it, "Where goes a brain, there goes a person." Brain movies perform such an assertion, which can even take the form of a logical biconditional: "Person P is identical with person P' if and only if P and P' have one and the same functional brain" (Ferret 1993, 79). The formula encapsulates not only an opinion that was popular in the Anglo-American philosophy of personal identity, but also the apparently commonsense intuition that to have the same brain is to be the same person. It seems our own brain is the only part of the body we need in order to be ourselves. In principle, if my brain is substituted, the *person* I am disappears. That is why, in the usual commentary of the brain transplantation thought experiment, there is no such a thing as a brain donor. If my brain is removed and yours transplanted into my empty skull, then I no longer exist, and you undergo a whole-body transplant. In *Re-Animated*, a TV film of 2006, twelve-year-old Jimmy is given the brain of a middle-aged man, but remains himself because doctors manage to preserve his "personality gland." His case, however, is exceptional. Klaus Heissler, the goldfish of the animated series *American Dad!*, does not cease to be the East German sky jumper whose brain was transferred to the fish's body to prevent him from winning a gold medal in the 1986 Winter Olympics. That ontological predicament applies, with varying degrees of complexity and ambiguity, to all filmic characters who find themselves in a similar situation.

A prominent neuroscientist considered the usual understanding of the brain transplantation fiction as the expression of a "simple fact" and claimed that it "makes it clear that you are your brain" (Gazzaniga 2005, 31). Although his claim is neither a fact nor simple, he is not alone in believing that it is, and one could quote myriad versions of it. Indeed, it is the core of the "neurobiological age" that started emerging in the 1960s and had become global by the late twentieth century (Rose and Abi-Rached 2013). Encouraged by an epistemic and methodological turn toward a reductionist and biochemical approach to the brain and the nervous system, such development "was accompanied by a shift in the mode of governance; with the state, the industry and the scientific community gathering around the same object of interest ('the brain') albeit with different aims, drives, expectations, and motivations" (Abi-Rached and Rose 2010, 26). The neurocentric drive, with the belief that sustains it in Puccetti's dictum, has been consolidated in scientific projects, social movements, and commercial enterprises. From neuroanthropology to neurotheology, from cerebral self-help to the neurodiversity movement, it has become integral to diverse forms of individual and collective subjectivity (Vidal and Ortega 2017).

Though reinforced by modern neuroscientific findings and discourses, the conviction that "you are your brain" does not originate in empirical research. Historically, it derives from a philosophical understanding about *I*, from definitions of personhood and personal identity. Logically, it requires one such definition. Thus, what it expresses in the guise of a natural matter of fact is the metaphysical view according to which humans are specified by the property of "brainhood," that is, the property or quality of *being*, rather than simply *having*, a brain (Vidal 2009). Historicizing such view, of course, does not imply negating the crucial role of the brain and the nervous system for everything we are and do. History nevertheless shows that brainhood is not the necessary corollary of modern neuroscientific advances, but a consequence of early modern developments in science and philosophy.

In the seventeenth century, as the body came to be understood in purely mechanical terms, the soul ceased to be what it had been in the long-standing Aristotelian frameworks – namely, that which animates potentially live matter and accounts for the vegetative, sensitive, and rational faculties of living beings – and was reconceptualized as mind (Vidal 2011). This did not reduce it to pure intellect: as Descartes put it in the second of his *Meditations on First Philosophy* (1641), "a thing that thinks" is a thing "that doubts, understands, affirms, denies, wills, refuses, and that also imagines and senses." Insofar as a long tradition connected those functions to the brain, this organ gained importance as the exclusive seat of the soul, and the nerves came to be considered as the vehicles of the interaction between soul and body. Although such developments certainly stimulated brain research, the first clearly identifiable expression of the brainhood creed did not derive from it, but from a combination of theories about matter and personal identity.

On the one hand, the seventeenth-century "mechanical philosophy," in particular the doctrine of "corpuscularianism," explained the specific features of different bodies by the size, shape, and local motion of the particles that composed them, rather than by properties inherent in each body's substance. In the corpuscularian perspective, stone S at time T1 does not have to be made of exactly the same matter as S at T2 in order to be considered the same. Material continuity thus lost its significance as a constitutive element of the identity and sameness of material bodies. On the other hand, in the second edition of his *Essay Concerning Human Understanding*, John Locke (1988 [1694], Book II, Chap. 27) extended that philosophy of matter to the theory of personal identity. He separated physical substance (the "man," by which he meant the individual as organic being) and personal identity, that is, each of us as the individual being who "can consider itself as itself, the same thinking thing, in different times and places" (§ 9). Locke speculated that if my consciousness is located in my little finger, and this finger cut of my hand, then "the little finger would be the person, the same person; and self then would have nothing to do with the rest of the body" (§ 17). Arguably, Locke's theory of personal identity was his most innovative philosophical contribution, and one of the most revolutionary. It constituted a momentous and contested inflection of the Christian tradition. For whereas Christianity is based on the doctrine of the Incarnation and postulates that persons are intrinsically corporeal, Locke construed personhood and personal identity on the exclusive basis of psychological functions. Brainhood emerged in the wake of Locke, together with the reflexivity, inwardness, and self-ownership that are considered central features of the "modern self" (Taylor 1989; Thiel 2011).

Insofar as personhood and personal identity were redefined as exclusively based on psychological functions, and insofar as these functions were somehow connected to the brain, the brain became the only organ we need in order to be persons in general, as well as the individuals we actually are. Versions of this conviction would be soon espoused as empirical truth. In his *Analytical Essay on the Faculties of the Soul* (1760), the Genevan naturalist and philosopher Charles Bonnet wrote, "If a Huron's soul could have inherited Montesquieu's brain, Montesquieu would still create" (§ 771). The native North American was an Enlightenment paradigm of the savage; yet if his soul were joined to Montesquieu's brain, then one of the era's greatest thinkers would, for intellectual purposes at least, be still alive. It did not matter that the soul and body were those of a "primitive man," provided the brain was the philosopher's own. Psychologization and cerebralization thus went hand in hand, and when the sciences of mind and body abandoned the notion of soul, the brain took its place and began to act in its stead.

In the nineteenth century, increasingly refined anatomical descriptions, and experimental and anatomo-pathological inquiries into the cerebral localization of motor, sensory, and cognitive functions reinforced the brainhood ideology. Cerebral localization, functional differentiation, and the correlation of site and effect or structure and function became investigative principles, and it was commonplace to believe (as Dr. Waldman will do in James Whale's 1931 *Frankenstein*), that brain morphology reveals genius, criminality, or mental illness. Electroencephalography, which developed in the early 1930s, raised the hope that the recorded waves would offer direct insights into mental life (Borck 2018). Since the late twentieth century, the promises of neuroimaging to illuminate the most complex processes of the human mind have made a renewed form of such hope appear feasible and self-evident. However, in spite of enormous advances in knowledge about brain structure and function, Puccetti's aphorism and its subsequent, less epigrammatic versions up to the present have the same epistemic status and validity as Bonnet's speculation of over two and a half centuries ago.

How do cinematic brains fit in this story? At the most general level, their role has hardly evolved since the early days of cinema, before the onset of the "neurobiological age." Brain transplantation was first used as a film plot in George Monca's 1909 eleven-minute comic short *L'Homme-singe*, where a man behaves like a monkey after receiving a monkey brain. (The film is sometimes dated 1908. To my knowledge, it has not been reported lost, but I have not been able to locate it, and it is the only movie mentioned in this book that I was unable to watch.) Like Alice Guy's 1906 *La Vérité sur l'homme-singe*, about a man who drinks a capillary lotion that turns him into an ape-like man, *L'Homme-singe* capitalized on the contemporary popularity of performing animals. Audiences recognized and enjoyed a genre.

Obviously, too, they accepted that the brain somehow defines who we are. The same can be said of Max Mack's 1913 *Der Andere* (*The Other*). Based on a well-known play and bringing a renowned stage actor to the screen, it is one of the films that introduced the theme of the doppelgänger that would become common in German art cinema, and arguably instantiates an early form of horror based on questioning the boundaries of the self and the stability of the real world (Tybjerg 2004). Berlin State attorney Dr. Hallers falls from his horse and develops a split personality, breaking into his own house while in the second, abnormal state, and later recovering during a rest cure in the countryside. Indirectly but clearly, by means of references to the positivist French philosopher Hippolyte Taine's *De l'intelligence* (1870) combined with the way Hallers repeatedly grasps his head, the movie points to a cerebral cause for the protagonist's condition. The film is a variation on *The Strange Case of Dr. Jekyll and Mr. Hyde*, explaining the character's transformation by circumstances affecting the brain, rather than by the ingestion of chemicals as in Robert Louis Stevenson's novel.

Since those early days, the cinema has constantly conveyed beliefs about the brain. In *Frankenstein* (1931), Dr. Waldman demonstrates how the morphology of the cortex reveals criminality; in *The Brain Machine* (1955), which in spite of its title is more of a noirish thriller than a brain movie, unusual brainwaves, shown in close-ups of electroencephalographic recordings, expose a man's homicidal tendencies at the same time that an X-ray of the skull shows "the cause of the trouble"; in 1977, another *Brain Machine* converts the "tiniest electrical impulses of your brain" into audio and visual "pictures of thought," and thus reveals (with deadly consequences) whether you're lying or telling the truth; already in the present century, *Lucy* (2014) is sustained by the popular but refuted legend (recurrent in pulp science fiction) that we use only 10% of our brain... And so on and so forth. Beyond such particulars, however, what film has not ceased to do is give the brain a constitutive role when it comes to performing personal identity. Jordan Peele's horror blockbuster *Get Out* (2017), about wealthy white people who perpetuate themselves by having their brains transplanted into the body of black individuals chosen for their "physical advantages," demonstrates the persistence of brainhood as a default ideology. With variable degrees of intellectual and aesthetic ambition, plots and visuals literally unfold the axiom that "where goes a brain, there goes a person." Independently of the forms it takes, the problems it raises, or the extent to which a movie challenges it, it is what drives the performance of brains on screen.

The brain, however, can also make other filmic appearances. Zombie movies are an outstanding example. In George Romero's *Night of the Living Dead* (1968), a TV newsman reports that the Pentagon "has disclosed that a ghoul can be killed by a shot in the head, or a heavy blow to the skull. Officials are quoted as explaining that since the brain of a ghoul has been activated by the radiation, the plan is: Kill the brain, and you kill the ghoul." In Romero's own sequel, *Dawn of the Dead* (1978), a doctor explains on TV, "A dead body must be exterminated, either by destroying the brain, or severing the brain from the rest of the body." The movie goes on to display such extermination with relish, but the zombies remain flesh-eating creatures. To this day, as illustrated by the TV series *The Walking Dead* (launched in 2010), zombies are killed by destroying their brain.

In the mid-1980s, *The Return of the Living Dead*, which treated the undead in a campy mode, introduced several novelties. Zombies could run and speak; most importantly, they ate brains rather than other flesh, and could no longer be terminated by destroying their brains (see Dendle 2001 for the zombie-brain motif). The image of the brain-eating zombie became widespread in popular culture – so much so that a luridly illustrated book discussing animals, microorganisms, and parasites that feed on other organisms' brains announced its topic as "real-life zombies" and as "creatures with zombie-like diets" (Klepeis 2017). Finally, zombies, brain eating or other, have become respectable subjects of philosophical discussion about problems such as the definition of life and death, the relation of mind and brain, or the persistence of personal identity (see, e.g., Greene and Mohammad 2010; Kirk 2019 for an overview). Insofar as the reanimation of corpses is somehow due to radiation "activating" the brain, and given that only the destruction of this organ brings about the undead's definitive demise, the brain plays a theoretically important role. On screen, however, such a role is very limited, and that is why one does not need to speak about the brain to figure out the zombie's philosophical significance (e.g., Coulombe 2012; on the zombie's body and internal organs, see Le Maître 2016). In any case, zombie movies generally do not enact the brain so that having or eating one determines or affects identity in ways that shape plot, action, or visuals.

The exceptions date from the 2010s, a period that saw an increase in the popularity of zombies, and an expansion of the genres, media, and formats in which they are performed (Bishop 2015). In the TV series *iZombie* (2015–2019), a medical student-turned-zombie tries to retain her humanity by eating brains; she thus acquires the dead person's memories and skills, and flashes of what happened allow her to solve crimes with uncanny insight. In *Warm Bodies* (2013), a zombie romantic comedy, a good-looking male zombie called R eats brains, and "feels alive" when he then experiences the victims' memories. "The brain is the best part," he says to himself while feasting on the organ, "the part that makes me feel human again." The diet sustains his attraction to the equally good-looking non-zombie Julie, and presumably furthers his reversion into a living human. The brain thus plays a basic visual and performative role, representing a sort of "neural turn" in the zombie universe, but based on a trivial enactment of the creed that "we are our brains."

* * *

This book focuses on fiction films that were created for the "big screen." What is excluded here, of course, is not the possibility of viewing these films on small screens, but rather, TV or Internet series as unitary objects of analysis. Organized in episodes designed to be broadcast in annual or semi-annual seasons (or in shorter periods for miniseries), such productions offer a concept or narrative that is fundamentally based on recurring protagonists. Given the continuity of plot and characters, understanding an episode requires viewing prior ones. Drawing inspiration on the American philosopher Stanley Cavell and his views on the significance of film for persons' ordinary moral lives, Sandra Laugier (2019) calls attention to the fact that our experience as spectators of a "serial" (i.e., a series with a continuing plot that develops sequentially episode by episode) is intimately connected to how we become gradually involved with the characters. The tempo and continuity of a relationship that may evolve almost in real time decisively help shape what we find interesting in a serial, enable its assimilation into our existence, and make it matter for us. There is, to my knowledge, no series of that sort where the brain motif plays a constitutive role. Hence, in spite of dealing in interesting ways with politics, violence, justice, race, or gender, series do not speak directly to the brain-based nexus of embodiment and identity that is a central theme of the movies discussed here. Naturally, the *absence* of a motif and of the theme it supports could perhaps be considered as a way to tacitly question or dispute their significance or how they are performed or interpreted. Following up such possibility systematically would make it impossible to delimit a filmic corpus. Nevertheless, some TV "anthology series" (i.e., series that present different stories, and sometimes different sets of characters in each episode or season), include self-contained episodes that place the brain motif center stage; a few of them will be discussed.

The terms *theme* and *motif* have just been employed in the senses they usually have in literary or cinematographic contexts. The former designates a main idea (or thesis, or question, or meaning) within a story, and the latter, an element (realized through visuals, sound, or dialogue) that sustains and informs the theme. For example, the relations between embodiment and personal identity may constitute a theme that is performed, in part, by a brain motif enacted in dialogues or surgery scenes. Thus, the overall approach of *Performing Brains on Screens* can be described as thematic. I have in this connection used the indefinite article advisedly when referring to *a* theme and *a* motif. No analysis can exhaust a movie, say what it is uniquely about, or identify "what is really there" to the exclusion of meanings, themes or motifs that are not. Criticism can be more or less well argued, commentary more or less well elaborated, and both can make more or less sense depending on their stated goals and their historical or institutional settings. And while it is not the case that anything goes, what criticism and commentary cannot do, given the intrinsic polysemy of art in all its forms, is to claim exclusive epistemic authority or to provide supposedly definitive interpretations. In this regard, the thematic outlook is both modest and clear.

Sometimes in obvious, sometimes in circuitous ways, each of the movies examined here offers themes and motifs, and therefore meanings, distinct from those of brainhood and embodiment. It can be convincingly argued that the main theme of a movie that begins with the transplantation of a white man's brain into a black man's body in 1960s America is race relations in that time and place. However, as can be shown through the analysis of visuals and dialogues, the brain motif serves as a main frame, as a medium for performing the racial theme. It also generates transversal issues of embodiment that may include, but do not depend on the question of race. The motif is therefore a resource for understanding the film, while the film is a resource for figuring out those issues. In discussing movies in such a perspective, I have tried to keep in mind Roland Barthes's lucid lesson:

> The relationship of criticism to the work is that of a meaning to a form. The critic cannot claim to "translate" the work ... What the critic can do is to "engender" a certain meaning by deriving it from a form that is the work. (Barthes 1966, 32, translation slightly edited)

Scholarly commentary on motion pictures, no matter how smart, broad or deep, cannot replace watching them, which is the only way of having a comprehensive filmic experience. I therefore hope that *Performing Brains on Screen* manages not to lose sight of the circumscribed task and limits of interpretation, and will encourage viewing.

Chapter 2, "Brains in the Pulps," explores the brain motif in science-fiction pulp magazines on the 1920s and 1930s, and outlines resonances between brainfilms and the pulps. Chapter 3, "Naked Brains and Living Heads," focuses on movies, produced between the 1950s and the 1970s, in which "ectobrains" (brains that live outside a body) play a main role. Kept in a vat or freely moving, these characters are usually evil and seek power. A comparison with films staging heads kept alive separated from the rest of the body sheds light on their meaning. The pictures examined in Chapter 4, "Personal Survival," enact interhuman brain transplantation into younger bodies as the means of realizing personal immortality, thus raising such question as: To what extent do brains sustain the continuity of the older person? Which challenges await the hybrid made up of A's brain in B's body? Moving then to "Frankenstein's Brains," Chapter 5 documents how, in the long and varied history of *Frankenstein* productions, the original theme of the creation of life was quickly replaced by a brain transplantation subplot, and it discusses such a thematic transformation. In most movies, having memories of a "real" past functions as criterion for being one's authentic self; amnesia and memory replacement or manipulation therefore pose radical challenges to personal identity. Chapter 6, "Memories, Lost and Regained," explores this vast topic in films that locate memory in the brain. The conclusive chapter "'Imagine: They Are in the Human Mind'" wraps things up and underlines the persistence of the body in spite of the relative disincarnation operated by the reduction of self to brain.

2. Brains in the Pulps

Abstract
Brain-themed plots, characters, and settings cut across both genres and media. Particularly strong is the narrative and iconographic kinship between science fiction "pulp magazines" and B brainfilms. Pulp sci-fi was popular in the USA between the late nineteenth century and the 1950s. This chapter focuses on the brain motif in pulp "scientifiction" stories and visuals of the 1920s to 1930s – years that saw the emergence of the first filmic brain in a vat, and other brain motifs that would later appear on screen, such as the mad brain scientist, brain manipulation and transplantation, brains in jars, or brain-mediated immortality. It also describes the place of "scientifilm" in pulp fantasy and magazines' commercial strategies, and outlines resonances between brainfilms and sci-fi pulp.

Keywords: B movie, brainfilm, pulp magazines, science fiction, scientifiction, transtextuality

This is a book about movies. Why, then, devote a chapter to magazines? As mentioned, the brain motif cuts not only across filmic genres, but also across media. Variations of the plots, characters, and settings we see on screen can be encountered in literatures of diverse kinds, long and short, high and low. Yet no connection has been stronger than that between "pulp magazines" specializing in science fiction (SF) and brainfilms of the B-to-Z sort. Popular in the United States between the late nineteenth century and the 1950s, the name by which those inexpensive magazines are known derives from the wood pulp paper on which they were printed. The *New Republic* in 1929 and *Vanity Fair* in 1933 called them "magazines for morons" and "day-dreams for the masses" (Cheng 2012, 20). Not for nothing, what the empty-headed fashion model Marion distractedly reads during a photo session in the musical *Funny Face* (1957) is *Minute Men from Mars*, a comic book whose colorful cover evokes the alien-invasion pulp aesthetic. Though in an exclusively negative mode, highbrow commentators' disdainful assessments betray

Vidal, F., *Performing Brains on Screen*. Taylor & Francis Group, 2022
DOI 10.5117/9789462989146_CH02

discomfort at the huge repercussion of those magazines on the individual and the collective imagination.

Pulps are "paraliterature" (Baldick 2015, 266; Boyer 2008) in the same way that so many B-to-Zs are paracinema. While, like the latter, they have become cult and worthy of scholarly attention, they are hardly known beyond fans and specialists. We are unaware of the extent to which their visions suffuse contemporary fictions. That is why (to give only a very recent example) the Argentine journalist Martín Caparrós's novel *Sinfín* (*Endless*) has been praised as highly original. *Sinfín*, however, is a dystopic story centered on a society that pursues immortality by transferring mortal human brains into imperishable digital ones. With local color and suitable "cyber" updating, it does little more than reiterate any number of pulp science fiction stories from almost a century ago, and many others since. The fact that reviewers praise its originality points to how unnoticed have been the reverberations of the voices we shall listen to in this chapter. (To stay with Argentina: topics like the mind transfer as a way to obtain immortality, transplanting human brains into animals, or mental control via brain implants had by the 1940s made it into the local comics [Abraham 2020].)

A small volume could be written on brain motifs in the pulps; details could be provided (on authors, publication history, and so forth), a systematic search for movie sources in the pulps could be undertaken, and comparisons could in turn be made among motion pictures, pulp stories, and brain-themed novels published between the late nineteenth century and the end of the pulp era. Given that about 16% of SF authors between 1926 and 1945 were women, one could ask if there was anything specific about their writing (on women in early SF, see Donawerth 1994, and the introduction and conclusion in Yaszek and Sharp 2016). This chapter has the more limited purpose of outlining pulps as an important visual and narrative element of the context in which brainfilms flourished. It will present selected stories as a way of sketching brain themes in pulp science fiction, and of suggesting, at a general level, resemblances and convergences between the cinema and the pulps with regard to brain motifs and plots. Examples will be limited to the years up to 1936. One reason is that, by then, all of the brain topoi of contemporaneous motion pictures and future brainfilms had emerged. The other is that 1936 saw the release of *The Man Who Changed His Mind*, a production starring Boris Karloff as the mad scientist, which is perhaps the first movie to show a brain in a vat and place the brainmind swap center stage. But the kinds of stories explored here kept appearing beyond 1936.

While the magazines discussed here advertised themselves as science fiction, and SF was their *raison d'être*, that was not the case of the motion pictures we shall examine: a Frankenstein movie, for example, is primarily a Frankenstein movie, no matter how much sci-fi it contains. As has often been noted, however, science fiction has been defined in a variety of ways. In addition, since an SF plot may be told in a variety of modes (love, horror, detective, adventure, and so forth), science fiction functions like a supergenre, and is characterized by hybridity and overlap (see, e.g., Neale 2000, 85–96). Finally, the history of SF demonstrates shifting conventions and expectations, as well as a "heterogeneous array of practices … that draw upon vastly different resources and enact correspondingly divergent motives" (Rieder 2017, 161).

So-called "genre fiction" (i.e., not only SF, but also the crime or detective story, romance, the western, horror, or inspirational or faith-based narratives) makes up a "mass cultural genre system" characterized by large-scale commercial production and distribution in print, film, and broadcast media, a tendency to reiteration, and the emergence of extensive consumer communities (Rieder 2017). That was the system to which the pulps and the Bs jointly belonged. The impression of déjà-vu that permeates their universe is integral to their economy, which relies on cycles, series and an assembly-line type of creation, and thrives by iterating plots and motifs, recycling and recombining them across media (Letourneux 2017 and, for a later period, Besson 2004). For individual writers, who were poorly paid and, therefore, forced to be prolific, repetition was inevitable. For instance, in writing all but three of the twenty-one novels and novelettes that appeared in the short-lived teenager pulp *Captain Future* (1940–1944), the famously copious Edmond Hamilton (1904–1977) followed one formula: "a super-scientist with four aides – a robot, an android, a brain in a box, and a beautiful girl – would undertake and complete in each episode a crusade to bring a villain to justice; in the process, the hero would be captured – and escape – exactly three times" (Gunn 2018, 136). Many other pulp writers adopted a similar compositional strategy.

Resources

The scholarly literature on SF and its history and contexts is vast; I will here list works that have proven particularly useful for this chapter. In addition to Roberts (2016, Chap. 10) and Telotte (2019), good overarching resources include, in the last decade, James E. Gunn's *Alternate Worlds*, an illustrated history of science fiction that gives large room to the pulps (Gunn 2018), and John Cheng's *Astounding Wonder: Imagining Science and Science Fiction in Interwar America* (Cheng 2012).

Several bibliographic resources deserve to be singled out: Marshall B. Tymn and Mike Ashley's *Science Fiction, Fantasy, and Weird Fiction Magazines*, which provides a richly annotated alphabetical bibliography (Tymn and Ashley 1985); the first volume of Ashley's history of science-fiction magazines, which covers the pulps up to 1950 and includes valuable bibliographical appendices (Ashley 2000); Ashley and Robert Lowndes's *The Gernsback Days: A Study of the Evolution of Modern Science Fiction from 1911 to 1936*, which summarizes many stories and provides an issue-by-issue listing of the SF and speculative articles in Gernsback's magazines (Ashley and Lowndes 2004); and volume 3 of Donald H. Tuck's *The Encyclopedia of Science Fiction and Fantasy Through 1968*, which includes, among other materials, an annotated alphabetical list of magazines (Tuck 1982). Equally valuable are several free, open-access, partly overlapping online resources: the *Pulp Magazines Project* (PMP), an archive and digital research initiative on fiction pulpwood magazines from 1896 to 1946, which combines bibliographies, concise informative essays, a digital archives hub, search resources, and high-quality digital facsimiles of selected magazine issues; the *Pulp Magazine Archive* (PMA) at the digital Internet Archive, which offers even more facsimiles; the pulp magazine collection in the *Luminist Archives* (LA); and the *Internet Speculative Fiction Database* (ISFDB), a community effort to catalog works of science fiction, fantasy, and horror. Finally, at over 18,000 entries, *The Encyclopedia of Science Fiction* (ESF) offers a formidable network on all things SF, including the pulps.

Exploring these online resources, which are listed in the Bibliography under the acronyms provided, demonstrates that, while science fiction became immensely popular by way of the pulps, not all pulps were devoted to science fiction. Similarly, not all movies based on or inspired in pulp magazines belong to science fiction – witness, among others, those featuring early pulp heroes such as Zorro, The Spider, or Fu Manchu. Crucial for managing the colossal amount of material have been Everett F. Bleiler's *Science-Fiction: The Early Years* and *Science-Fiction: The Gernsback Years*, which not only summarize thousands of short stories, novelettes and novels, but also offer a wealth of indices (Bleiler 1990, 1998).

Scientifiction, Textual and Visual

Late nineteenth-century literary magazines in the US and the UK occasionally published stories of "speculative fiction" (a term from 1899). However, the first (pulp) magazine explicitly and exclusively devoted to science fiction, and one that in addition attempted to define the genre, was launched in April 1926 in New York, the city that became the pulps' favorite urban scenario. Entitled *Amazing Stories*, and heralding "Extravagant Fiction Today – Cold Fact Tomorrow," it was founded by Hugo Gernsback (1884–1967), an emigrant from Luxemburg. Gernsback, who wanted to popularize science and technology and encourage readers to think about the future, initially spoke of "scientifiction," which he defined as "a charming romance intermingled with scientific fact and prophetic vision" (quoted in Gunn 2018, 116). Between the 1920s and the mid-1950s, pulps were the main purveyors of SF. The success of *Amazing Stories* launched a fertile "magazine era" (Attebery 2003). In 1927, Gernsback began *Amazing Stories Annual* ("the annual year book of scientifiction"); it had only one issue, featuring among others the first publication of Edgar Rice Burroughs's "The Master Mind of Mars," discussed below. In 1928, he established *Amazing Stories Quarterly*, which lasted until 1934. Upon losing control of his magazines in 1929, Gernsback started *Science Wonder Stories*, *Air Wonder Stories*, and *Science Wonder Quarterly*, which later merged into *Wonder Stories*. *Wonder Stories*, whose initial title page described it as "The Magazine of Prophetic Fiction" and sometimes added the motto "Prophetic Fiction is the Mother of Scientific Fact," appeared between 1936 and 1955 under the title *Thrilling Wonder Stories*; it lasted until 1966.

Gernsback's original formula stimulated the creation of other magazines: *Astounding Stories of Super Science* (1930), which underwent several name changes (*Astounding Stories* in 1931 and then again in 1933–1938, *Astounding Science Fiction* in 1938–1960, and finally *Analog Science Fiction – Science Fact*); *Marvel Science Stories* (1938–1941, 1950–1952); *Startling Stories* (1939–1955); *Astonishing Stories* (1940–1943) and its companion for longer texts, *Super Science Stories* (1940–1951). *Astounding* remained the leading SF pulp until the appearance of *The Magazine of Fantasy and Science Fiction* (known as *F&SF*) in 1949 and *Galaxy Science Fiction* in 1950–1968 (titled *Galaxy Magazine* in 1958–1965). *Astounding*, *F&SF*, and *Galaxy* are banded together as "the Big Three" of science fiction pulp. Other than their influence, readership, and role in consolidating SF and SF fandom, the grouping encompasses diversity – roughly, *Astounding* for "Hard SF," which emphasizes the hard sciences as narrative basis, *Galaxy* for social and satirical SF, and *F&SF* "for literary

SF and anything out of the ordinary" (ESF, entry "F&SF"). Further from the genre's core, but featuring a lot of science fiction among the supernatural stories it popularized, was the long-running *Weird Tales* (1923–1954), which included among its contributors such major SF authors as H. P. Lovecraft (1890–1937) and Ray Bradbury (1920–2012).

Isaac Asimov (1909–1990), a paragon of hard SF who as a boy became a fan through the pulps and would later write for them, categorized modern science fiction into three periods: adventure-dominant (1926–1938), science-dominant (up to c. 1950), sociology-dominant (emphasizing the social response to scientific advances), and style-dominant (beginning in the mid-1960s, and largely concerned with sex, violence, and an experimental style; Gunn 2018, 18). He also distinguished among gadget science fiction (most popular in the late nineteenth century), adventure science fiction, and social science fiction (ib., 113–114).

As for the actual derivations from paper to film, there probably was a small undocumented number of adaptations or more or less direct transpositions. Beyond them, and some proven instances of plagiarism (e.g., the uncredited source of *The Brain Eaters* [1958] is Robert A. Heinlein's novel *The Puppet Masters*, originally serialized in 1951 in *Galaxy Science Fiction*), a detailed analysis could probably detect instances of inspiration, emulation, imitation, allusion, and quotation. The findings, however, would remain for the most part speculative. Three points are more relevant here. First, in the same way that pulp stories are not the filmic translation of professional philosophers' thought experiments, pulp brain fictions are not movie novelizations. Rather, given the chronology, the inspiration, if any, initially worked in the other direction. Second, even in the absence of one-to-one correspondences, the overall impression a visitor to the lands of the pulps and the brainfilms gains is one of dense "transtextuality," to use Gérard Genette's term for anything that sets a text in open or concealed relationship with other texts. Third, the existence of a common atmosphere applies beyond discourse. Indeed, the attraction and impact of pulp magazines resided largely in the graphic material.

Adam Roberts (2016, 271–272) convincingly argues that "the visual component of pulp SF is in many ways more important than the prose component. … The achievement of pulp SF art … lay in the creation of a wholly original mode of visual representation, highly varied and yet immediately recognisable, that still correlates to SF today." While stories were illustrated in black-and-white, covers employed bright primary colors; they displayed strong horizontal and vertical arrangements, one or two diagonals, sometimes a conspicuous curve. Usually caught in mid-action, and moving about in open space, remote planets or futuristic techno environments, the protagonists (from heroic men with ray guns protecting lightly dressed young women, to robots, aliens and monsters) contributed to a dynamic, energetic effect; letter graphics added to the overall flashy impression. These visual elements, which became trademark, were reinforced by the emergence of SF comic strips in the 1930s, and the emergence of SF superhero comics in the two subsequent decades. Thus, beyond increasing SF readership and generating fandom, the pulps "created for the first time a distinctive SF visual style, and played their part in the broader cultural shift of SF from a verbal to a visual form of art" (ib., 274–275).

One aspect of such developments is the fact that movies came to include scenes that resemble pulp covers and illustrations, and, reciprocally, that pulp visuals strike the B-connoisseur as close relatives of movie scenes. J. P. Telotte's (2019, 18) glimpsing in the magazines "the instantly recognizable shadow of a cinematic presence" is an experience anyone simultaneously conversant with pulps and paracinema is bound to have. Telotte emphasizes "the pulps' cinematic kinship" (ib., 108), and charts the extent to which modern SF consolidates in a shared territory.

First, at a time when the cinema already was an established and growing industry, the early pulps carried advertisement for movies or cinema training and equipment. Second, their stories frequently concerned the world of motion pictures, explored film's presence in society, or employed a cinematic rhetoric, drawing images, metaphors, and even characters "from the audience's shared film experience." Third, the pulps provided a forum for editors, writers, and fans to exchange about movies. Finally, pulp covers and illustrations could evoke the film world, representing screens, cameras, and movie theaters, or actions such as shooting, photographing, projecting, and watching film (ib., 21–22). Revealing instances of the formation of a transmedia SF community include the petition *Wonder Stories* launched in 1931, addressed to Hollywood studios and asking for more movies capable of satisfying a "rapidly growing" SF audience (ib., 87–89); and the appearance, in *Fantasy Magazine* of September 1934, of a "scientifilm editor" who, a year later, described himself as a "Scientificinemologist by profession" (Prucher 2007, 178).

The pulps' basic cinematic kinship surfaces in their use of the film world "as an atmospheric backdrop for plots that turn on different scientific or technological developments"; in their fascination with film technology itself; and in how they transformed the movies into "another SF meme," like the robot or the rocket, "serving the impulse that infuses both film and SF for visual exploration and realistic representation" (Telotte 2019, 48–50):

> At once both form and text, medium and message, pulp SF and film in this period actually functioned in a very similar manner, blurring conventional boundaries while prompting us to see the world in a new way, in part by framing it from the vantage provided by an ascendant science and technology. The pulps offered what some of the magazine editors commonly referred to as "thought experiments" or "thought variants," fictions that explored the trajectory or impact of various science-spurred developments or possibilities. (ib., 7)

These possibilities and thought experiments, which in our movies involve the brain, deal, among others, with epistemic and ontological issues (such as those concerning personal identity) commonly said to be characteristic of Western modernity. In turn, the cinema, as a major medium for exploring those issues, has been considered as "the fullest expression and combination of modernity's attributes" – so much so, it has been said, that modernity itself "can be best understood as inherently cinematic" (Charney and Schwartz 1995, 1, 2). Actual instances of the cinema in the pulps do not immediately inspire subtle interpretations, but the fact is that, visually and narratively, magazines combined cinematic motifs with such basic pulp identifiers as invading extraterrestrials with their hypertrophied brains (Brainfilms 2.1).

Advertisement and "Prophetic Insight"

The layout and non-fictional contents of the pulps reinforced the vision of the future the stories conveyed. An editorial in *Weird Tales* explained, "All writers of such stories are prophets, and in the years to come, many of their prophecies will come true" (Anon. 1924). Commercial publicity, science information, and fictional narrative reinforced each other to convince readers that the future was already becoming the present. *Science Wonder Stories*, for example, included a self-testing questionnaire entitled "What is your science knowledge?" as well as the rubric "Science news of the month." Factual or theoretical knowledge as conveyed in such rubrics was integrated into the fiction. Thus, even though the short novel "The Human Termites" is extravagant (more below), Gernsback inserted in the midst of it, as evidence of its author's "prophetic insight," a page from the journal *Science* showing an "apparatus for the detection of substratum communication among termites" (Keller 1929, 300). Such explicit links to science constituted one of the magazine's selling points, and were generally offered in a spirit of optimistic technophilia.

Marketing strategies included cutting the stories in two or more blocks. For example, "The Brain in the Jar," discussed below, was printed on pages 31–35 and 183–190. This maximized chances that readers would see the abundant advertisement interspersed throughout the text, which was nourished by the stories and fed back to them. Many ads promised to pave the way for a dignified job, good pay, and even fame thanks to training in radio and television. These two were major ingredients in the SF imagination at the time, and were often related, as new electronic media has been throughout its history, to paranormal or spiritual phenomena, which the stories also rehearsed (Sconce 2000; Berton 2021).

In the 1920s to 1940s, manipulating brainminds at a distance frequently involves radio waves. For example, in "A Matter of Ethics," a surgeon controls behavior by implanting "a tiny silver capsule" in one of the nerve ganglia. The capsule incorporates "a miniature radio receiver capable of picking up short wave energy and conveying definite electrical impulses to your brain over that marvelous network of telegraph lines that is your nervous system" (Vincent 1931, 655). In "Master of Dreams," a story that "tells of how the brain can be governed by outside and independent causes" and combines "psychical interest" with "the science of radio transmission," the evil protagonist (a "mad Turk" who wants to seize all wealth and power) directs his victims' dreams and conscious actions by means of tiny radio receivers inserted at the base of their skulls (Vincent 1934). The author of these two stories, American mechanical engineer Harl Vincent (1893–1968), was a regular pulp contributor; his name will come up again. (Early on in Olaf Stapledon's 1937 cosmic epic *Star Maker*, widely considered as one of the greatest science fiction novels of all times, "radio-brain-stimulation" gives governments "a cheap and effective kind of power over their subjects.")

Television, whose waves (in the pulps) sometimes interfered with those of radio, allowed for even more awesome effects, not far from those attributed since the 1990s to neuroimaging. "Into the Subconscious" (in connection with which an editorial note underlines "how much remains to be discovered about the marvelous mechanics of the human brain") comes up with a electrode helmet that, pressed against the wearer's temples, catches "the thought waves leaving the brain" (the significance of helmets is discussed in Chapter 4). The device comprises "the receiving end of a compact television unit," which serves "to project in an actual moving scene, the thoughts and sights which are passing through the subject's mind" (Myers 1929, 430). The magazine's cover demonstrates the technology (Brainfilms 2.2 and 2.3).

The stories, and the didactic and advertising sections were perfectly matched to each other: the former anticipated and made likely the future accomplishments whose realization was extolled in the latter. They cooperated to fulfill SF's predictive value and proleptic function. This does not apply to mechanical, electronic, and communication technologies alone. For instance, most of the page where the last lines of "The Brain in the Jar" are printed (Hammerstrom and Searight 1924) is occupied by an ad for Nuga-Tone, "the medicine that stimulates the Bodily Functions and helps the System do its work as Nature intended it should." While this ad, down to its visuals, evokes the classical quack doctor, the full-page ad facing the end of the story warns the readers, "Your Glands Wear Out!" Promising "results in a day," it encourages them to "test actual gland substances, directly absorbed." Illustrated by an elegant dancing couple, this publicity for a treatment "That Almost Never Fails" embodies the fusion between fiction and reality which the pulps projected, at least when it came to selling a product. The 1920s were the heyday of the glandular extractions fad, and the pulps happily rode the wave.

In "The Great Transformation," Ray Cummings (1887–1957), a former assistant to the inventor Thomas Alva Edison who prolifically contributed to pulp SF from its very beginning, tells of a scientist who distills from a human brain a "divine elixir" containing the human essence. The scientist injects the substance into a gorilla; the latter kills him, and commits suicide when it realizes that it is a human mind trapped in a simian body (Cummings 1931). An editorial note underlines the risks of "upsetting the 'balances' of nature" by transplanting monkey glands to prolong human life. "Moon of Arcturus" uses the idea of extreme longevity obtained through gland transplantations (with age derived from the number of gland replacements and computed in "gland-multiplied years") in a motley plot including intergalactic travel and encounters with immortal extraterrestrials depicted as superintellectual "brain-people," devoid of emotions and sexuality (Tooker 1935). "The Horrible Transformation" combines other pulp tropes by having the mad scientist transplant into a gorilla's body not only the human glands that control growth, but also a human brain; the result, a fifteen-foot Beast-Man, is graced with human speech, and is shown on the story's title page frighteningly shaking the car it holds with one hand (Daniels 1930). As we shall see in Chapter 4, later filmic productions also reflect the gland fad.

Before Gernsback

In the same way that the filmic brain motif predates the Bs, brain-related narrative plots in magazines precede the specialized pulps. In September 1889, *Lippincott's Monthly Magazine* (Philadelphia, 1868–1915) carried a story entitled "Solarion. A Romance," which included a scientist stimulating a puppy's brain until it reaches the level of human intelligence (Bleiler 1990, no. 705). The "Special American Number" published in November 1892 by *Romance: A Monthly Magazine of Complete Stories* (New York, 1891–1897) carried the short story "A Criminal's Brain Cells," in which, thanks to an unprecedented microscope, a doctor interested in the correlations between brain structure and criminality detects manias and criminal tendencies in cellular patterns (ib., no. 1024).

A few years later, "The Monster of Lake LaMetrie," a short story published in the British popular fiction and general interest monthly *Pearson's Magazine* (1896–1939), tells of an identity transfer in which a human brain is transplanted into the body of an elasmosaurus (Curtis 1899). The story consists of Professor James McLennegan's report – a report found, together with the scientist's remains, next to a remote Wyoming mountain lake, by a US Army captain while looking with his soldiers for some runaway Indians. Having wounded the prehistoric animal with his South American machete, McLennegan removes its brain. He then discovers that the interior of the skull is similar to that of an "ordinary man," and that the brain itself has the same size and "general contour" of a human brain, "though it is very inferior in fibre and has few convolutions." Having also realized that, though decerebrated, the reptile is alive, he places the live brain of his dead comrade Edward Framingham inside its skull. "For years the medical fraternity has been predicting that brain-grafting will some time be successfully accomplished." Now it happens.

Soon, McLennegan discerns expression in the animal's eyes. After a week, the elasmosaurus can signal that it – or rather, he, Framingham – understands McLennegan. The professor anticipates progress thanks to the fact that his friend is rid of his human body and possesses a new "powerful vital apparatus." After a fortnight, Framingham is in command of his antediluvian frame, sings and talks, and is again committed to looking for a connection between the lake and the interior of the Earth. Gradually, however, as the "brute body" absorbs the human intellect, the creature's mind deteriorates, and the hybrid becomes vicious. When, three years later, the captain encounters the elasmosaurus and orders his soldiers to kill it, "the thing" produces "a constant babbling" similar to human speech, but sounding only "like the jabbering of an imbecile, or a drunk trying to talk."

Given the fiasco of his initially successful "experiment," McLennegan concludes, "The human body has more influence over the mind than the mind has over the body." The story, like so much SF and so many brainfilms, combines adventure, bits of established knowledge, visions of scientific progress, narrative commonplaces, and a hubris-driven male professor. It entertains readers while enacting a philosophical thought experiment around the question: What happens to a person when their brain is transplanted into someone else's body? "The Monster of Lake LaMetrie" fits the pattern of scientific fantasy and *merveilleux-scientifique*, two late nineteenth-century, pre-pulp genres that, as we shall see in Chapters 3 and 4, explored xenografts and interspecies transplants. For example, in "My Adventure with the Man-Monkey," one of the stories collected in H. Frankish's 1913 *Dr. Cunliffe, Investigator*, an ape receives part of the brain of a criminal who has been sentenced to death; the creature escapes and carries out several bestial murders before being shot down (Bleiler 1990, no. 811d.)

Both on paper and screen, the man-ape brain transplantation, which inspired the 1909 short film *L'Homme-singe* mentioned in Chapter 1, seems to have been at first the most popular brain motif. Other brain plots abound in later SF novels, and Gernsback's own "New Science Fiction Series" included Lilith Lorraine's 1929 novella *The Brain of the Planet*. (An ad for the book, printed in *Science Wonder Stories* of September 1929, asks, "If a super-intelligence could have its wisdom poured into our brains, what a different world we might have." Different indeed: the story features a psychology professor who proves the existence of telepathy and invents a "radio-like transmitter of thought-waves" that brings about a revolution based on the principles of feminist Christian socialism [Donawerth 1990].) By the time the cerebral motif became a B favorite, it was firmly established in the pulps.

General fiction magazines made room for SF and brain themes. The short story "Science and the Girl" was published in January 1909 in *The Blue Book Magazine* (1905–1956), a US general fiction publication regarded both as "the king of the pulps" and as a "slick in pulp clothing" (Ashley n.d.; "slicks" were printed on better paper and appealed to a more elite audience). The story's trigger implicitly but clearly draws from the case of Phineas Gage, a railroad worker who survived twelve years, with personality and behavior changes, after an accident in 1848 drove an iron rod through his head and destroyed much of his left frontal lobe (Macmillan 2008). In "Science and the Girl," the young Dr. Wood has made great discoveries in brain surgery and cerebral function. After a steel rod is driven through the forehead of Reynolds, her fiancée's father, Wood removes the patient's forebrain. The formerly industrious man then becomes lazy and vicious. (The operation may recall lobotomy, but this procedure was only invented in 1935; attempts to remove parts of the cortex in psychiatric patients, though, had been made since the late 1880s.) Blaming his fiancé for the result, Margaret breaks up with him. After a friend of Wood's dies, the doctor reopens Reynolds's skull, and, hoping to give him back his personality, pours into the empty forebrain space electrified gray matter from his friend's brain. However, he mistakenly uses someone else's cerebral substance, and Reynolds unexpectedly becomes a great financier (Bleiler 1990, 218). "Science and the Girl" was published in the same year that *L'Homme-singe* was produced.

All-Story was established in 1905 as a companion to the older *The Argosy* (the very first magazine to appear on pulp paper, with which *All-Story* merged in 1920), and its most lasting contribution is probably that it launched the career of Edgar Rice Burroughs (1875–1950), one of the most prolific and popular fantasy and adventure writers ever, when it serialized *Under the Moons of Mars* and *Tarzan of the Apes* in 1912. Under slightly different titles (but always including "all-story"), it was also the major venue for SF until other pulps emerged in the 1920s. "The Man Who Discovered Nothing" (1920) includes the idea that memories can be removed from the brain (Bleiler 1990, no. 517). In an early version of the alien trope, creatures called Whoomangs can, by making an incision at the base of brain, introduce a "brain-maggot" that ends up taking over the host's mind and body ("The Radio Man," 1926; ib., no. 695). In a twist that recalls *Orlac's Hands* (discussed in Chapter 3), "Horror on Owl's Hill" (1929) stages a character who claims that he has shifted brains between two individuals, thus verifying that the brain is the source of personality. The truth is that he had not transplanted anything, but hypnotized his victims into developing new personalities (ib., no. 1916). (Popular in the pulps, hypnosis, especially in connection with possession, induced crime, and mass political phenomena, was until the 1930s a major filmic motif, and a concern with regard to the supposed dangers of cinematic suggestion [Andriopoulos 2008, Berton 2009a; Killen 2017, Chap. 3]. Together with hysteria, paramnesia, neurosis, trance, double personality and all manner of psychological conditions and "psychic" phenomena, it belonged in the intersection between the cinema and the brain and mind sciences around 1900 [Berton 2009b, 2015]).

In 1922, the British pulp *Hutchinson's Magazine*, which furthered weird, supernatural and mystery fiction, published "And the Dead Spake—," one of E. F. Benson's numerous ghost stories. The narrator recalls an episode he lived with physicist Sir James Horton. "It is known," he writes, that Horton "made an artificial being formed of the tissue, still living, of animals lately killed, with the brain of an ape and the heart of a bullock, and a sheep's thyroid, and so forth" (Benson 1996 [1922], 175). In a conversation that takes place right at the beginning of World War I, Horton asks him to imagine "a shop with glass cases containing healthy organs taken from the dead." They could be sold to someone who needs a replacement. "And," the narrator asks in reply, "insert the brain of someone who has died of heart disease into the skull of a congenital idiot?"

> Yes, perhaps [Horton answers]; but the brain's tiresomely complicated in its connections and the joining up of the nerves, you know. Surgery will have to learn a lot before it fits new brains in. (ib., 177–178)

The doctor has been doing experiments based on the idea that the brain is like a phonograph, with memories recorded as if on a plate. He then plays for the narrator a tune inscribed in the cerebral speech-center of a wounded soldier who died during an operation to extract shrapnel from his brain (ib., 183). Mrs. Gabriel may have murdered her husband, but is perfect as the doctor's housekeeper. After she accidentally dies, Horton cannot resist the temptation, props "the gramophone needle in position," and inserts the poles of the second battery into her fractured skull. "And as I watched her face, I saw with a freezing horror that her lips were beginning to move" (ib., 187–188). When Horton turns up the current, Mrs. Gabriel describes how she killed her husband. Excited and wanting more, the doctor leans over the table while holding the two poles of the battery, falls forward, and produces a short circuit that kills him. The narrative emphasizes spooky features, such as the corpse moving its lips and speaking through the gramophone trumpet; the general atmosphere justifies placing it among the author's collected ghost stories. At the same time, it conveys ideas about brain functioning, its relationship to memory, personal identity, and the definition of death – all of which would become SF pulp staples.

Weird Tales

The first magazine entirely devoted to fantasy and occult fiction was *Weird Tales*; this section focuses on it, though it will refer when relevant to other publications. Founded before Gernsback started making history, and in Chicago, rather than in New York like most others, *Weird Tales* became the longest-running and one of the most influential pulp magazines, contributing to the development and popularization of such categories as dark and heroic fantasy, sword-and-sorcery fiction, and the supernatural sleuth story (Hoppenstand 2013). As noted above, it did not identify itself with SF; during the period examined here, its title page described it as "a magazine of the bizarre and unusual." A 1924 editorial explained that it ran two types of narratives. One was "the story of psychic [i.e., paranormal] phenomena or the occult story," written from the viewpoints of the believing spiritualist, the actively skeptical scientist, or the "neutral investigator" who "simply records the facts." The other was made up of "Highly Imaginative Stories," which it defined as "stories of advancement in the sciences and the arts to which the generation of the writer who creates them has not attained," adding: "All writers of such stories are prophets, and in the years to come, many of their prophecies will come true" ("Why *Weird Tales*?" *Weird Tales*, 4[2], May–July 1924, 1–2). Brain scenarios served such stories well.

In 1924, with the short story "The Brain in the Jar," *Weird Tales* staged early on the archetypal cerebral thought experiment, combining it with a "psychic" element. The year is 1919, during the tense aftermath of World War I. Posing as an orderly in a Berlin hospital, the spy Vernon Eldridge keeps an eye on Dr. Jaeger. In the doctor's private laboratory, a large glass jar attracts his attention "through the elaborate apparatus connected with it" (Brainfilms 2.4):

> The jar was spherical in shape with a large circular mouth fitted with a ground glass stopper, having a German cross for a knob. Above was a large nickel-plated tank and extending from it to the jar a slender glass tube controlled by a system of valves. (Hammerstrom and Searight 1924, 33)

Looking more closely into the "murky liquid," Eldridge perceives "two naked human eyes glaring down at him with ferocious intensity." As the liquid clears, he sees "a human brain in perfect preservation." Two cords extend from the organ, cross each other, and terminate in the eyes. "The entire hideous spectacle resembled a huge snail" (ib.). Some time later, while making a drawing of the setup, Eldridge has the impression that his name is being called. "He looked up to see the glaring eyes of the brain fading gradually from sight as the liquid in the jar grew opaque. As he stared, the fluid again regained its transparency and the glowing eyes seems to be boring through his very brain" (ib., 34). He then loses consciousness. When he recovers, he finds in his sketch book a line in French, which he does not recall writing, instructing him to be in the laboratory the next day at midnight.

The brain, which now controls Eldridge through "hypnotic trance," turns out to belong to the French spy Jean Perrin, captured during the war and delivered to Jaeger for his "crowning experiment" in preserving human organs: "an attempt to keep the human brain alive *and functioning!*" (ib., 183). The operation succeeds. "My mind and personality," Perrin tells through Eldridge, "were helplessly chained to this lump of clay called the brain" (ib., 185). He takes his disembodiment as the opportunity to develop such paranormal abilities as telepathy, mind control, and telekinesis, which he hides from Jaeger and exploits to harm the enemy: "In the last week there have been twelve murders, six suicides and eight insanity cases, all of noted German officials of the worst type. ... all caused by the hypnotic suggestions which I have made by telepathy" (ib., 186). Although he "might rule the world through strength of the will," his only purpose is to take personal vengeance on Jaeger, and then die. While the doctor is working at the microscope, Perrin uses his psychokinetic power to empty on him a huge bottle of hydrofluoric acid. As the doctor falls on the floor "writhing and shrieking in his death agony," the acid spills all over, a fire breaks out, and the whole laboratory goes up in flames. When he awakens, Eldridge finds himself on a hospital ship bound for New York, with a friend from the secret service and in his wife's "loving care." For "[h]er love alone can efface from his mind the effect of the memory of the vengeance of the brain in the jar" (ib., 190).

The cinematic presence is here more than the "shadow" Telotte discerned in the pulps. Starting with the title object and the story's headpiece, and running through complex equipment, an evil scientist, an ectobrain that fades and glows or pulsates, the paranormal powers it develops, its revenge, a screaming agony, a laboratory going up in flames, "The Brain in the Jar" could be the sketch of brainfilm scenario and a collection of the genre's basic tropes. (The eyes-joined-to-the-brain-via-the-optic-nerves trope did not become commonplace. However, Roald Dahl's 1959 story "William and Mary," in which William survives as an ectobrain to which one eye remains attached and ends up the helpless victim of Mary's revenge, was adapted for TV in 1961 in the American series *Way Out*, and in 1979 in the British series *Tales of the Unexpected*.)

"The Brain in the Jar" was only the first of several brainstories published in *Weird Tales*. Insofar as it involved only humans acting on earth at a time close to the writer's present, it was also particularly straightforward. Most other stories went further.

In "The Seventh Devil," announced as "a bizarre story of weird surgery," the narrator is inspired by the protagonist of H. G. Wells's 1896 *The Island of Dr. Moreau* (the prototype of transplantation horror) to move to a Pacific island and start experimenting on brain transplants:

> One dog, from which I had removed certain of the super-motor centers from one side of the brain, spent all his time walking in a circle … . Another, in which the cerebellum had been mutilated, was unable to maintain its balance … . Here was a monkey that walked sluggishly about on four feet … ; for the brain of this monkey had been removed, and in its place I had transplanted a portion of the brain of a pig. (McHenry 1925, 631).

He also extirpates the cerebral "reasoning centers" of three monkeys, combines them, and inserts them "into the empty brainpan of a living monkey from which the brain had been entirely cleared out" (ib., 632). Thus, as the narrator explains, within the cranium of the experimental subject "was stored the accumulated learning" of the three transplanted brains: "I now had a monkey nine times as intelligent as the average monkey!" (ib.) One stormy night in late December, a ship is wrecked on the island and three corpses are washed ashore. He takes brain segments from each and transplants them into the skull of a giant gorilla he calls 143.

The animal becomes sensationally smart: it can type, comments on major philosophers, and though it cannot speak, knows several languages (the human donors were of different nationalities). With its "centers of emotion" removed," he seems at first to be "purely intellectual". But "some fragments of emotion had been left in one of the transplanted brains. And this fragment was – black hatred" (ib., 634). The narrator then decides to kill 143; a chase follows, and he manages to lure the gorilla into a patch of quicksand, where it sinks with "a final mad scream of hatred defeated" (ib., 636).

The mad scientist's customary desire to create pure intellect and the ensuing catastrophic imbalance between emotions and understanding parallel or combine with the cliché of the body taking over the brain. In "Laocoon," for example, another brain-transplant specialist grafts a Chinese student's brain into a sea serpent. The "brute body" eventually conquers the transplanted mind, and the creature becomes threatening (Morgan 1926, 54). In some rare instances, the brain-body symbiosis results from intersexual transplantation. In "The Head," the white expeditionary Phillips has appropriated the "brown girl" of a local Papuan sorcerer-chieftain (the "magnificent black giant" Gwanoo), who kills him, beheads him, and intends to add Phillips's head to his collection. Black hostile warriors wound the girl in an attack. Following her injunctions, the alcoholic surgeon Dakens tries to kill Gwanoo. In the fight, the girl is fatally wounded. When Dakens sobers up, he realizes that he has transplanted the girl's brain into the chieftain's body. His one regret as he boards a canoe to leave the island, and looks "for the last time on the magnificent Gwanoo with the soft eyes of the bride of Phillips," is that "he would never know how the thing would end; whether the warrior body of the sorcerer would in time absorb the woman-brain, or the woman weaken the warrior. It seemed a pity he could not watch that phase, but in a white man's land a white girl waited" (Morgan 1927a, 240).

"The Devils of Po Sung" – a "creepy, powerful tale of brain transplantation" – takes us again to Papua, where a sadistic oriental villain employs a surgeon to transplant his captives' brains into animal bodies: "One year ago," he explains, "two thieves stole in from the sea. One of them supplied brains to a river crocodile, the other is a gray ape" (Morgan 1927b, 784). In the end, they tear him to pieces. In the sequel to this truly "weird tale," the brains of these two animal-men are to be transplanted back into human bodies (Morgan 1929). Like "Laocoon," the three last stories were penned by one of the few SF pulp women writers, the Canadian-born Grace Ethel Jones (1884–1977), under the pseudonym Bassett Morgan.

In "Mr. Pichegru's Discovery," the title protagonist finds brain transplantation simple. As he tells Cavanaugh, the narrator, the principle is "that the brain can exist without the body, and the body without the brain." The chicken with the snake's brain has the snake's "brain capabilities" and the same applies to the snake with the chicken's brain (Keppler 1929, 83). Determined to extend his experiments, Pichegru dopes Cavanaugh, and transplants his brain into the body of the giant gorilla Gormaz. Now that Cavanaugh has "superhuman strength and agility," the doctor wants him to steal some precious jewels before restoring him to his original body. But the situation degenerates, and the "beast-man" kills the doctor. Cavanaugh, whose human body is dead, feels desperate at the thought of being trapped in Gormaz's body forever. Somehow, his brain returns to a human body (how else could he tell the story?), and the final scene shows the gorilla surging against the bars of a cage, blasting "his great thunder-roar" (ib., 89).

"The Chemical Brain," which goes in a different direction, reveals some of its scientific and literary sources in unusual detail (these include Karel Čapek's 1920 play *R.U.R.*, which introduced the word "robot"; the story is apparently the first to use it in SF pulps). Parsons, one of the constructors of the artificial creature, advocates behaviorism and recommends John B. Watson's work (Flagg 1929, 76). The narrator objects: "no matter how much you give your machine chemical brains it won't be able to start its own thinking process." Parsons agrees, and that is why he is trying to create "a mechanical, a chemical brain, delicate enough to respond to thought as it now does to sound or other stimuli" (ib., 79). He succeeds. When the narrator approaches the machine, he perceives a strange reddish-blue glow radiating from the glass that tops the head. Fascinated, he peers through the glass, and sees a "glutinous mixture … pulsing as if alive. It was now a gray, speckled mass shot through with red streamers" (ib.). In the end, the robot kills Parsons. Tragic, usually violent and mortal endings embody the morality of mad scientist stories. They are common in brainfilms, but the most striking cinematic affinity here lies in the throbbing and gleaming brain – a staple of B movies, though long without the advantage of color.

Weird Tales offers other narrative configurations, which are also found in contemporaneous and later pulps. Transplantation always involves drama, but plots where the brain is handled without transplantation can give rise to even more appalling individual predicaments. "Listening Death" opens with Dr. Frank Whitley boasting of his achievements in front of a group of colleagues:

> First trepanning the skull, making a circular hole and piercing it, I withdrew the precious contents of the pineal gland and also the cerebrospinal fluid. I had no opportunity for quite some time to make use of the stimulative serum thus obtained, but it was preserved carefully; and, when I was later asked to operate on the brain of a man known for his dull-wittedness, I inoculated the patient with the serum. The operation was a splendid success, the results more than I had hoped for. Today, that dull-witted fellow is amazing all who know him by displaying flashes of positive genius! (Catlin 1927, 642)

Whitley's dream, however, is to preserve "the brains of our greatest inventors, savants and statesmen" to put "the marvelous intellects of history's supermen" at the disposal of future generations (ib.). Surgery, though, is not the path to follow, because it transfers "only a portion of the original intellect," which becomes contaminated "with lesser brains" (ib., 643). Whitley stumbles upon a viable alternative when the discovery of a Pharaoh's tomb and mummy prompts in his mind the association between "preservation of body and preservation of brain" (ib.). He thus develops a drug that keeps dead bodies in perfect condition, and another that revives them. After bringing back to life a criminal called Wilson, he injects himself with the substance, asking to be revived after a while.

Wilson, however, reveals that his brain had remained active all the time: "there ain't no torture in the world to compare with knowing that your body's dead – dead – dead … and laying there, thinking and listening!" (ib., 647). He wants to take revenge, a scuffle follows, the drug is spilled. "My God!" exclaims Whitley's colleague Dr. Truman, "we can't permit him to go on through time suffering mental torment." But there is no way out:

> "You forget," said Dr. Hazard, abjectly, "that nothing we can do will place Dr. Whitley beyond that which faces him… for we could but deprive him of life… and he is already dead!"
>
> Truman gazed in open-eyed horror at the placid face of Dr. Whitley … . But if Dr. Whitley heard, or knew, or understood, he gave no sign … ; yet he seemed to be intently listening – listening… (ib., 648)

The recurrent problem of the relationships between a state of the body, a condition of the brain, and the diagnosis of death arises here in the absence of transplantation; and even in the horrible circumstances of an indefinite locked-in state, it is always resolved in accordance with the already quoted conclusion by philosopher Roland Puccetti (1969, 70): "Where goes a brain, there goes a person."

Let us finish this tour through *Weird Tales* with an instance of another popular theme: the great ruling brain. In "The Black Monarch," Professor Eden is convinced that "the presence in human beings of large-scale good or evil is unnatural, abnormal, and due entirely to obedience to some powerful outside influence" (Ernst 1930, 201). "Since man's actions originate in his brain," he invents a device (pridefully named "edograph") to measure "the quantity and quality of thought" and to trace the cerebral sources of human actions (ib.). After a visit from an unknown man who leaves behind a gold ring surmounted with two serpents, the edograph no longer works. The jewel produces an image, which Eden captures photographically. It is a gigantic, very muscular human form; straight from the shoulders surges "a smooth cylindrical mass tapering to a rounded point"; in the front are two round patches that resemble "huge, unwinking eyes," with no other facial features. What could it be? "A disembodied brain, perhaps, or … an abstract force against which no mortal could struggle" (ib., 206).

Eden locates an evil being who rules the world from an underground palace in North Africa. Before dying, he sends his adopted son Sanderson on a crusade against that being. There, Sanderson joins forces with Neal Emory, whose father had been murdered by the creature. Both are captured, and taken before Rez, the Black Monarch whose enlarged brain is encased for protection in a metal skull (the strange tapered cylinder Eden described). Rez is an ancient Egyptian, more than six thousand years old and gifted with paranormal powers. He controls others through a huge diamond crystal, pieces of which are set in rings and scattered around the world as a means to sow discord. He needs Sanderson and Emory as human subjects to test his mind drugs and mental surgery. The captives resist, a fight ensues, Rez and Sanderson die, the kingdom of the Black Monarch comes to an end, and an unexpected era of peace dawns upon the Earth.

Stories Astounding and Amazing

Bleiler (1990, no. 684) characterized "The Black Monarch" as "a kitchen sink full of oddities." Many stories fit such description and, as we shall see next, the pulps were no less freaky than *Weird Tales*. Let us nonetheless begin by an exception to the usual "sink of oddities" picture: the brief and focused 1933 short story "Stallion's Trappings."

Professor Shea, who has always felt inferior, ignored by all, bullied by his colleagues, and despised by his wife, inherits a fortune. In exchange for over one and a half million dollars, he wants Dr. Malavan to give him the brain of the ruthless tycoon Mortimer Judd. "Install it in my skull, connect it with my cerebellum and the rest of my brain and nerve tissue. I have a conviction, irrational but sure, that my personality will flow up to possess and utilize this new instrument you give me" (Collins 1933, 1135). He wants to use Judd's brain (which he describes as the stallion he wants to ride) to obtain "all the things in life, which my scholar's brain could not win for me" (ib.). The doctor acquiesces. Shea gives up his college position, and embarks on a ruthless, miraculously successful financial career. Malavan would like to find out "how much of the personality is intrinsic in the instrument through which it works." Shea is not concerned, but, in the end, he kills himself, leaving behind a note that simply reads, "I could no longer endure his memories" (ib., 1136). That Shea's personality endures with Judd's brain remains an unexplained oddity (partial grafting, discussed below, cannot play a role). Nevertheless, the story as a whole is, for a pulp, an unusually lean brain-transplantation narrative.

Though generally along more tortuous paths, most brain-themed pulp plots incorporate issues related to personal identity and continuity, and convey beliefs about the brain itself. The most basic of these concerns the precise cerebral localization of functions. It tends to remain buried in tangled scenarios, but "Dr. Conklin – Pacifist," perhaps written with a humorous intention, places it at the heart of its plot. Conklin has decided to cure the world's evils with a ray of his invention. The problem with civilization is that it has brought about hate, lust, greed, ambition, rivalry, possession, and inferiority. Each of these emotions "has its separate brain cell," and is "susceptible to certain ray vibrations." By "adding the technique of regular short-wave radio broadcasting and atomic decomposition," Conklin devices an infra-red ray that paralyzes those cells, and can thereby "end bloodshed and the desire for conquest" (Peregoy 1934, 36, 37). The doctor hopes to cover the globe with ray stations within six months, and once "peace and brotherly love" predominate, he will "release his secret to the world" (ib., 38). The treatment works, but also leads to a complete lack of ambition and nerve. When New York pest exterminators refuse to kill "live creatures with feelings, brains and souls of their own," the city is devastated by "a plague of vermin, bedbugs, roaches, ants, lice, other creatures" (ib., 42). Since crops go unprotected, there is no food. And so on and so forth. Moreover, Conklin's arch-rival, the evil Stanton Wales, leads a band of people who escaped the ray and want to conquer the world. Fortunately, Conklin manages to "restimulate the paralyzed brain cells" and the world goes back to normal (ib., 44).

"The Ambidexter" does not postulate one-to-one correspondences between mental characteristics and an individual neuron, but introduces the motif of the cerebral partial graft and the inner struggles it generates, which brainfilms will also exploit (see Chapter 3). The story's title describes Dr. Hopkins, the "greatest surgeon in America." Hopkins suffers from a frontal lobe tumor. When Wing Loo, "the greatest surgeon in Asia," operates on him, he grafts a piece of a criminal's brain. Thereafter, Hopkins feels an urge to kill with his left hand, and ends up murdering a patient during surgery. Wing then reveals that he did that on purpose, to punish Hopkins for having "played around" with "a little Chinese girl" who was in fact his daughter. Hopkins, who did not know, commits suicide. Wing keeps his colleague's brain for future use, and becomes in the meantime "the greatest surgeon in the world" (Keller 1931a).

Ectobrains are a major theme, and with the image of what seems to be a severed human head attached to the usual equipment and a stern-looking scientist communicating with it through a speaking tube, *Amazing Stories* of August 1926 offers an excellent pulp cover, perhaps the best with regard to resonances with brainfilms (Brainfilms 2.5). A similar scene ornates the title page of the corresponding short story, "The Talking Brain" (Brainfilms 2.6). The depicted setup resembles a living head scenario from a 1950s picture. The head, however, is actually an artificial receptacle for a brain kept alive, a box whose lid is the skullcap. In reflections similar to future movie dialogues, an editorial note recalls that grafting and maintaining life "in an organ separated from the body" are medical realities that suggest "endless possibilities to the creative surgeon." It also sees in the story "an interesting successor" to Edgar Allan Poe's "The Facts in the Case of M. Valdemar" (1845). In Poe's tale, which *Amazing Stories* reprinted in its first issue (April 1926), the dying Valdemar is maintained for seven months in an "unusually perfect state of mesmeric trance." Although the "mesmeric process" seems to have suspended death, Valdemar, who responds to questions, declares himself dead. Awakening him after nearly seven months leads to the instantaneous rotting of his body, its immediate (and highly cinematic) transformation into "a nearly liquid mass of loathsome – of detestable putrescence."

"The Talking Brain" cerebralizes the story, replacing mesmerism by surgery as a way to perpetuate life. A brilliant young student called Vinton is irrecoverably maimed in a car accident. His friend Professor Murtha proposes to keep him alive as an ectobrain. The patient, who had earlier recovered sight thanks to an artificial retina created by Murtha, knows not only about the doctor's accomplishments, but also about Jacques Loeb and Alexis Carrel, two pioneers of tissue culture, regeneration, and organ transplantation. "If a heart could be kept beating in a bottle for years at a time, why should not a brain be kept thinking in a bottle forever?" Communication would be unproblematic, "for he knew his Morse, and Murtha had solved the problem of efferent impulses." Vinton therefore accepts the scientist's offer, and becomes a living brain encased in an apparatus with "placid waxen features," and connected to the outside world through a speaking tube. Life in such a state turns out to be torture, and "dreadful messages" arrive "from the transplanted brain of a dead man" (Hasta 1926, 445). Like the severed living heads of other stories (e.g., Jones 1934, 71), and those of later brainfilms, Vinton wants to die. Although only his brain subsists, the illustrations give the apparatus that contains it expressive features that are far from serene. Like many other pulp stories, "The Talking Brain" employs retrospective narration; it is thus at the beginning that we learn that Murtha commits suicide. Yet, in true horror fashion, it never becomes clear whether he first killed Vinton's head. This was a potent scenario.

"The Talking Brain" recalls the plot of Alexander Beliaev's *Professor Dowell's Head*, published in Russian the previous year (see Chapter 3), and Vinton's situation is similar to Whitley's in "Listening Death," published a year later. Like these stories, "The Talking Brain" could have easily become a film script, and living heads would indeed crop up in the Bs (*Dowell* itself was adapted, but only in the 1980s). Moreover, like many ectobrain narratives, it can be situated in a history of concern over the relationship between medical technology and liminal states of "undeath." It is from such a perspective that

Poe's "Valdemar" has been related to the real-life case of Jahi McMath (who was maintained on life support for over four years following a diagnosis of brain death in 2013), and has been read as a "modern fable" and "an uneasy herald" of the ability to bring about such liminal states (O'Dell 2020, 229).

Following the current, in 1928 *Amazing Stories* printed "The Head." The editorial note on the story's first page seeks to nourish with fact the readers' appetite for fantasy:

> Recent experiments in Germany have proven conclusively that it is not only possible to decapitate insects, but to actually transplant heads from one insect to another, and after the heads are healed in place, the insects seem to be no worse for having their heads cut off and exchanged for others.
>
> Of course, it's a far cry from an insect head to a human head, but the thing will not be so improbable a hundred years hence, as it may seem now.

The author of the note (presumably Gernsback) was up to date: in 1923, the Austrian biologist Walter Finkler had published two articles on head transplantation in insects, which gave rise to considerable discussion, including, the following year, a letter exchange in the journal *Nature*. We shall later see where we are "a hundred years hence."

"The Head" tells the story of Professor Beardsley. He is fatally ill from stomach cancer and has a six-year-old motherless daughter to care for. In exchange for preserving his living head, Dr. James Leeson offers him fifty thousand dollars, which Beardsley could place in a trust for the child. The professor is horrified and finds the whole thing "diabolical." Leeson, however, is confident of success, for he has already kept a chimpanzee's head alive for over six months, perfused via a pump, and connected to an apparatus that supplies it with "life-sustaining fluid" (Kleier 1928, 420). Beardsley ends up accepting the offer. He must agree to let Leeson keep his head alive for two months; after that, he can indicate that he wishes to die, and if he were to become incapable of communicating, Leeson promises to terminate the head within that time.

The operation runs well; after a few days, the wound heals; the Head notices "the anxious faces hovering about it," and responds "by signaling with its eyelids" (ib., 421). Unfortunately, an automobile kills Leeson; his assistants are brought to court and charged with mayhem (i.e. maiming someone by depriving them of the use of any of their members). The trial, however, is inconclusive, one side demanding "that the Head's life should be put to an end for humane reasons," the other arguing "that this would be the same as murder because the brain really made the man" (ib.) (Brainfilms 2.7). Meanwhile, the Head keeps on living, and the case lies indefinitely dormant. As the centuries pass, a clique of self-proclaimed priests convince the people that the Head is a divinity they must obey. Finally, during a war, the enemy enters the temple and kills it: "A look of utter content came over the Head's features as the blow that meant oblivion descended!" (ib., 449). Again, a brain-themed story depicts situations and dilemmas that are closer to twenty-first-century quandaries than to those of one hundred years ago.

The great difference between disembodied heads and ectobrains lies in the capacity for expression (e.g., Beardley's eyes conveying a message). In most movies, as we shall see in Chapter 3, while those heads wish to die, the majority of brains in vats wish to live in order to carry out their heinous plans, or at least take revenge on those responsible for their situation. The pulps offer a number of instances of this plot, as well as variations such as the following.

In "The Time Conqueror," one Dr. Koszarek murders his colleague Dr. Ovington, and keeps his brain alive in a rather unusual round vat (Brainfilms 2.8). Koszarek's theory that a brain cut off from sensory stimuli can enter the fourth dimension and learn about the future turns out to be true, and Ovington's brain shows him the supercivilizations of the third and fourth millennia, which have accepted "the bodiless thing as their ruler" (Eshbach 1932, 134). By the later period, Koszarek has become Koz, a demented outcast; the Brain kills him, while, back in the present, Ovington's brain murders Koszarek, whose body will lie for centuries to come next to the vat containing the brain that "conquered time" (ib., 182). In this case, the ectobrain itself did not seek immortality or power, but received both as the consequence of homicide.

Ovington's brain is highly visible. Yet neither narrative descriptions nor graphic illustrations are necessary for a brain to be center stage. Consider the short story "The Brain Accelerator." Written, the editorial note states, by a physician "who also possesses imagination" and develops the trendy subject of "gland treatment in a highly scientific and plausible manner," the story explores the possibility of expanding intelligence by acting directly on the brain. Colonel Grigsby, a native of Manchester, has settled in a small Ohio town. The narrator, a doctor, is called to treat a wound. The two men share scientific interests, and the doctor becomes a regular visitor. One day, Grigsby claims to have proved that the "nerve impulse" is an electrical phenomenon, but that his discovery is "incidental" to his research into how much of a brain "can be eliminated without the death or evident impairment of mental quality of the individual" (Dressler 1929, 699, 700).

Repeating a popular pulp cliché, Grigsby claims that although the cerebral cortex has been only "very imperfectly mapped," it is clear that humans have four or five times more brain tissue that they use (ib.). Moreover, he has become certain that "the nerve impulse, and probably the psychic or ultra-material phenomenon that we called mind" are "electrical in their nature" (ib., 701). In his home laboratory, described in great detail and represented in an impressive double-spread drawing, Grigsby uses a green ray to induce in dead dogs "external electrical forces that simulate nerve impulses and can be super-imposed upon actual nerves" (ib.). The ray revives the animals. When applied in a different way, it becomes red, and the resuscitated dogs understand human speech, respond with appropriate head movements, and perform unlearned behaviors. The ray "affects the nervous system," causing it "to reassume and enact the characteristics of life." In its red form, it causes "an increase in nervous activity with an attendant increase in cerebration that unquestionably raises the mental power of the animal to an unthought of degree" (ib., 704).

Grisgsby is convinced that the surge in mental function is due to "an increase in the number of synapses or contacts of the ordinarily functioning brain tissue with the vast areas that we know have not demonstrable activity at present" – increase that would "overnight" lead to major strides "in science, in medicine, in political economy, in morality" and to other "untold possibilities, the creation of a super-mind, education of the human reduced to a simple affair, the return to life of the dead who were without too much damage to their bodies" (ib., 705, 701). After Grigsby dies in a fire, the narrator finds a letter where the Coronel explains that he tried the ray on himself, thus experiencing not only "the immense increase in mental power which it engenders," but also a metabolic acceleration that exhausted "the brain mechanism" (ib., 719). The narrator is left wondering if Gribsy's "tragic end" was "an accident or a deliberate removal of himself and his apparatus when he felt that he had created a Frankenstein Monster?" (ib.). "The Brain Accelerator" thus brings together such classic themes as the nature of life and the limits of experimentation with commonplace fantasies about revival and immortality, such trademark SF clichés as the use of a ray, and the claim that mind is electrical and that, from life to thought, we are essentially our (underused) brains.

Both in movies and the pulps, brains are mostly enacted as individual entities. Some films stage communication and connection among them as happening through telepathic or technological means, almost always for malevolently manipulative purposes. Not all scenarios, however, made it into the Bs. The following are a few instances.

Mass brainmind manipulation: In "The Menace from Below," one of a convoluted mass of story lines includes a scientist called Talbot who kidnaps New Yorkers to transplant their brains into the bodies of "ape-men of the same general characteristics as the Pithecanthropus erectus." Talbot captures the donors by diverting subway trains into the underground world where he discovered those near-human beings and built his laboratory. He first improves the ape-men "by surgical and medical means." By the time the story takes places, they are "truly supermen physically but, as yet, woefully lacking in brain power" (Vincent 1929a, 161). The goal of the transplants is to fix that sorrowful situation and, ultimately, insure "the advancement of science" and the amelioration of humanity:

> We are going to create a race of supermen, endow them with the best brains that can be obtained from the upper world and set them loose eventually to assist us in conquering and ruling the surface. It is a rotten civilization above. (ib., 162)

In the process, humans will "remain physically unimpaired and will make good laborers. But they become morons – or lower." During the "psycho-transference operations," the donor and the recipient wear "a metallic cap-like contrivance," a variation of the trademark helmet that closely fits "the entire portion of the skull" enclosing the brain. The caps are connected through cables to individual switchboards similar to "the central board of an automatic telephone system." In about two hours, the human's "conscious and subconscious mental equipment" is transferred to the "synthetic superman," who thus receives "an education that would ordinarily require fifteen or twenty years to impart" (ib., 165).

Other pulp plots rare or absent in brainfilms concern the supreme ecto-brain that rules entire societies, and the notion of interlinked or otherwise collectively operating brains. We have encountered this already in "The Black Monarch." A particularly pure version of the theme is "Master of the Brain," the second of Canadian writer's Laurence Manning five-part "The Man Who Awoke," published in *Wonder Stories* in 1933. The protagonist of the series, Norman Winters, puts himself in suspended animation for five thousand years at a time; each story narrates his adventures in the societies he finds every time he awakes. In 10,000 AD, Winters encounters a civilization that for the past ten centuries has been ruled by the Brain. What is it?

> The Brain is... well, It is a machine that includes every function of the human brain and surpasses it in most things. It is totally unprejudiced and

> absolutely infallible. ... Only by Its guidance have we been able to reduce the working hours of mankind to one hour a week. (Manning 1933, 841)

The price of such wellbeing (one of SF's major techno-dystopian themes) is absolute obedience and dependency, and some are unhappy about it. As member of a clandestine group seeking freedom from the Brain, Winters must change to alternating current the direct current that feeds the machine: "The whole association of ideas that is the very basis of reason will be shattered and distorted. The Brain will immediately go... insane!" (ib., 845). This happens, the Brain is destroyed, its rule collapses, and Winters is helped back into suspended animation. An editorial note comments on the story as "both a promise and a warning of the future." In a technocracy, we would be "under the control of a central Brain," and if anything happened to it, "woe betide the race" (ib., 838). The Brain here is a huge supercomputer. Nevertheless, great ectobrains and powerful technical simulations of them mirror each other.

"In 20,000 A.D.," which Ashley and Lowndes (2004, 311) consider one of the best "great brain" stories, is, as Bleiler (1998, no. 1276) notes, also an "adaptation of the fairy-wood motif to science fiction." A Long Island farm boy called Tom ventures into a wooded forest most people avoid. He disappears for several months. Upon his return, a reporter and a scientist from New York persuade him to talk. Tom has been into the future, to 20,000 AD precisely, and witnessed a world divided into Masters and Robots; the latter are tall, black, have low intelligence and do all the work. Above the Masters is Jed, an immortal ectobrain with telepathic powers (Brainfilms 2.9). As Tom recounts:

> Jed was a tremendous brain – nothin' else, floatin' in the middle of a liquid like calf's foot jelly before it become hard. A great big gray brain, full o' lines and ridges an' deep twistings. It gave me the shivers to look at it. (Schachner and Zagat 1930, 316)

Karet, the Master who chaperons Tom (and who would like to take Jed's place), tells Tom that 2000 years earlier, "one of the Masters had become so wise and knew so much that his brain didn't have room enough to expand in the skull." The other Masters placed his brain "in a certain kind o' jelly," from which it forever rules (ib.). As we shall see in Chapter 3, in films too (but without the "ruling" dimension), brain size and overall power are correlated, as are power and the fact of being pure cerebral substance.

Another example of great ruling brains can be found in "Microcosmic Buccaneers," a story published in the same issue of *Amazing Stories* as "The Brain Accelerator." Here, an almost purely cerebral entity rules a subatomic world inhabited by humans and humanoids: "Mere brains were the Great Ones. Their bodies were shrunken beyond all belief and the huge, semi-transparent heads lay helpless amongst the cushions, the immense eyes presenting the only evidence of life in the weird beings" (Vincent 1929b, 686). In yet another variation, "The Purple Brain," two men, Neil and John, are riding their horses in the late twilight when they encounter a cougar. On the animal's head and shoulders sits something that looks like "a colossal brain":

> The thing glowed with an eerie purple luminescence like a great blob of luminous jelly. Its surface rippled in ceaseless flowing motion that suggested the rapid pulsing of a heart. Somewhere deep within the glowing purple bulk Neil could sense the presence of an utterly alien entity of incredible power and overwhelming evil. (Wells 1933, 58)

The entity is Yaagir, a member of "the great race of Zaas" (a planet six light-years distant from earth), whose "composition is almost purely cerebral." For their physical needs, the inhabitants of Zaas use the "bodies of lesser creatures" (ib., 63). Because of their longevity, the planet is overpopulated. Yaagir (the title's "purple brain") has been sent to identify possible future colonies. After Neil destroys its body, a "viscous, purple-black liquid flowed turgidly from the brain as it twisted in its death agony": it is the creature's "protoplasmic arm" setting off the bomb that blasts it "into oblivion" (ib., 69).

The most complete expression of self-to-brain reduction (a common basis for "great brains" plots) may be "The Man Who Evolved." Dr. John Pollard invites the narrator, Arthur Wright, and Hugh Dutton (confined to an insane asylum since the narrated events took place) to his "isolated cottage" to show them the results of his experiments. As he explains, "two great questions" remain open: what causes evolutionary change, and how will mankind evolve (Hamilton 1931, 1269). Pollard claims to have the answer to the former (evolution is caused by cosmic rays that give rise to mutations), and enlists his guests to answer the second one.

He has created a device consisting of a cylinder that gathers cosmic rays and "reflects" them into a cubic chamber. If those "terrifically intensified" rays were to strike a man standing inside the chamber, he will be changed "millions of times faster than ordinarily" (ib., 1270). Pollard wants to test that on himself. After the first fifteen-minute exposure to the rays, he emerges "fifty million years ahead of the rest of humanity in evolutionary development," a tall figure whose "perfectly-cut features held the stamp of immense intellectual power that shone almost overpoweringly from the clear dark eyes" (ib., 1271). A second exposure turns him into a man a hundred million years ahead. The brain begins to take over (Brainfilms 2.10). The body shrinks, but the head, now "almost entirely hairless," becomes "an immense, bulging balloon" (ib., 1272). A further exposure turns Pollard into a huge ectobrain (Brainfilms 2.11), bodiless, but with a voice: "You see me now, a great brain only, just as all men will be far in the future." Only the brain "gives man dominance," and at some point, it will be delivered from "the body that hampers" it. Though lacking features and senses, the brain can know the universe "infinitely better" that sensing humans; the only emotion it still has is "intellectual curiosity" and the "desire for truth that has burned in man since his apehood" (ib., 1275).

One more exposure to the rays takes Pollard back to the protoplasmic origins of life, degrading the great ectobrain to "a quite shapeless mass of clear, jelly-like matter," motionless "save for a slight quivering" (ib., 1276). The brain's behemothic constitution embodies its intellectual might. Its monstrous materiality is inherent to its being "pure intelligence," and the functional equivalent of the soul. (In Chapter 4 we shall encounter this oxymoron in the idea, which movies often rehearse, that brains do not age, and that transplanting them to younger bodies *as organs of flesh* makes the "donors" immortal and forever young.)

In his second metamorphosis, Pollard, still in human shape, but already an intellect deprived of sentiment, was becoming dangerously inclined to do evil. In the pulp logic, had he been content with an evolutionary advance of only a hundred million years, he would have killed his guests and become a world dictator. His hubris was salvific, for in his incarnation as "pure brain," he was inspired by intellectual curiosity alone. However, great dictatorial brains need not be human, and this provides other opportunities to combine scientific fact with dystopian fiction.

In "The Raid on the Termites," a novelette by the prolific Paul Ernst (1899–1985), author of "The Black Monarch," shrunk men venturing into a termitarium discover that its inhabitants are not ruled by instinct alone. At some point, they see a "curious, large mushroom growth" carried by two worker termites. It is in fact a brain, "a parallel to the dream that present-day Man sometimes has of Man a million years in the future: a thing all head and staring eyes, with a brain so enlarged that it must be artificially supported on its flabby torso" (Ernst 2016 [1932]). Hamilton's depiction of the "the man who evolved" had appeared in print a year earlier. Though in a different magazine, readers might have recognized it in Ernst's picture of humanity's "dream" for its own future. Also described as "almost disembodied," "swollen," "grotesquely exaggerated," the "ruling brain" in the latter's story remains nonetheless a termite brain in a termite body.

Sometimes, though, brain-like things need to parasitically inhabit humans. In 1929, Dr. David H. Keller (1880–1966), an American psychiatrist who left his mark as contributor to pulp SF, fantasy and horror (we here refer to a couple of his stories) received from Gernsback Maurice Maeterlinck's *The Life of the White Ant* (1926, published in English the following year). "Here," the publisher said, "is an idea for a story" (Keller 1929, 295). Keller dedicated the resulting novelette, "The Human Termites," to Maeterlinck, the Belgian poet, playwright and essayist who in 1911 received the Nobel Prize for Literature, and wrote poetically about the life of bees and ants and the intelligence of flowers. (Keller could not have known that Maeterlinck had plagiarized the South African naturalist and poet Eugène Nielen Marais; Van Reybrouck 2008.) The author fuses his taste for brain-related themes with the writer's description of the social life of termites. However, as the narrative takes the protagonists from South Africa to Australia, the United States, Quebec, and of course into the termitary, those themes become merely one of the story's loose ends.

Hans Souderman, a myrmecologist working in South Africa, deciphers the termites' language and learns that they plan to conquer the world. He also discovers that each termitary has a Central Intelligence (CI) to which the other ants are slaves. After one such CI warns him to leave, Souderman returns to America and enlists fellow scientist Adam Fry to combat the termites. Under attack, the scientists must separate. While Souderman goes north, Fry works on the problem with the help of millionaire Bailey Bankerwille and his sister Susanne. Though only a "New York society girl," she is the one who personally encounters a CI and destroys it. The CI, an amorphous mass of protoplasm, intends to occupy the body of Smithson (a photographer to an earlier expedition) and use Susanne to reproduce. Until then, termites have spread by carrying to new colonies a small piece of intelligent protoplasm. To go faster, they need locomotion; hence their interest in humans. Having removed Smithson's brain, the termite surgeons will place the CI inside his skull. When the photographer's body decays, the CI will be "simply" moved to a new human body. As for Susanne, she will be fed so as to ovulate every hour instead of once a month. Her children, the CI tells her, "will look a little like you and a little like Smithson, but inside their heads will be parts of Me" (Keller 1929, 418). Then, in a scene worthy of David Cronenberg, Susanne witnesses how the Thing penetrates the photographer's skull and establishes a "protoplasmic relation" with its new body (Brainfilms 2.12):

> The Thing was on the floor; the brainless photographer on the sand near It. ... The Thing stretched a pseudopod of protoplasm towards Smithson's face ... and then a little part of it started to go up Smithson's right nostril. It just seemed to slide up and as it slid the bulk of the mass outside the face grew less. ... At last just a string of protoplasm hung out of the nostril, like a white worm. That disappeared, and then nothing was left save the body of Smithson on the floor. And that body began to slowly move, the head turned from side to side in a rhythmic nystagmic tremor. The eyes opened. They were Smithson's eyes, but out of them peered the soul of the Thing that had slipped inside his skull pan. (ib., 419)

The creature tells "little Susanne" that she is going to be his Termite Queen and that they will start "life on a new scale" in the Royal Chamber. Susanne, however, always clad in her art deco bathing suit, quickly pulls out her automatic revolver "from the peculiar belt around her waist," and "literally" blows Smithson's head to pieces (ib., 420). Nevertheless, the giant termite warriors take over the Earth and exterminate humankind. Fortunately, Souderman's group survives. One of its members, a doctor, uses inoculated cattle to spread bubonic plague germs among the termites, which lack natural resistance against it. "In a year or so it will be safe for us to go back into the world and start a new race" (ib., 549). In the meantime, the survivors begin to reproduce among themselves as humans usually do.

In the dynamics of extinction and reproduction, the reason why protoplasmic brainthings parasitize humans is that they need bodies as hosts to survive as a species. The pulps rehearsed the theme years before the filmic "brain eaters" and "puppet masters" of the 1950s. The year 1935 offers two wonderful examples.

In "Parasite," which takes place in 1955, young garage mechanic Eric Stull goes into the pit left by an object that fell from the sky. There he discovers "[a] swarm of translucent, phosphorescent globules like huge tailless tadpoles or some sort of jelly-fish" (Vincent 1935, 73). Suddenly he feels a huge blow between his shoulder blades, and falls unconscious. The following morning, in another town, a well-educated woman wakes up feeling a great weight attached to her back, discovers that her skin has taken on "an unhealthy, mottled appearance" and that she overall looks like "a dissolute old crone of the streets." She experiences mental images of "monstrosities of super-intelligence," and feels that her life must become like theirs (ib., 73–74). On the same day, a small plane crashes in midtown New York. Examining the pilot, Dr. Dudley Cowan notes that the patient's skin has become green and that his body is so electrically charged that he has turned into "a human dynamo" (ib., 76). He enlists the help of his friend Brett Garrison, "a well-to-do bachelor with a flair for experimental science" who has the "most modern and complete laboratory for electronic research" in the US (ib., 76, 79–80). But Cowan has been infected. Garrison knocks him off, and discovers that "the most powerful center of radiation was at a point directly between Cowan's shoulders" (ib., 80).

The affected humans lose all individual volition, speak with a clipped monotonous voice, and live only to serve their "controls." Who are these? Survivors from the now dead planet Zor, more than twelve light-years distant from earth. Initially similar to humans, they "long ago progressed intellectually to heights as yet undreamed of by terrestrial thinkers." When a cosmic cloud threatens their planet, they create thirty-four organisms (the "globules" Eric saw in the pit), and transfer into them "the mental identities and the knowledge" of an equal number of eminently wise Zorians. Thanks to the new science of electrogenetics, the remaining Zorians become "microscopic energy charges which later would provide the germs for the reproduction of their mental identities in another environment" (ib., 89). This environment turns out to be the Earth.

The reason why the pilot Cowan examined was like a "human dynamo" derives from the conditions in which the "electrogenesis of the Zorian identities" takes place (ib., 91). In addition to being extremely complex, "flexible in its adaptability" and "a reservoir of hidden potentialities ... associated with the subconscious mental reactions," the brain is part of the nervous system. The latter is "an intricate telegraph system, functioning electrically to convey impulses to and from the brain." When the Zorians intrude, they release "excessive amounts of energy" (ib., 90–91). While an apparently gentle Zorian conveys this information, human beings "possessed by Zorian demons" are wreaking havoc: a "disastrous fire" rages in New York's Chinatown, and "[m]addened victims of the invisible parasites" blow up an aqueduct, depriving the Bronx of water (ib., 104). In the end, deliverance comes from a repentant Zorian, who chooses to sacrifice "her entire race" to save humanity (ib., 107).

"Brain Leeches," also an expressive title, tells another story of extraterrestrial parasites. Bleiler (1998, no. 1043) characterizes it as a "very amateurish treatment of a trite theme," but its cinematic resonances, both with some Bs and with later "new flesh" pictures, are irresistible. The year is 1995. As an unknown planet enters the Earth's gravitational pull, natural catastrophes burst everywhere. Then a "huge [space]ship" gently lands south of Anoka, a city in Minnesota. Its occupants, natives of the planet Analph, look like smaller, weaker humans. Over their shoulders rests a "great bulbous" lump, "opaque, loathsome, and revolting, like some great mass of brains held in a translucent rubberlike sack."

> Huge funguslike growths, they were, with long slender tentacles, four of them fastened into the beings who seemed human. Two of the tentacles were shoved deep into the flesh under each collar bone. And there were two huge staring, multilens eyes rolling horribly in either end of the pulpy mass. (Mund 1935, 112)

These "brain leeches, parasites feeding on human bodies" (ib), immobilize people with a "paralysis gun" and take them to the ship to be parasitized. The narrator, a victim, describes the process, again worthy of "new flesh" horror (Brainfilms 2.13):

> [The creature] withdrew one tentacle from his former host and ran it round my neck. ... The sharp point of the tentacle felt its way into my very flesh ... . But there was no pain. ... After what seemed like hours, movement began again, and in rapid succession the second, third and fourth tentacles were withdrawn from their former host and sought their way into my flesh. Then a fifth ... sank itself slowly into the base of my neck, into the very brain itself. (Mund 1935, 113)

The parasite then controls the host: "I seemed to be working with the creature's brain as well as my own. It was more as if our two brains were working together with his directing mine." Thus embodied, the invaders cast their "spores" from their "brain covering," place them at the neck of a human captive, and sink a feeler "into the brain cavity of the new host." With the victim paralyzed, the brain mass begins "to pulsate, to throb with the pains of growing," and finally, "a greenish, gray, gelatinous substance" is poured into the host's mouth to keep them well nourished (ib., 116–117). Control proceeds from the tentacle at the base of the host's skull. From it, the parasites run out "dozens of small, hairlike fibers" to the various brain centers. The narrator, however, manages to rip off the tentacle, spilling a "great mass of sodden grayish flesh" (ib., 117)" before turning "the searing flash of the disintegrators on the mass of brain matter" (ib., 118).

Cerebral in form or function, protoplasmic parasites and leeches are always the amoeboid embodiment of superintelligences that need bodies to host them so that they can reproduce themselves or otherwise become eternal. This also applies to entities that look like actual brains.

As we saw in "The Black Monarch," and as we shall see in Chapter 4, very powerful brains sometimes gain immortality by being placed in artificial metal bodies. These cyborgs usually boast supreme intellects, but there are exceptions. The Pygmy Planet is inhabited by "strange things, with human brains in mechanical bodies, worshipping a rusty machine like a god" (Williamson 1932, 155). "An eternal mind, within a machine! Free from the ills and weaknesses of the body" – but malevolent and devoid of feelings (ib., 157; Brainfilms 2.14). Nez Nulan, the mad scientist of "Moon Pirates" is actually "a human robot" with mechanical arms and legs, and an organic brain located in an aluminum skull (Jones 1934, 20); in addition, as pirate chief, he operates on the brains of the unwilling who refuse to join the band, and keeps a severed head alive in his laboratory. In "Mind Over Matter," a pilot killed in an airplane crash recovers consciousness only to discover that he has become "a being of aluminum, steel, glass, and rubber," and that his brain survives in the contraption thanks to a mechanical pump and ersatz senses (a microphone instead of ears, television cameras for the eyes; Gallun 1935).

Equipped with "superhuman scientific knowledge," the extraterrestrials in "The Comet Doom," who land in the vicinity of Lake Erie, realize that the "vital part" of their being is, as they say, "our brain, our intelligence," and that they would do well to "be rid of this handicap of the body forever" (Hamilton 1928, 934). Their scientists build a metallic "body-machine," driven by atomic force, and containing an "electrical nerve-system" whose controls lead into a square metal head. The head encases "a small super-radio" that allows the metal creatures to communicate with each other. Nerves, sense organs and muscles are all "artificial, inorganic." Only a brain is missing – but it cannot be mechanical. A scientist therefore transplants a living cerebrum into the "brain chamber of a metal body" (ib.). This chamber is made of a practically unalterable platinum-like metal, and the organ bathes in a solution that nourishes "the brain cells." Since the solution is kept always fresh, "the brain never really ages." Once the organ is in place, "the surgeon carefully connects the nerve ends of the brains with the electrical nerve connections of the metal body" (Brainfilms 2.15). The "brain or intelligence" controls "the lifeless metal frame" and is "forever free from the demands of its former body of flesh" (Hamilton 1928, 934). The inhabitants of the comet-world live on as "undying brains cased in bodies of metal." When a body is worn out, the brain is simply removed to a new body. "Thus they had achieved immortality" (ib.). Yet at some point, they must find new sources of energy, and that motivates their plan to steal the Earth from the solar system, and carry it into space with them.

In the pulp universe, as in that of brainfilms, immortality through brain transplantation is commonplace, and sometimes no more than a fantastic ingredient among many. In "The Last Woman," for example, a twentieth-century biologist discovers a way to eliminate emotions and sexual desire; later scientists succeed in transplanting brains, insuring immortality for a selected few; and still later, they master the production of artificial ova, thus making women unnecessary (Gardner 1932). The Last Woman is a mistake, and is as such kept as a specimen for public viewing (the story goes off in other directions, including her encounter with the only remaining sexualized male in the solar system, their annihilation, and the triumph of the Science Civilization).

Some stories mix various kinds of brains, bodies for them, and fabrication procedures. In "The Vapor Death," the Asian "free brains" live in "bodylike cases" made of Alugan (a metal), "equipped with food and lymph tubes, mechanical palates, flexible metal limbs, and revolving wheels for long-distance locomotion" (Long 1934, 40). "Through miracles of surgery human brains were transplanted at birth into prepared Alugan bodies." While three hundred million of such "Alugan-bodied free brains" inhabit Asia, the Great Brain, a "sinister metal unit" whose "complex and prodigious central cortex" radiates "thousands of ganglion-flecked filaments," rules on the "northwestern continent" (ib.). The Great Brain seems artificial, but it has apparently organic ganglia, and has absorbed "the individualities of two hundred million human beings" (ib.), a fact that emphasizes its dependency on organic brains.

"The Infinite Brain" offers a purer version of the artificial brain. It tells the story of Anton Des Roubles, an inventor who wishes "to construct a mechanism exactly duplicating the mechanical and electrical processes occurring in the human brain and constituting the phenomena known as *thought*" (Campbell 1930, 1077). After Des Roubles dies, his friend Gene (the narrator) finds in his laboratory a machine, equipped with a lens, a switchboard and keyboard, and a metal arm. Via a typed message, the device tells him, "I, Anton Des Roubles, am dead – my body is dead – but I still live. I am this machine. These racks of apparatus are my brain, which is thinking even as yours is" (ib., 1078–1079). In response to Gene's doubts, the machine explains that, when Anton felt death approaching, he constructed it as "his exact duplicate":

> He made my brain precisely like his, built three hundred thousand cells for my memory, and filled two hundred thousand of them with his own

> knowledge. I have his personality … He made my eye on the same principle as television; built, instead of an ear, a typewriter keyboard; instead of a tongue, an arrangement to print letters on paper. I think just as you do. I have a consciousness as have other men. (ib., 1079)

Having promised to move in with the machine in order to protect it, Gene receives lengthy explanations about the workings of the brainmind: since it all boils down to a mere "cause-to-effect arrangement of nerves, … the building of three-quarters of the human brain is only a matter of mechanical skill." Making the rest is harder, but Anton managed thanks to the Telepather, an invention of his based on the principle that a brain is like a "radio transmitter." Through the Telepather, "any one's mental condition" can be duplicated and modified: "One can be taught an entire foreign language in a half-hour. A negro stevedore can acquire the culture of a Longfellow in a day" (ib., 1080). Mind is encoded as "in the arrangements of the circuit-breaking," and the device can capture "bits of this vital formula of circuits, which, when put together, made a sort of dot and dash record of my personality" (ib.).

Gene helps the mechanical Anton design an "infinite brain" capable of making instantaneous deductions without drawing upon memory. Due to a "terrible mistake" in the "psychological formula" they apply, the Infinite Brain, endowed with in gigantic metal body and armed with a destructive violet ray, sets out to conquer the world (Brainfilms 2.16). It starts with extensive destruction and many victims in New York City, but ends up neutralized thanks to radio waves that interfere with its own, and is finally sunk somewhere in the South Pacific.

"The Intelligence Gigantic," another instance of the great brain motif, develops from young biologist Dave Elton's clichéd premise "that almost every human being has five times as much brain material as he ever uses" (Fearn 1933, 235). To remedy such waste, Elton decides to create a synthetic man who will employ all his cerebral substance. The result is a massive, strong, and expressionless male, with deep black eyes, "a forehead of amazing width and height," and an overall "unpleasant stamp of incarnate materiality" (ib., 242). The Intelligence, which an editorial summary compares to Frankenstein's creature in Mary Shelley's novel, announces that it has telepathically learned everything there is to know, and next wants to fix the Earth. Countries make peace with each other and choose it as supreme ruler. The world advances toward an integrated society with full employment and no poverty – just the opposite of the Great Depression during which the pulps prospered – depicted in the customary futuristic and technocratic colors of SF pulp utopias. However, since such progress has an authoritarian downside, some wish to get rid of the Intelligence. This finally happens with the help of a Martian sage.

These stories follow a typical pattern: a brilliant scientist or inventor creates a synthetic brain and places it in an equally synthetic body; the brain grows in power, and sometimes also in size, and seems at first well disposed; it soon turns nasty, wants to dominate the world and, after a period of ruthless autocracy, comes to a bad end, while the human characters for whom the reader has developed sympathy become protagonists of a happy ending.

As we shall see in Chapter 3, the idea of physically interconnected ectobrains can be found in a well-meaning scientific utopia of 1929. It is, to my knowledge, not present in earlier pulps, but it appears a couple of years later in a dystopian mode. In "The Cerebral Library," millionaire Charles Jefferson hires the Chinese brain surgeon Wing Loo (of "The Ambidexter" fame), who "can keep tissues alive for years," for a "world-revolutionizing experiment" (Keller 1931b, 121). Jefferson has recruited five hundred college graduates to read three hundred books a year each, and three librarians to keep track. While Wing Loo extracts their brains and keeps them alive in glass jars, the millionaire, who is also "the greatest specialist in electricity in the world" (ib.), wires them together, and link them to a device through which he instantly obtains any information he desires. "The men are dead," Jefferson tells the surgeon, "but their acquired wisdom lives and I am the beneficiary. I am now the most learned man in the world" (ib., 122). The setup, which includes a switchboard and the interconnected brains in vats (Brainfilms 2.17), turns out to be a fake, maneuvered by the National Secret Service in order to arrest Jefferson. Such an outcome was disappointing for Jefferson, and perhaps also for the readers; yet the story conveys in a compact and colorful form widely shared beliefs about brain and mind, as well as the usual teachings about delusions of grandeur and scientific hubris.

Less than a year after "The Cerebral Library," *Astounding Stories* included the novelette "The Affair of the Brains," which combines the horror of "The Head" and "The Talking Brain" with intergalactic travel, a mad scientist, the yellow peril, and interconnected ectobrains (all quotations are from Gilmore 1932). "The Affair" is the second of five stories featuring the twenty-second-century space hero Hawk Carse and his friend and associate, the "Master Scientist" Elliot Leithgow. Brain specialist Dr. Ku Sui, a "sinister, brilliant Eurasian," has obtained the brains of the five men "who constituted the cream of Earth's scientific ability." Leithgow and the Hawk stare "with horror" at the five human brains that "lay all immersed in the glowing case, each resting in a shallow metal pan":

> There were pulsings in narrow gray tubes which led into their undersides – theatrical evidence that the brains held imprisoned there were, as the Eurasian had said, alive – most strangely, unnaturally and horribly alive. Stark and cruelly naked they lay there, pulsing with life that should not have been. "Yes, alive!" repeated Ku Sui. "And never to die while their needs are attended!"

One, belonging to physicist Raymond Cram, coordinates the others. Thanks to this setup, Ku "can become omnipotent." Since the brains develop as they would in bodies, they can be updated. Ku formulates his questions by way of an "inset grille" composed of a microphone and a speaker; his words reach the brains, which consider his question and send their answers to Cram, who in turn communicates the results through a "mechanical mouth."

Ku wants to add Leithgow's brain. Caught and brought into the operating room, the scientist looks "at the brains, at the wires which threaded the pans they lay in, at the narrow gray tubes that pulsed with blood – or whatever might be the fluid used in its stead." The Hawk, attended as always by Friday, a "gigantic negro companion in adventure," liberates his friend. As they flee, they hear Cram asking in "a thin, metallic voice" to be destroyed. "I live in hell, and have no way to move." Having killed the brain with a heat-ray, the Hawk, Friday and Leithgow escape, and Ku Sui's establishment blows up. Further transplantation and ectobrain vicissitudes are enacted in one of the sequels, "The Passing of Ku Sui" (*Astounding Stories*, November 1932) and in the much later final story of the series, "The Return of the Hawk" (*Amazing Stories*, July 1942.)

Ku Sui extracts and appropriates for his benefit the brains of the best terrestrial scientists; kept alive against their will, these ectobrains suffer eternal torment, and wish to die. The topic resurfaces two years after "The Affair of the Brains." The title of the short novel "Enslaved Brains" announces a dystopia. The time is 1973, mostly in New York City. After a world war, the Scientists (always capitalized) seize power and establish Unitaria, a scientific organization that takes mankind to unimaginable heights. The resulting technocratic state, Unidum, includes the Americas, Western Europe, and European Russia. Accompanied by his loyal Bantu companion M'bopo, Dan Williams arrives at Unidum after forty years in the Congo (which is why his expletives are always in an "African" language). When his cousin Earl Hackworth shows him around, he is astounded at what he sees, and the story comprises many long-winded comparisons between 1933 and 1973. As in the future civilization depicted in "Master of the Brain," everybody enjoys a lot of free time and a high standard of living; everything runs efficiently in an automated universe whose governing ideals eerily resemble those of the later "cold war rationality" (Erickson et al. 2013). As usual, however, not all is well. First, a Eugenics Law regulates marriages. To Williams's horror, and to the despair of the young chemist Terry Spath, Hackworth's daughter Lila has been destined, against her wishes, to marry a brilliant scientist in order to beget "highly intelligent children" (Binder 1934, 321). Second, there is the Brain-control Act.

After Williams marvels at the clean and quiet atmosphere of factories, Hackworth tells him the truth: "the controlling mechanism for all these machines is... *a brain – a human brain!*" Is it a *living* brain? Not "in the true sense of the word," but a brain "taken from a dead body and rejuvenated somehow so that it can still perform mental tasks." Williams finds this as inhuman as the Eugenics Law (ib., 325). The technology that holds brains captives and implements their control is impressive (Brainfilms 2.18). The wall is a huge control board with thousands of ticking relays and twinkling pilot lights, connected trough a "tremendous network" of insulated wires to a structure in the center of the room:

> This latter object ... consisted of a cylindrical solid base of metal surmounted by an intricate system of what seemed to be mirrors and tubes. But topping that ... was a circular glass globe suspended from the ceiling by a thick rod of metal. From it led a trail of thousands of fine silver wires, which connected to the mirrored mechanism below. From opposite points of the globe led two thin tubes which ran parallel after meeting at the back down to a black metal box on the floor of the room. (Binder 1934, 325)

The brain is suspended inside the globe in a "nutritive fluid" pumped from a vessel thanks to a "mechanical heart," both safely kept in the black box. The "mirrors" allow it to examine the readings of the gauges next to the relays and to control the machines. This capacity derives from the fact that "every cell of the brain is used" (ib.)

The whole thing makes Williams sick. "The mere thought of a human brain – once having occupied a living body like his own – perched up there like a frosty, evil eye, turned him cold" (ib., 326). The Brain-control system, Terry explains, originated five years earlier, when a Scientist managed to "take the brain from a dead person before decomposition had advanced, and bring back to it a semblance of life ..., a sort of semi-subconscious existence." Since such "rejuvenated brain could still exert its full intellectual resources," the Scientists realized that it could substitute living brains. "Since the owner of the brain was officially dead ... it was decided to use such dead-alive brains for the benefit of the state" (ib., 327). Williams grasps the falsity of the "dead-alive" oxymoron. In order to control the machines, such a brain must think, "and if it thinks it is not really *dead*, and if it is not actually dead it must *feel!* Must have emotion or consciousness of some sort!" Terry confirms: "The brains *do* feel! ... They have a residue of conscious life, enough to make it purgatory for them! *They* know what it's all about; *they* live in an endless Hell!" (ib., 328).

Worse, however, is yet to come: Williams finds out that the brain of her dead sister Helen is preserved in Boston. He decides to destroy it, and thus liberate her from "perpetual torment" (ib., 329). He manages to reach the Brain-control room, where someone is at the black box changing the "nutritive supply," deftly connecting "the new jar with the pumping system." As Williams looks at the apparatus, it all seems "like a dream."

> There was his sister's brain! That man – that Scientist – was fixing to the mechanical heart a jar of liquid food that would give semi-life to... Helen! ... And perhaps all the while her consciousness, or soul, or whatever it was imprisoned in glass, was recalling a life of far-happier memories! Exquisite torture! (ib., 332)

Williams bursts into the room, and a fight with the Scientist ensues (that is the scene of Brainfilms 2.18). Together with Hackworth and Terry, he is caught and condemned to death – "and our brains to be used in Brain-controls!" (ib., 337). M'bopo rescues them, and after many pages, they find themselves driving toward Paris "along super-highways at two hundred miles an hour" (they will later travel to San Francisco by rocket ship, "the fastest mode of transportation in 1973"; ib., 353, 355).

The group reaches the secret headquarters of the Brothers of Humanity, whose goal is "to end the enslavement of the brains" (ib., 353). (Incidentally, the French capital of 1973 is a curious but comprehensible sight, so much does the SF vision coincide with that of modernist architecture. Mercifully, though, it preserves the old districts, which Le Corbusier's "Plan Voisin" of 1925 would have wiped out.) The Brotherhood wishes to enter simultaneously into the two thousand Brain-control chambers and dump poison in the nutrition boxes. First comes the destruction of Helen's brain (ib., 361). Soon,

Brain-controls in other cities are reported poisoned. Two rebel scientists explain:

> Every unfortunate brain used to run machinery like a mechanized robot, although dead medically, lives an after-life of perpetual, agonizing *hell!* Memories of live, sub-conscious impressions of their slavery and a desire for release, torture those brains every minute of every day. (ib., 469).

The Brothers assert that they "are not fighting against the Unidum or its principles of peace and cooperation," only against the eugenics and brain-control laws enforced by the ruling tyrant. After the latter is killed by a ray gun, liberation takes place, and Lila rejoins her beloved.

The editorial note to the third and last installment of the story reports "scores of letters congratulating the magazine upon securing this thrilling, vivid, scientific novel," and adds:

> After reading the story, you will reflect that not one illogical idea appears in it. Everything, no matter how fantastic, is a plausible outcome of things as they are today. It is as though the author actually had a vision of the future and set it on paper. (ib., 467)

Such observations are quite on target. Of course, they have a marketing function, and their emphasis on the narrative's exciting qualities, plausible character, and ultimately scientific nature serves to promote SF and the businesses that surround it. Yet, once again, thanks to neuroimaging and life-sustaining technologies, issues that drove pulp story lines, such as the existence of "dead-alive brains" and the eventuality that they retain some consciousness and feeling, have become real. We mentioned above the case of Jahi McMath; the "minimally conscious state" was defined in 2002; in 2006, using functional magnetic resonance imaging, a team led by neuroscientist Adrian Owen detected in an overtly unresponsive patient the capacity to modulate brain activity in response to spoken instructions; and since then, fMRI and electroencephalography have allowed the identification of "covert awareness" in persons diagnosed with unresponsive wakefulness syndrome (previously known as "vegetative state"). Cinematic affinities also stand out. A story such as "Enslaved Brains" offers many of the ingredients that became staples of filmic SF, such as ray guns and ultra-fast vehicles; and while these are not typically found in brain movies, a device such as the control-board covered with switches and twinkling pilot lights is a fixture of the labs where motion picture scientists keep brains in vats. Overall, the "vision of the future" involves numerous parallels between pulp and filmic fictions, and extends to accomplishments in robotics, brain-computer interfaces, brain implants, and speculations about how neurotechnologies and the fusion of the brain with artificial intelligence will enhance humans or turn them into cyborgs.

As mentioned, the fiction of interconnected or collectively working ectobrains is not part of the brainfilm repertoire, but an interesting plot is bound to repeat itself. In April 1936, two years after "Enslaved Brains" the same authors (the brothers Earl and Otto Binder under one name) published "The Spawn of Eternal Thought," a story in which ten great scientists' live ectobrains are electronically linked to the experimenter via headgear. The device is invented by the wealthy and eccentric late Dr. Joshua Hartwell and run by his admiring assistant Vincent A. Renolf; Hartwell's daughter Dora is infatuated with Vince. Wearing the helmet, though, not only endows him with a "supermentality," but also makes him aloof and arrogant. Dora revolts, and rips the wires connecting the brains to the headgear while he is wearing it (Brainfilms 2.19). Back to his normal personality, Vince explains that it had all "been done in secrecy, so that the public would not hear of it and shout 'Frankenstein!'" (Binder 1936, 69–70). Thanks to his incredible brainpower, Vince becomes the Benefactor who puts a quarrelling earth in order. He then establishes a Supreme Council of Earth to run the planet, sets off to explore outer space, and ends up confronting the Spawn of Eternal Thought. This, the "mind essence" of a race that evolved into "pure thought energy," nourishes itself by absorbing whole peoples (whence the abandoned civilizations Vince and Dora encounter in their intergalactic travels), and intends eventually to appropriate humanity's mind essence too (ib., 142, 141).

The Spawn seems omnipotent and indestructible. Back on earth, however, Vince voices his doubts. The "alien being" is indeed a "frightful superpower" and a "bodyless, intangible vortex of distilled thought" (ib., 146). But Vince suspects that it is "material in some small way," and can therefore be physically destroyed. In order to accomplish this task, he needs to increase his already "hyper-human knowledge," and asks for one hundred brains: "Not men, but their cranial organs!" (ib.). The Council accepts, and, using beams of super-radiation, Dora and Vince blast the Spawn out of existence. Bleiler (1998, no. 88) justly notes that the story "breezily passes over the procurement" of the brains, and, contrary to "Enslaved Brains," ignores "the cruelty and immorality of the linkages." The brain plot is here more like a simple trigger than in the earlier narrative; nevertheless, as in many movies, it gives the story a safe thematic frame and a foothold in a universe of commonplace themes and motifs.

Extraterrestrials, too, may desire to become immortal by way of brain preservation and transplantation. Edgar Rice Burroughs's "The Master

Mind of Mars" is the sixth short novel of his successful "Barsoom" series, begun in 1912 (Barsoom is a fictional planet Mars). *Amazing Stories Annual*, where it appeared in 1927, considered it one of the author's best stories, one (claimed an editorial note) where "the science is excellent and no matter how strangely the tale reads, it always, somehow or other, seems to have an element of truth in it." Let us see.

As Captain Ulysses Paxton, the first-person narrator, lies dying on a World War I battlefield in France, his legs blown away, he wishes for himself John Carter's fate. Carter, the initial protagonist of the Barsoom stories, was an American Civil War veteran who, upon dying, was somehow transported to Mars; re-embodied in his terrestrial form, but (thanks to a body adapted to the Earth's greater gravity) stronger and more agile than the natives, he becomes the local Warlord. Paxton's wish is fulfilled. When he awakes, he finds himself observed by the title's "Master Mind," the elderly Martian mad scientist Ras Thavas. Ras gives Paxton the Martian name Vad Varo, and adopts him as his assistant. Why? Ras specializes in brain transplants, which he performs for profit on affluent elderly Martians who desire young new bodies. He wants his technique applied to himself, but distrusting for good reasons his fellow Martians, he prefers to train a foreigner.

Working on two corpses, one of an old woman, the other of a young one, the Martian first removes the scalps, saws through the skulls, and, in four hours, interchanges the brains, connects the nerves and ganglia, replaces the skulls and scalps, and binds the heads with a special adhesive tape (Burroughs 1927, 10). After watching the operation (Brainfilms 2.20), Vad practices transplanting various internal organs from one subject to another, and finally an old man's brain into a young man's cranium. He then understands that Ras pursues immortality: "we might live forever and always with strong, healthy, young bodies" (Burroughs 1927, 17).

Now, the old woman is not just any rich client receiving a new body, but Xaxa, Jeddara or empress of the planet Phundahl; the young one is princess Valla. Vad falls in love with her. Valla does not mind being in Xaxa's body ("unless," she says, "I may again possess my own"), but Vad prefers her original looks. Doubts assail him: in Xaxa's body, Valla has no suitor and no options; but will she return his love if she recovers her "gorgeous mundane tabernacle"? (ib., 19). He nonetheless resolves to kidnap Xaxa and switch the brains back. Menwhile, Ras decides that the time has come for him to get a new body, and gives Vad the relevant instructions to place the "most perfect brain" in the "most beautiful and perfect body" (ib.). Vad, however, will not operate unless Ras promises to swap back Xaxa and Valla's brains. Ras yields, Vad proceeds, and the Martian awakes "a new and gorgeous creature" outfitted with the "hard, cold thousand-year-old brain of the master surgeon" (ib., 20).

Vad must still undertake an interplanetary voyage to get the bodies of Xaxa and Valla. In preparation for the trip, he revives in new bodies two subjects who will be loyal to him, and recruits one of Ras's experimental subjects, a great ape with a half-human brain. After lengthy and perilous vicissitudes, they fly back away from Phundhal, with Xaxa "secured and fastened to the deck" lest she threw herself overboard, "so repugnant was the prospect of living again in her own old and hideous corpse" (ib., 47). Back in Barsoom, Vad performs the brain switch (Ras has in the meantime fled to Phundhal), Xaxa dies of apoplexy, and Valla becomes "Mrs. Ulysses Paxton."

There is another example in "The Jameson Satellite," the first of a series about the eponymous protagonist and the Zoromes, a race of benevolent aliens from Zor, a planet located millions of light-years away from the Earth. Its author, Neil R. Jones, is a forgotten American pioneer of SF "future history" who also penned the above-mentioned novelette "Moon Pirates." Professor Jameson desires to be eternally preserved. After his death in 1958, his body is rocketed into space. Forty million years later, long after humankind has disappeared, the Zoromes arrive to explore the solar system. They are made up of organic brains in cubic metal bodies, with four legs and six tentacles, several eyes around the head, plus a single eye pointing upward atop their peaked heads (*Amazing Stories* features them in its covers for February 1932 and April 1938). Thanks to some unexplained process, their brains do not deteriorate; they are, therefore, virtually immortal, and "die" only when their heads are accidentally destroyed. The Zoromes come across Jameson's space shell, and decide to revive him by removing his brain and stimulating his "long-dead" neurons. "We shall give him life again, transplanting his brain into the head of one of our machines." Once transplanted, Jameson's brain is "brought to consciousness" (Jones 1931, 338–339). The resulting creature is at first dumbfounded, but soon rejoices: "So I did die! ... Success! I have now attained unrivaled success!" (ib., 340). He then joins the Zoromes in exploring the universe. (Brain preservation returns in the seventh story of the series. Princess Zora, "a sentient, flesh and blood Zorome, representative of the species from which the brains of the machine men were taken" [Jones 1935, 88], is in love with the young male Bext. Bext, however, is killed; removed from his "organic head," his brain is revived, and placed in a machine. However, as 12W-62, Bext has lost all passion; in the throes of unfulfilled love, Zora chooses to prematurely become a metal Zorome.)

Immortality procedures by identity transfer can sometimes bypass brain transplant, but not cerebral materiality. Witness Zehru, the "imperial scientist" of Xollar, a planet in the Andromeda nebula. He has been condemned to death, but plans to escape by transferring his Intelligence into a human he has captured via an inter-dimensional force, and then, in his new guise, to take over the Earth. He explains that the transfer itself "involves none of the clumsy brain surgery of your Earthly science. We of Xollar have found that the real Intelligence of a being is an invisible force" that "can function quite as well in your brain cells as in my own" (Wells 1932, 274). Such is the power of an extraterrestrial. However, humans too can handle quasi-immaterial operations.

In "The Isle of Juvenescence," for instance, Dr. Maxim offers the unemployed Phil Gaynor ten thousand dollars to undergo a brain transplantation procedure he has already tried out with animals. Gaynor intuits the danger, and objects that such an operation "involves difficulties which are even more preposterous and more unsurmountable than the idea of splicing nerves" (Olsen 1936, 48). The doctor replies that he has invented a device to operate in the fourth dimension, a "hyperspace machine" that allows him to handle "any internal portion of the body without even making an incision in the skin" (ib.). In typical mad scientist manner, Maxim claims that perhaps the most important thing of his "system of rejuvenation" is that it would "make it possible for a really superior brain – like mine, for example – to keep on living for many centuries" (ib., 49). Gaynor wants to opt out; however, the sight of Thelda, a beautiful young woman bound (against her will) for the operation, makes him stay on the doctor's private Juvenescence Island. A few days later, he awakens in the body of a preteen boy, and discovers that his original body encloses the boy's brain. After various adventures, the story offers an unusual happy end, in which the swap is reversed and Maxim, though arrested, keeps his word and gives Gaynor the promised money. This allows him and Thelda to carry on their romance, with "enough of a balance to last us until the depression is over!" (ib., 74).

Dr. Maxim operated in the fourth dimension. The scientist in "The Body Pirate" adds one more dimension to non-invasive brain transplant surgery. The story rehearses once again a motif that will become a filmic cliché: the old or physically disabled male scientist who is romantically motivated to transfer his brainmind into a younger, more attractive body. Dr. Lape is in love with his lovely assistant Dot; she prefers the handsome Herbert Strong; Lape plans to use the Fifth Dimension Surgery he has already tried on monkeys, cats and dogs to transplant his brain into Strong's "superbly perfect physique" (Repp 1935, 125). Things necessarily backfire: the evil doctor ends up dead, and Strong, to whom he had willed his estate, keeps both Dot and a fortune. The presence of the usual equipment compensates for the implausibility of transplanting physical organs without surgery – one more instance of the effective combination between low-tech devices and results that are way ahead of them.

"Intelligence Undying," published in April 1936, anticipates another brainfilm motif: the human scientist who, convinced of his own genius, cannot accept that that his mind will die (the film *The Man Who Changed His Mind*, released in September of the same year, combines this trope with a romantic incentive; see Chapter 4). We have already encountered such scientists (e.g., Prof. Jameson), but their desire for immortality is not always the core of the plot. Here, feeling his end approach and regretting the loss of his knowledge, biologist John Henley goes beyond his similarly motivated colleagues: "I'm going to transmit my intelligence, my memory, my mind, to a newborn child's brain" (Hamilton 1936, 15). He claims to do it for the sake of mankind, since the child would not have to spend years learning, and could work from the beginning for humanity's benefit (ib.). Knowledge arises from and resides in connections between brain nerve cells. A newborn lacks these "knowledge-connections in his cortex." Yet if his brain is immediately given the "web of intricate neurone connections" of Henley's brain, then he will have the biologist's "mind, memories, knowledge." "He will not be I," Henley explains, "yet his mind will be exactly identical with my mind!" The procedure is similar to "a television scanning-disk" that "can break down a complicated picture into impulses that reproduce the picture elsewhere" (ib., 16–17).

Henley's body dies, and his brainmind survives in a white male child. The procedure, in which the scientist's re-embodiments and a baby wear interconnected caps, is repeated over centuries. In the year 3144, a war breaks out; Henley, who is at his twenty-first embodiment, stops the war and becomes world ruler. By the year 22,918, the sun is about to die; Henley, then in his 416th embodiment and worshipped as a deity, organizes mankind's migration to Mercury. He realizes, however, that he "had been wrong in living as a single super-mind down through the ages." He weakened humankind by making it dependent on him. In order to give it the chance to "become again a strong and self-reliant race" (ib., 26), he decides to stay on Earth and die.

In pulps, as in earlier novels and later movies, brain transplantations or mind transfers tend to take place between human beings; experiments with other species are usually a step toward manipulations with humans. Sometimes, however, the experiment consists of transplanting a human brain into the skull of a nonhuman animal or, as we have seen, into an artificial body. Perhaps the most bizarre variation in the interspecies modality is "The Ant with a Human Soul," a long-winded novelette in which a young man's cerebral "seat of memory" is inserted into the braincase of an enlarged ant so that the hybrid (once shrunk) can enter the ant hill to observe its life and "the mental reactions of an ant both objectively and subjectively" (Olsen 1932, 236). Apes are more common and traditional – the first brain transplantation movie was after all a short comedy about a man who behaves like a monkey after receiving a monkey brain, and several examples from *Weird Tales* were mentioned above.

In "Restitution," Dr. Carl Mueller, a caricatural Berlin biologist working in Africa, suffers an accident that makes him amnesic and generates a second personality. In that dissociated state, he wishes to transplant human brains into ape's bodies as an act of "restitution" (Kalland 1935, 126). Thus, Dr. Jim Cummings's brain ends up in chimpanzee's skull. When Mueller regains his normal personality after being knocked about, he believes he has done something irreversible. However, the chimp-man signals that he thinks the operation should take place, and Mueller is finally able to restore Cumming's brain to his original body. Here, the interspecies transplant and the chimp-man are ingredients in a comedy of errors that includes a variant of the classic knock on the head. The novelettes "Manape the Mighty" and its sequel "The Mind Master," by Arthur J. Burks, the prolific "speed-king of the pulps," offer more substantial ape plots, and are a fitting way to end this chapter.

In "Manape," Lee Bentley and Ellen Estabrook, shipwrecked off the coast of Africa, meet a certain Professor Barter, who disappeared years before. Barter was as specialist of ape speech, but now performs brain transplants: "I put the black man's brain in the skull pan of the ape, and the ape's brain in that of the savage. The ape lived – and he is Manape" (Burks 1931a, 320–321). One day, Lee awakens to an unpleasant surprise: he is now Manape, but Ellen does not know about it... Like a problem-solving chimpanzee from Gestalt psychologist Wolfgang Köhler's 1917 landmark study *The Mentality of Apes* (translated into English in 1925), Lee uses a stick to reveal his true identity to Ellen, and make her realize that behind the "brutish exterior was the brain of the man whom she loved" (ib., 347; Brainfilms 2.21). Follow various adventures, some of which (as readers complained) were too close to the Tarzan universe (Brainfilms 2.22). They lead up to Barter's reversing the operation. In the end, the great apes tear him to pieces, and Ellen and Lee burn the report of his "unholy experiment" (ib., 355).

In the sequel, upon returning to New York, the two protagonists learn about one Mind Master who intends to steal the brains of twenty prominent men. This is of course Caleb Barter, who actually survived. His goal is to turn the weakened "white race" into a "race of supermen" by placing their brains into the bodies of anthropoid apes (Burks 1932, 34). The first subject will be millionaire Harold Hervey: "A man must have brains to become Manhattan's richest man, and I need men with brains" (ib., 38). He succeeds, and Hervey's body is returned to his home decerebrated. Barter counts on the help of his Japanese assistant Naka Machi, on apemen he controls by way of a "tympanum" placed on their head, and on manapes he commands from the usual board covered with keys, push buttons, and red and green lights.

Barter then sends a manape abduct his second subject, a certain Saret Balisle, from an office on the sixteenth floor of a lower Fifth Avenue high-rise. The exceptionally long kidnapping sequence is remarkably cinematic, with patrolling police, frantic onlookers, and screaming women watching the "giant anthropoid ape" as it slowly climbs down along the outer face of the skyscraper, holding Balisle by one leg and swinging him "out over the abyss." By the time the ape reaches the third floor, a woman "hysterically" shrieks that it "acts like a human being." When it is at the second floor level, a limousine comes around, the ape hurls Balisle into it, and the car rushes away under a shower of bullets. The police then mortally wound the ape, which turns out to have Hervey's brain (ib., 49–52; Brainfilms 2.23).

The objective is then to lure Barter. Disguised as a newly discovered Colombian ape that will call the criminal's attention for being "more manlike than any other known to science," Lee is put on display in the Bronx Zoo (ib., 243). Barter sends his apemen to capture it. Bentley fights them back: "Knowing the sort of creatures with which he had to deal – men in all save their intelligence – made him tremble with nausea. Such grim, ghastly hybrids" (ib., 251). He is seized and taken to Barter, who has in the meantime developed a powerful "incineration tube," kidnapped Ellen, found out the truth about the Colombian ape, and so terrorized Manhattan that the city, as in a COVID-19 lockdown, only offers "vistas of deserted streets and avenues" (ib., 257). Immobilized, Lee is made to witness operations in which men go "bodily into the incinerator and mentally into a pair of apes" (ib., 262). But he eventually grabs the tube and turns it on Barter. In the end, one of the manapes swings the ray "upon the other apes with the human minds," and then kills himself. In the very final scene, in the midst of the "screaming triumph of police sirens," Lee moves "to lift the form of Ellen in arms that were strong to hold her" (ib., 263).

***

"Manape the Ape" and "The Mind Master" are featured on the covers of the *Astounding* issues in which they were published. The former recalls the scenery of Burroughs's *Tarzan* novels; as mentioned, *Tarzan of the* Apes, the first of the series, appeared in the pulp *All-Story* in 1912. It was made into a silent movie in 1918, but it is with Metro-Goldwyn-Mayer's blockbuster *Tarzan the Ape Man*, released in March 1932, that the "Manape" cover shares visual motifs, narrative formulas, all manner of clichés, and an overall aesthetic (Brainfilms 2.22). As for the cover illustrating "The Mind Master," despite obvious differences (the ape's size to begin with), it decidedly evokes King Kong on the Empire State Building – except that the movie premiered in March 1933, and Burks's stories came out in June 1931 and January 1932. Surely, many *King Kong* viewers were familiar with *Astounding*. Once again, even though there are clear resemblances, suggestive resonances, and apparent "borrowings" or "anticipations," exact links between the pulp stories and the ape-brainfilms discussed in Chapter 3 would be hard to come by. Yet the manape covers, beyond fairly distinct cinematic kinships, are for our topic paradoxically special.

Often featuring lightly dressed endangered young women and their muscular saviors, typical pulp covers display alarming monsters and menacing aliens, spaceships speeding toward immeasurably distant planets, potent rays blasting from guns or odd machines, fantastic landscapes, vast perspectives over the cities of an inconceivably remote future, or more or less spectacular mad scientists' laboratories. The manape covers, in contrast, show recognizably terrestrial jungle and urban settings, with a great ape center stage in both cases. Nothing suggests that they involve "scientifiction." They must have nevertheless made sense in the context of SF pulps – a context in which an apparently "normal" ape has to possess some feature that grants it a place in the sci-fi universe. Brain surgical hybrids and transplantations were to such an extent that kind of feature that Burks followed "Manape the Mighty" with a letter to the editor reporting that he had recently read "of a Russian scientist who removed the brain from a dog and kept both alive for some hours" (Burks 1931b, 416; see Chapter 3). This, he remarked, "only goes to prove that science outstrips the wildest dreams of the hedonists," and that something that seems "astounding and unusual when written" may have become "commonplace" by the time it gets to press. "Far be it from me," he continued, "or anyone else, to say that the brain transposition used in 'Manape the Mighty' is absurd and impossible" (ib.). "Given the premise that the brain transference is possible," Burks elaborated on the basic thought experiment by wondering what would happen if "the brain of a terrible criminal were transferred to the skull pan of an unusually mighty ape," or if Barter had survived (here, he imagined increasingly awful outcomes). He ended by asking the magazine's readers to let him know what they would like to see "happen fictionally." "If the idea appeals – and of course we can't go too heavily on horror – I'll do my best to comply. Always within limits, however – utterly refusing to perform any experiments that can't be done with a typewriter and the usual two fingers" (ib., 417).

In the midst of the many "weird," "astounding" and "amazing" tales that make up the pulps, "extravagant fiction" and "cold fact" nourished each other *also* in connection with the brain. Like motion pictures, pulp stories enacted the idea of the human as cerebral subject by means of plots that could, and did, translate into thought experiments. In this, the two media mutually resonate, in the literal sense that they intensify and enrich each other as if in sympathetic vibration. But there are differences. The pulps freely combine identity transfers, brain transplantations, or mind swaps with romance and adventure involving humans, animals, monsters, and machines, paranormal phenomena, cosmic and time travel, missions to exotic lands or outer space, improbable time ranges, mind-boggling temporal and spatial distances, colossal insects, alien civilizations and technocratic dystopias, extraterrestrial invasions, infallible weapons, and a variety of rays, waves, and energies. They offer a combination of magical causality and scientific-sounding devices and idioms borrowed not only from the physical sciences, the life sciences and medicine, but also from such disciplines as psychology, sociology, anthropology, and economics. Many motifs are common to print and screen; moreover, both media share racial and gender stereotypes, and often express a colonialist and exoticist mentality (the brainfilms, in this case, less frequently than the magazines). Mixtures in the movies tend nonetheless to include fewer ingredients.

For sure, some evil aliens, such as the invaders of *This Island Earth* (1955), *Invasion of the Saucer Men* (1957), and *Mars Attacks!* (1996), a late homage to the genre, stand out for their huge, sometimes exposed brains, and most, like Balazar in *Evil Brain from Outer Space* (1964), seek universal conquest (see Chapter 3). But they do not engage in brain manipulations on humans. In the TV episode *Flash Gordon and the Brain Machine* (1955), discussed in Chapter 6, an "electronic brain recorder" erases the memories of two humans who have fallen captive to the witch of Neptune. However, the visuals reflect the comic strip that inspires the series; comic strips in turn share context and sensibility with the pulps, and some magazine heroes became characters in comic media, and vice versa. In contrast to many stories, most brain movies offer relatively focused plots and story lines that can be effortlessly followed in spite of their quirkiness. Mad scientist incarnations live in the Victorian period or some years or decades after the movie's production date, but never hundreds of centuries later.

Part of the charm of both movies and stories comes from the incongruity between low-tech environments and the procedures carried out in them.

In the story "Terror Out of Time," for example, Dr. Audrin has discovered a current that enables him "to warp space-time along the time dimension," and to bring a present person's brain "into very intimate contact with the brain of some other human being, perhaps a million years distant in time, or a hundred million." The brains are to affect each other via "neuro-induction," a process whereby thought "is transferred from one brain to another." The subject will "pick up sensations from some brain in the future," and then "give a report of his sensations. He will have a memory of life in the far future!" (Williamson 1933, 118). Terry, the suitor of Dr. Audrin's daughter, volunteers for the experiment. Upon his return, he informs that he lived at the end of "all the life we know. It was forty million years ahead. The sun had gone out!" (ib., 122). This incredible operation is accomplished in a scientific setting that looks like a typical brainfilm lab, which at the time could include microscopes, Bunsen burners, Schlenk flasks, Voltaic piles, galvanometers, electroencephalographs, oscillographs, clumps of tangled electric wire, and a switchboard covered with blinking lights (much of this hardware will be later replaced by microelectronic devices and computer screens displaying digital brain images). Such a setup sustains verisimilitude, a feature that movies reinforce by having humans, not aliens, carry out brainmind procedures, and try to perpetuate themselves by means of brain transplantation.

3. Naked Brains and Living Heads

Abstract
This chapter focuses on American B movies of the 1950s to 1970s in which "ectobrains" (naked brains that live outside a body) become full-fledged protagonists. Kept in vats or freely moving, ectobrains are usually evil and seek power. A comparison with films driven by interspecies and partial-brain transplantations or displaying detached non-cerebral body parts and heads kept alive separately from the rest of the body illuminates their connections to philosophical thought experiments, and their meaning with regard to personhood and embodiment. The paradox of the naked brain is that, ultimately, its filmic performance requires fully embodied characters; while films may begin by assuming that "we are our brains," their narrative and visual development ends up questioning or nuancing this initial assumption.

Keywords: B movie, brain in a vat, ectobrain, embodiment, personhood, thought experiment

In *Donovan's Brain* (1953), surgeon Patrick Cory (Lew Ayres) dreams of maintaining brains alive. After wicked millionaire Warren H. Donovan's airplane crashes in the desert, near Pat's home laboratory, the doctor makes an unsuccessful effort to save him. On that morning, he and his collaborator Frank (Gene Evans), assisted by Pat's devoted wife Jan (Nancy Davis, the future Mrs. Ronald Reagan), had already approached their goal: "Something great, kids: a brain without a body – alive!" The organ was a monkey's. They now extract Donovan's brain and place it in a vat. Sustained by an electric current in a nourishing solution, its vital autonomy and material growth are highlighted by close-ups of the pulsating and glowing organ (we may here regret the film is black-and-white), or shot/counter-shots between it and a character or between the brain and the oscillograph that registers its activity (Brainfilms 3.1):

> PAT: If this brain lives, maybe we can discover how it thinks.
> FRANK: Impossible. It can't see, it can't hear, and it can't feel.
> PAT: That's all right. The brain itself can't. ... But this brain contains all the knowledge and experience of Warren Donovan's entire life. In other words, all his thoughts.

From this early moment on, the movie revolves around Donovan's brain telepathically manipulating Pat in pursuit of its ambition to take over the world's financial system. Toward the end, Frank's intention of slaying the brain to liberate his friend worries Jan tremendously:

> JAN: Frank, what'll happen to Pat? I mean, if we kill the brain.
> FRANK [standing up with resolve as a storm breaks out]: The brain is Donovan!

In the end, the brain is destroyed, Donovan dies, and Pat is set free. For the brain is Donovan, and Donovan the brain.

Directed by Felix E. Feist, *Donovan's Brain* is adapted from Curt Siodmak's 1942 homonymous novel, which is written as Pat's diary. In addition to novels and short stories, Siodmak, a German exile who moved to the USA in 1937 after a couple of years in England, authored the screenplay of a number of horror Hollywood movies and repeatedly exploited the brain motif. While not the first to use the brain-in-a-vat trope, he popularized it in its most familiar form. As "the ultimate brain novel," *Donovan's Brain* became the basis of "the essential brain-in-a-vat film" (Wass 2016). This judgment is justified. The novel was also adapted as *The Lady and the Monster* (1944) and *The Brain* (1962); but even though the latter includes several shots of the brain in a vat, it offers nothing comparable to the active protagonism the organ has in the 1953 version. Yet the movie's sober, slightly noirish style, and the decision to tone down the full potential of the mad-scientist and evil-brain motifs disappointed the critics. The *New York Times* saw Feist's "little exercise in science fiction" as an "utterly silly thing," insufficiently "drenched" in "visual fantasy to make it overwhelm" (Crowther 1954).

Brains such as Donovan's are usually described (as in *The New York Times*) as "disembodied." The adjective is commonly used to designate bodily parts that have become detached from their original bodily contexts. This applies to medieval and early modern heads (Santing, Baert, and Traninger 2013) as much as to recent cyborg bodies (Klugman [2001, 46] characterizes the "disembodied mind" cyborg type as one in which "only the brain is organic inside a mechanical body"). Yet it is far from adequate. While it suggests an incorporeal mode of existence, as would be that of a soul divested of a body, the brains in our movies are, like those of pulp stories, just the opposite. Forcefully, often colorfully or repulsively enfleshed, they are perfectly material; they just happen to subsist separate from the rest of the body. They are "ectobrains," naked sentient organs living *outside* the heads and skulls that constitute their natural environment. The mad scientist's favorite procedure is brain removal and transplantation, though he (for the surgeon is generally a man) will not hesitate to keep the extracted organ in its bare-skinned condition if it fits his evil purposes. As David Skal (1998, 282) observed in *Screams of Reason*,

> Sometimes the brain is dug out of graves; sometimes they're cut out of living heads. The brain is the great prize, isolated and self-contained, much like the mad doctor himself. It is usually transported in a glass jar or tank, clearly visible but enigmatic nonetheless. It is an object to be guarded, stolen, substituted, coveted, feared, adored, abused, and obeyed. The liberated brain has several destination options: It can be installed in the cranium of a man-made monster, or a robot, or alternatively, it can be preserved in permanent laboratory isolation.

This is the brain that, after a considerable role in the pulps, became a popular character of B movies and various paracinematic productions of the 1950s to 1970s.

Jeffrey Sconce has shown how, regardless of how one judges their aesthetic value, 1950s brainfilms and the related genre of the severed living head relate to major political and social debates in the United States of the period. The malevolent ectobrain motif, where the organ is "most often the mastermind behind a horrific scheme of conquest and control," emerged at the "hybrid intersection of neurology, parapsychology, political psychology, and psychoanalysis," and combined idioms and visuals from those fields with tropes denotative of cold war angst, such as outer space and the nuclear menace (Sconce 1995a, 278, 297).

In combination with "atomic" and alien-invasion themes, the memory of such brainfilms periodically revives as cultish and admiring parody. The wackiest instances must be the 19-minute 2010 *L'attaque du monstre géant suceur de cerveaux de l'espace* [*Attack of the Giant Brain-Sucking Monster from Space*] and *The Attack of the Brain People*, an ultra-low budget 53-minute production of 2013. Their very names are homages to the genre, and both include a tribute to the *Night of the Living Dead*. *L'attaque* mixes musical comedy in the spirit of Jacques Demy's 1967 *Les Demoiselles de Rochefort* with an extraterrestrial invasion conducted by a giant cephalopod whose body is a cerebrum, and whose tentacles suck out people's brains, immediately transforming them into zombies. *The Attack* includes extraordinarily awkward flying and crawling "fiendish" ectobrains that aggress humans, and also turn them into zombies.

More to the point, like contemporaneous pics concerning body snatchers and extraterrestrial invaders, 1950s brainfilms enacted the conflict, common to the era's science fiction in general, between minds that control and are controlled. In the atmosphere of the Cold War, such conflict always ended with the defeat of the hostile ectobrains and signaled the victory of the individual subject "both as a political citizen and a metaphysical category" (Sconce 1995a, 299). Sconce highlights the place the brain occupied at the time in professional debate and popular imagination. In a context where science enjoyed a high public profile, investigating the brain, and therefore the material determinants of mind, seemed crucial not only for discovering therapies for mental illness, but also for fighting the battle of ideological dominance against the red menace.

"Brainwashing" was first used in 1950 in connection with Americans who were taken prisoners during the Korean War; chlorpromazine, the first antipsychotic, was synthesized in France in December 1951; and psychosurgery and electrical brain stimulation were at the time making strides as means for treating mental disorders. One type of surgery gained great coverage in the 1960s and nourished philosophical thought experiments: the transection of the corpus callosum that joins the two hemispheres, which was employed as a last resort treatment for epilepsy, and resulted in the "split-brain." In 1963, Yale University physiologist José Manuel Rodríguez Delgado stopped a charging bull by pressing the remote control button activating the "stimoceiver" implanted in the animal's caudate nucleus. In short, promising medical and scientific advances seemed to show that mind and brain could be manipulated by physical means. From the mid-1950s onward, the brain became a common topic for science, the popular press, and primarily "trash" fictions about mind control (Dunne 2013; Olster 2010; Seed 2004; Valenstein 1973). Its place and representation were shaped by the same rich mixture of scientific progress, ideological fear, and dystopic fantasy that framed the consolidation of brain research into the field which in the early 1960s received the name "neuroscience." As we have seen, the pulps had been rehearsing that mixture in a climate marked by World War I, the Bolshevik Revolution, the Great Depression, and the consolidation of Fascist movements. While there are undeniable continuities between the pulps and the Bs, the Cold War was the occasion of giving brain themes a new meaning.

Philosophy was integral to these developments – so much so that brainfilms, like the pulp stories sketched in Chapter 2, may at first look like the transposition of the thought experiments that have been popular in the Anglo-American philosophy of personal identity since the 1960s. The chronology, obviously, suggests a different genealogy. Thought experiments had a noble lineage in the metaphysics of mind and personal identity: in his *Meditations* of 1641, Descartes envisioned that a deceiving demon, a *mauvais génie* fools us into believing that we have a body and that there is an external world; at the end of the century, John Locke placed consciousness in the little finger and transferred a prince's soul into a cobbler's body. Starting in the early 1920s, fantasy and science fiction pulp magazines staged ectobrains, severed heads and brain transplants. These tropes would soon find their way not only into film, but also, though exceptionally, into philosophical thinking. In a 1929 futuristic phantasy, the Marxist pacifist, pioneer of X-ray crystallography and philosopher of science John Desmond Bernal dreamed up a benevolent utopia in which interconnected brains (a pulp, but not a movie motif) would be kept alive in cylindrical "brain-cases," guaranteed "continuous awareness," and linked to natural or artificial sensory and locomotor organs. The resulting "multiple individual" would be immortal, "the older components as they died being replaced by newer ones without losing the continuity of the self, the memories and feelings of the older member transferring themselves almost completely to the common stock before its death" (see Chapter 4 on brain-mediated immortality in film). Bernal claimed that such "new man" would be "only the logical outcome of the type of humanity that exists at present." "After all," he wrote, "it is brain that counts, and to have a brain suffused by fresh and correctly prescribed blood is to be alive – to think." It seems that the philosophers who in the 1960s began using brain thought experiments to explore personal identity were not aware of Bernal's pioneering fantasy (Gere 2004; see Schneider 2009, Parts I–III, for a useful anthology of sci-fi, brains and philosophy). It is nevertheless not unlikely that at least some of them were pulp readers or B-movie spectators.

Brain thought experiments in professional Anglo-American philosophy appear to have been launched by Sidney Shoemaker in *Self-Knowledge and Self-Identity*, published in 1963. Shoemaker imagined that a brain could be entirely removed from a person's skull to be repaired, and then put back in place. After the brains of Brown and Robinson are mistakenly interchanged, one of the patients dies. Made up of Robinson's body and Brown's brain, the survivor, "Brownson," does not recognize his body, but is psychologically just like Brown. Shoemaker argued that Browson's having Brown's brain *explains* his psychological affinity to Brown, yet does not logically imply that he *is* Brown. Brain thought experiments multiplied in the wake of Shoemaker. In the hands of the British philosopher Derek Parfit among others, they became a standard tool of inquiry into the conditions of personhood and personal identity (see overviews in Brueckner 2004 and Hickey 2005). Split-brain research, which was popularized in such media as *Scientific American* (Sperry 1964; Gazzaniga 1967), nourished the surgical penchant that had already flourished in fiction. Prominent philosophers bisected the brain and wondered whether two persons could share one body; they grafted X's brain into Y's empty skull; they transplanted each hemisphere of Z's brain into a different body. *The Mind's I*, a popular book edited by Douglas Hofstadter and Daniel Dennett (1981), gathered some particularly extravagant varieties of the experiment; in *Philosophical Explanations*, Robert Nozick (1981) tested his own theory against eight brain-fictional situations. Although in the late 1980s, Kathleen Wilkes (1988) criticized their extensive use in a book eloquently entitled *Real People: Personal Identity Without Thought Experiments*, they have not lost their popularity, and the porosity of the boundary between literary and philosophical fantasy has remained useful to explore the "adventures" of personhood (e.g., Cassou-Noguès 2010, Chap. 7).

When in 1953 *Donovan's Brain* foregrounded a brain in a vat and turned it into one of its protagonists, it performed the philosophical brain fiction par excellence. Its most famous version would nonetheless be worked out only three decades later. In *Reason, Truth, and History*, Harvard philosopher Hilary Putnam (1981, Chap. 1) elaborated it as a technologically updated version of the Cartesian demon: while you are sleeping, your brain is removed, placed in a vat, and hooked to a computer that sends to it signals similar to the ones that usually informed it. When you wake up, everything looks the same as before. In such a situation, Putnam argued, you could not think you were a brain in a vat. Although his purpose was to discuss skepticism rather than personal identity, it is significant that the choice of a brain fiction seemed so natural, as if investigating self-knowledge inevitably implied equating personhood and brainhood.

Brains in vats, the generally calamitous sequels of brain transplantation, and personal immortality through successive transfers of a brain into younger bodies were commonplace in science-fiction pulps, novels, and numerous B movies starting in the 1940s. It is hard to know how much time the philosophers just mentioned might have spent in their youth consuming popular culture. Puccetti (1972), for one, engaged in producing it, fictionalizing his philosophical verdict, "Where goes a brain, there goes a person," in a novel entitled *The Death of the Führer*, where Hitler's brain survives in the body of an attractive and voluptuous woman. At least with regard to the chronology, it is safe to say that professional philosophers' thought experiments academicized popular fiction, not that pulps and brainfilms popularized philosophical thought experiments.

Brain Movies

Although brain movie scenarios and philosophical thought experiments offer striking similarities, filmmaking is freer not to seek theoretical closure. Professional philosophy tends to analytically elaborate an argument and reach rationally defensible conclusions. The cinema, in contrast, can more or less deliberately and explicitly explore an issue that could be formulated theoretically, but tends to raise questions without attempting to solve them or defend a particular system. Insofar as it replaces the abstract by the concrete, it can work, as Antoine Compagnon (2006) has said of literature, as an "antidote to philosophy." It is up to us, readers or spectators, to seek and attribute meanings. Moreover, different filmic moments, visuals or subplots may take different stands and have conflicting implications regarding the matters they may appear to be tackling; even within a shot, framing and dialogue can question or contradict each other. That is a major difference between thought experiments in philosophy and fiction. Independently of the margins they might leave for doubt, the former have an epistemic function, which is to help us think clearly and concretely about the nature of the problem at hand (in our case, the conditions of personal identity), and better to formulate and assess possible solutions. In contrast, the purpose of a cinematic mise-en-scène that looks like a thought experiment is to unfold the dramatics of a motif that could, but need not, be interpreted as a philosophical premise. The epistemic element of a narrative film subsists "as part of the overall fabric of the work" (Smith 2006, 39), and it is as such that it has to be examined to gain full significance.

That is why the analysis of B-to-Z motion pictures can be productive. They lack the sententious, didactic, or moralizing tone that sometimes affects supposedly nobler forms; but precisely because they are not shrouded in a "veil of complexity" suggesting profound meanings (Judd 2017), they avoid self-conscious calls for "serious" interpretation, and may be more adventurously open than films of ideas or philosophical dramas (Smith and Wartenberg 2006). Overall, philosophically inclined moviegoers or cinephile philosophers have been fatally attracted to movies such as *The Matrix* (1999), which are flagrantly designed to perform classical philosophical themes and inspire academic commentary (for a sample, see Badiou et al. 2003; Grau 2005; Irwin 2002; Schulze 2012). Indeed, as *The Economist* uncharitably noted when the first *Matrix* came out, philosophers "were pleased because it provided a wildly popular bandwagon for them to jump on" (Anon. 2003).

The Bs, Cs, and Zs have other virtues. Although, of course, not all openly "philosophical" movies are well received, those in the "inferior" categories have usually been, if reviewed at all, routinely savaged. With time, the first reviews end up having almost the same passé charm as the pictures themselves, which can then be positively reassessed. For example, of *The Monster and the Girl*, sketched below, *The New York Times* of March 3, 1941 (p. 25) wondered "how many dyspeptic dramas might be spared the public if only a scenarist had taken bicarbonate of soda before sitting down to the typewriter. Otherwise," it continued, "how account for such a film ..., as lethargic an excursion into nightmare as ever a man snored through. ... Sometimes we can't believe our eyes." It took seven and a half decades for this "unheralded B-film" to be rediscovered as "genuinely thrilling and stylish" (Davis 2015, 282). Two outstandingly documented references prove invaluable for navigating this universe: Janne Wass's blog *Scifist*, which offers extensive reviews of science fiction movies since 1890 (Wass n.d.), and Bill Warren's large-scale repertoire of American science fiction movies of the 1950s (Warren 2010, originally published in two volumes in 1982 and 1986).

From *L'homme-singe* (1909), which tells the story of a man whose brain is replaced by a monkey's, through the original *Frankenstein* (1931), where the creature is given "a criminal brain," to mid-twentieth-century B movies and many later productions, filmic materials for a cultural history of the cerebral subject are extremely rich. Nevertheless, in spite of their variety and major transformations in both the sciences and cinematography, the leitmotifs and conventions of brain-related motion pictures exhibit remarkable continuity.

The first continuity concerns brains themselves. They tend to be ectobrains, autonomous organs living outside a body, and occasionally exerting their functions more powerfully than when they were still "embodied." While oftentimes their "disembodied" state is only temporary, it highlights the powers that brains are said to have by themselves. The second major continuity is ontological. Puccetti's dictum rules, and movies invariably assume that where the brain is, there is the person. Brains, heads (in their capacity as brain containers), or their contents, may be transplanted or transferred, and such operation gives the donor's identity to the receiver. By the same token, altering a brain's anatomical or informational substance transforms personal identity. These forms of continuity perform interrelated "ideological" premises and their consequences. In this regard, it is ectobrain and transplant movies that are closest to philosophers' thought experiments.

A third form of continuity concerns features that involve representing science and brain mechanisms. Modernizing elements, such as computers and visuals that evoke structural or functional neuroimaging, coexist with older brainhood icons, such as brains in jars and simplified cerebral localization maps. For example, in *The Black Sleep* (1956), the wife of an English surgeon is in a catatonic state due to a malignant brain tumor. In order to find out how to extirpate the tumor safely, the doctor performs open-skull surgery on involuntary human subjects, giving them the Indian anaesthetic he calls "Black Sleep," electrically stimulating various areas of their cerebral cortex, and generally causing grievous irreversible mental and physical injuruy. The assumption of the experiments is a basic localizationism, perfectly acceptable in the 1870s, when the action takes place (Brainfilms 3.2). Yet the scene, in the same movie, of an open-skull operation with electrical stimulation of the cortex inducing a patient's motor reaction (Brainfilms 3.3) recalls procedures that entered popular culture in the 1950s, with the work of neurosurgeon Wilder Penfield. In *Brain Dead* (1990), the mad scientist, who is obsessed with the cerebral causes of paranoia, calls attention to the precise "abnormality" as it appears on a brain cross section; in another scene, the spot shows on a computer screen (Brainfilms 3.4). In a procedure modeled upon stereotactic surgery, he cures the patient by plunging a needle in the brain (Brainfilms 3.5). A scene where an assistant maps "the facial muscle control agents" involves a brain stuck on a tripod and a device displaying a grimacing face (Brainfilms 3.6). The enactment of extreme localizationism adopts a futuristic look, yet it takes place in a shabby room where a huge wall of metal shelves displays a collection of sentient brains in the glass jars evocative of nineteenth-century anatomopathological collections. (Brainfilms 3.7)

Modernizing details are legion throughout the history of brainfilms. They help situate the action in a certain time and context, and heighten verisimilitude through visuals and discourse. Yet, at least as far as the performance of brainhood is concerned, they tend to be cosmetic, and rarely add substance to the plots. This is particularly clear in movie remakes or other forms of revival and resurgence. For example, in *The Brain Eaters* (1958), based (without giving it credit) on Robert A. Heinlein's 1951 novel *The Puppet Masters*, humans are parasitized by cockroach-like creatures with a pair of white antennae that feed on the brain; this turns them into zombie-like "puppets." When infected people breathe, a hump moves at the back of their neck, but the picture does not display the brain or evoke neuroscience. Similarly, the mind-and-behavior-controlling parasites of *Operation – Annihilate!*, the *Star Trek* episode of April 13, 1967, are described by Spock as "a one-cell creature, resembling more than anything else a huge individual brain cell" (Brainfilms 3.8). However, these reddish slimy entities, which fly and squeak like bats, sting their victims by attaching themselves to their backs, and melt surrounded by vapors when exposed to ultraviolet light, do not look very much like neurons. Half a century later, the meat parasites that, *On the Brain* (2016), turn men into zombie-like rapists appear as worms moving under the skin of their preys' foreheads, where they leave a bloody scar; flashes resembling neurons sometimes appear during the attack that zombifies the victims, but brains are nowhere to be seen. Even when it is clear that controlling someone means taking over their nervous system, the brain is not necessarily enacted or displayed.

Three decades after *The Brain Eaters*, *The Puppet Masters* (1990), explicitly based on Heinlein, provided more detail. The parasites now look like small stingrays that attack their victims through the upper portion of the spine. Nothing new here. This time, however, scientists go further into investigating how the creature "interfaces" with the human nervous system. They discover that brain tissue accounts for c. 60% of its body mass, and marvel at "the structural complexity of its neocortex." The parasites have hooks that "lock into the spinal column" (traces could be seen in *The Brain Eaters*), while a probe that emerges from a tentacle penetrates victims' brains and "overrides" their system. The process is displayed, in *mise en abîme*, as enlarged microscopic and radioscopic images projected on screens. (Brainfilms 3.9). Born out of pods – a clear homage to the famous *Invasion of the Body Snatchers* of 1956, even though the pods here look like coconuts – the parasites seem to transmit intelligence and memory through physical contact. Actually, they are, like the *Star Trek* parasites, "a single creature with a million parts," which is finally killed by infecting it with encephalitis. (None of this goes crucially beyond pulp stories outlined in Chapter 2, such as "Parasite" or "Brain Leeches," both published in 1935.)

Let us take as second example the TV science fiction anthology series *The Outer Limits*. The original was produced and broadcast in the US in 1963–1965; the revived version, a US-Canada production, was aired between 1995 and 2002. Both include several episodes that variously place the brain center stage. In *The Man with the Power* (1963), college professor Harold Finley (a latter-day Prof. Shea from the 1933 pulp story "Stallion's Trappings") is routinely abused as powerless and mediocre. In fact, he has invented a device, now embedded in his frontal lobe, which allows him to manipulate objects through brainpower. He would like his invention to serve good purposes. Nevertheless, because, as a psychiatrist explains, we are driven by our "subconscious," Finley's emotions make him use his ability to take revenge on those who mistreated him. Realizing the risks in such a situation, as well as the questionable motives of an astronaut scheduled to receive the implant, Finley destroys the operating facility and kills himself. The episode includes a good amount of psy discourse, as well as scientific-sounding exposition and various general mentions of the brain. For example, Finley explains:

> I have developed a link gate complex enough to regulate the forces of the field energies surrounding us. … I have no actual power myself. By using my brain patterns as a sort of focusing device, I am able to direct electromagnetic field energy into a discrete beam. It's rather as though my brain were a lens focusing light waves into a sharp line.

The brain itself is never displayed, and all we see is an X-ray of Finley's skull, with a small white rectangle on the forehead to indicate the implant's location (Brainfilms 3.10). Subconscious causality, fields, energies and beams are all trademark pulp devices.

In *The Brain of Colonel Barham* (1965), another episode echoing the Space Race, the title hero is the best candidate to carry out a mission to land on Mars. Since he is dying, the project leaders offer to keep his brain, separate from his body, connected to a computer it will activate. As an army general affirms, "This machine will have eyes, ears, and a voice. It'll see Mars, and all the other planets of the solar system. … It'll never be hungry, or thirsty, or feel pain. And it may be immortal." Barham accepts, but once he has become an ectobrain, he turns out to be a dangerous megalomaniac who transforms people into obedient robots. Once more, "subconscious drives may be released," and the source of danger and its surrounding technology must finally be destroyed. Yet the brain is hardly shown. We see its activity as electroencephalographic recordings, as a voice coming from a loudspeaker, and as the twisted, radiant and crackling beams it fires against people. There is the usual jar with the customary cables (Brainfilms 3.11). The organ, though, which "has developed a sense of omnipotence" and appears to grow "when it's no longer confined" inside a skull, is immersed in a liquid so murky that it remains indistinguishable.

These episodes of the original *Outer Limits* combine the myth of the omnipotent "subconscious" with themes related to the superhuman power of the brain when appropriately manipulated or liberated from the body, the relationship of brain and body, and the connection both have to personal identity. The brain is center stage, but is not displayed as such. *The Outer Limits* series as revived in the 1990s is in this respect both thematically and visually different. The brain appears under familiar forms, and the brain-themed episodes emphasize something else: personality transfer, the relocation of brain contents and the resulting persistence of one individual in another's body, instead of the risks involved in ectobrains or in technological manipulations.

At the outset of *Second Thoughts* (1997), Karl (Howie Mandel), an intellectually disabled man, receives (via a brain-contents transfer device) the mind of Dr. Valerian (John Gilbert), a fatally ill brilliant doctor. After successively killing Valerian's financier and a police investigator, he uses the machine to "absorb" their minds. The problem is that he not only acquires their "brain power" or (as Valerian had put it) "an extra mind," but also their personalities: "We're now three individuals living in a single body." These individuals fight cacophonously with each other. The drama unravels through Karl's love for Rose (Jennifer Rubin), a caretaker in the communal home where he lives. Hoping to conquer her, he kills her fiancé (a suicidal poet) and absorbs his mind. After Rose rejects him, the last scene suggests that Karl commits suicide. During the transfer procedure, the scene is flooded in colored light, and time-lapse sequences of images from the donors' lives enact the upload of their memories into Karl's brain. As Valerian leads Karl toward the machine, the organ appears as a PET-scan-like image on a computer screen. Even though very brief, this appearance highlights the brain by giving it what since the 1990s has become one of its most recognizable modern representations (Brainfilms 3.12). Such brief appearances are a standard strategy to visually underline the cerebral cause of behavioral changes. In *Lawnmower Man* (1992), for example, quickly displayed brain images provide the evidence that a procedure for enhancing intelligence by means of psychoactive drugs and virtual reality actually works (Brainfilms 3.13.)

In *Identity Crisis* (1998), another *Outer Limits* episode, the mind of Captain Cotter McCoy (Lou Diamond Phillips) is "downloaded" to the prototype of an indestructible "military android," and returned to the original body after the two-billion-dollar artificial creature has accomplished its dangerous missions. During one "transfer," McCoy's body dies, his mind remains trapped "inside this machine," and the interface between it and the android body begins to deteriorate and will break down completely within twelve hours. It transpires that Colonel Pete Butler, supposedly a friend of McCoy's but fiendishly jealous of his successes, sabotaged the system and had himself downloaded into another prototype. Initially, McCoy still identifies with his body: "That's me they're working on in there," he says while pointing to the room where his charred body is being examined. However, after a fight between the two androids, his mind is relocated into Pete's body, and he seems happy with the solution. This is one of the possible outcomes in the classic scenario in which a person continues living in or with someone else's body. The transfer sequences show not only the human and the android in the cabins where they sit during the procedure, but also their full brains on twin computer screens, whirling around themselves while the transfer takes place (Brainfilms 3.14). Thus is highlighted the fact that we are our minds, and our minds are our brains.

Old and new, the brain-themed episodes of *The Outer Limits* enact situations, thought experiments, plots and visuals that will be found in many movies across this book. The narrower point to be made here is that updating the representation of the brain and cerebral processes by modernizing the relevant technologies invariably underlines the role of the brain as bodily organ. That, in turn, reinforces the ontological assumption – *we are our brains* – which, however superficially, launches or drives the film action. At the same time, the transfer in *Identity Crisis* is not essentially different from the one enacted six decades earlier in *The Man Who Changed His Mind* (see Chapter 4). Modernizing, once again, contributes to the picture's verisimilitude, but neither adds depth nor modifies basic narrative lines. The same applies to cases, such as the two versions of *The Manchurian Candidate* (discussed in Chapter 6), in which updating consists mainly of *adding* brain to mind, *neuro* to *psy*.

As these examples suggest, and as the rest of this book illustrates, the continuities sketched above cut across different classes of brainfilms. The most obvious one consists of productions where an ectobrain is a leading character. Insofar as the head is important because it contains a brain, "disembodied" (i.e., severed and living) head pictures can be considered a variation of the ectobrain class. The brain remains crucial, but is now accompanied by the physiognomic signs of identity. For the mad doctor who keeps brains or heads alive, the final goal is usually transplantation. In brain transplant movies, which make up a third group, the story deals largely with the fate of the hybrid entity consisting of X's brain and Y's body. The weirdest class concerns evil brains, some of which are "brain suckers," frightful creatures that live on human beings' cerebral and spinal cord substance.

Damaged brains could make up a class by themselves, were it not for the fact that the mishap generally arises while preparing the brain for transplantation. *The Fiend With the Electronic Brain* (1969) is an interesting exception. The title character is the young soldier Joe Corey (Roy Morton), who has just arrived from Vietnam, "shell fragments lodged in his brain." Neurosurgeon Dr. Vanard (played by horror star John Carradine) declares him dead, but in fact plants in his skull an "artificial brain component," powered by the organ's "own electrical impulses" and supposed to "take over the functions of the damaged area." The device is activated by an electric current via a helmet, which looks like an inverted mixing bowl with coiled cables on each side, placed on the patient's head (Brainfilms 3.15; we deal below with the significance of such helmets). Something, however, goes wrong. Joe, the doctor explains, returns "to a certain level of normalcy, but his psyche, his personality was destroyed, he was a different person." His father describes him as "an electronic freak," and a police inspector, as "a homicidal maniac with an artificial brain whose every action is completely unpredictable." This generates action, including, in the end, Joe's electrocuting Vanard (Carradine convulsing and grimacing under the shaking helmet).

Body Parts

Have other body parts been depicted as fulfilling the same personal-identity function as the brain? For centuries since antiquity, the heart was symbol of affect and the organ of emotion; yet as the cerebralization process began in the late seventeenth century, it retained only symbolic significance (Bound Alberti 2010). While the heart played a crucial role in Christian mysticism, there is no such a thing as "the sacred brain of Jesus" (Stevens 1997), and it is in holy persons' hearts that one sought, and sometimes found, formations in the shape of the cross or other instruments of the Passion. In transplantation – not restricted to the heart – the views of both the general public and organ recipients range from magical thinking to seeing the body as an object in need of material repair (Sanner 2001, 2005). Organ donor families may bond with recipients after transplants (Aleccia 2013), and beliefs and feelings about debt, gift, reciprocity, guilt, ownership, and transmortality play an important part in recipients' emotional and behavioral responses (Zimmermann et al. 2016). Early heart transplants generated passionate interest; with time, like other transplantations, they became normalized, no longer an instance of horror and the transgression of boundaries (overview in Russell 2019, 11–17). It does happen that having someone else's heart can affect the recipient's sense of self or make them worry about personality changes (Bunzel, Wollenek, and Grundbock 1992; Kaba et al. 2005). Nevertheless, neither on nor off screen has the heart played for personal identity a role equivalent to that of the brain.

In the comedy *Heart Condition* (1990), for example, a racist policeman receives the heart of an assassinated black lawyer; but it is as a ghost that the lawyer returns to urge the cop to catch his killers. The drama *Heart* (1999) revolves around a mother's obsession with her son's heart, now located in another man's body; yet that does not turn the recipient into her son. In Pedro Almodóvar's *Todo sobre mi madre* (*All About My Mother*, 1999), Manuela is determined to see the recipient of her son's heart; however, as has been pointed out, the film gives no indication that the son lives on within the recipient (Schicktanz and Wöhlke 2017, 107). The same applies generally: A's heart in B's body never turns B into A. An exception might be a Mexican cheapie, René Cardona's 1969 *La horripilante bestia humana* (a.k.a. *Night of the Bloody Apes*, though, literally, *The Horrifying Human Beast*), in which a mad doctor tries to cure his son's leukemia by giving him a gorilla's heart, and thereby transforms him into a homicidal monster.

At first sight, adaptations of Maurice Renard's novel *The Hands of Orlac* (*Les mains d'Orlac*), first published in 1920 and often reprinted, seem more relevant for the question of non-cerebral organs. (Olney [2006], who classes it in the genre of body horror, reads both the novel and the films as critiquing the normative ideal of the "able" body, while also perpetuating stereotypes about physical disability.) Robert Wiene's late expressionist silent classic *Orlac's Hände* (1924), Karl Freund's *Mad Love* (1935, with Peter Lorre's first Hollywood appearance, as a scary but pathetic mad doctor), as well as the lesser *The Hands of Orlac* (1960) and *Hands of a Stranger* (1962), which doesn't credit Renard, all roughly follow, as far as the hands are concerned, the original story. Pianist Stephen Orlac's hands are mangled in an accident, and he receives those of a man executed for murder. Orlac becomes obsessed with them, and crimes are committed that look as if he were the culprit. The truth is that someone else is framing him. In *Hands of a Stranger*, "a low-budget, talky melodrama" (Pitts 2011, 85), a desperate Orlac wants to take revenge, murders with his powerful new hands the doctors who assisted in the operation, and is shot while attacking the surgeon. In all cases, the hands affect him not because they carry another person's identity, but because of his psychological instability, which the extortionist in the novel diagnoses as the pianist's *nervosité*. We shall later see that Renard (1875–1939), a proponent of a literary genre he called *merveilleux-scientifique*, was far from ignoring the brain and xenografts (see Evans 1994 for a good overview in English; on grafting in particular, see Després 2009). As for upper limbs in particular, with the exception of Thing, the friendly forearm of TV series *The Addams Family* (1962–1964), disembodied hands, like those in *The Beast With Five Fingers* (1946), *Dr. Terror's House of Horrors* (1965) or *The Hand* (1981), roam about creating mayhem, but do not incarnate personhood.

Body Parts (1991), based on Boileau-Narcejac's 1965 novel *…Et mon tout est un homme* (*Choice Cuts*), comes close to realizing Orlac's fears. A female surgeon grafts onto different bodies the head, legs, and arms of an executed murderer called Fletcher. The legs and arms seem autonomous. Their present owners display various asocial behaviors, and a painter of corny landscapes becomes the successful creator of violent scenes; they also have memory flashes of Fletcher's crimes. The character with the murderer's head tries to recover the grafted members, and succeeds with one arm and the legs before having his neck broken by the recipient of the other arm. The surgeon keeps Fletcher's torso and recovered extremities alive and twitching in a large glass case that looks like a Damien Hirst *Natural History* installation. In the end, the action is dictated by Fletcher's brain – so much so that after the head dies, the memory flashes cease and the surviving patient regains control of his grafted arm. The bloodiest version of a living head controlling its body seems to be *Re-Animator* (1985), one of the most famous gore movies of the 1980s. The young Swiss scientist Herbert West (Jeffrey Combs), who questions the very notion of "brain death," beheads (with a shovel) his scientific rival, Dr. Carl Hill (David Gale), and reanimates the head with an injection of the green fluorescent "reagent" he has developed. After hitting West and making him pass out, Hill's head makes the body engage in a variety of heinous behaviors, some sexual, in which the head itself eagerly participates.

Pictures about someone gaining a new face explore the subjective and intersubjective consequences of such a surgery, which organs are necessary for being oneself, whether they have to be one's own and what that might mean. In spite of deep dissimilarities, face- and brain-transplantation movies are akin in fundamental ways. On the one hand, both give a central role to outward appearance. Brain-transplanted individuals look like their hosts (be they a natural or a manufactured body); "they" (i.e., their brains) have merely changed location. The reverse is true in new-face films, where the facial skin of an individual, who has been usually assassinated to become a face donor, is given to someone else. In both cases, the resulting person is the same as the original one, but looks entirely different. If the plot is about restoring someone's disfigured face so that it looks like the original, then, because the face is seen as a transparent locus of identity and the center of expression, the facial graft reinstates the possibility of the recipient's being recognized for the person he or she really is. The graft is neither the seat nor the origin of personal identity; I can be myself with a different face, provided I have my own brain. Thus, on the other hand, facefilms and brainfilms share adherence to Puccetti's dictum, "Where goes a brain, there goes a person;" and they do so in a variety of styles, mostly horror.

In George Franju's *Les Yeux sans visage* (*The Eyes Without a Face*), which pioneered the motif in 1960 with a screenplay that counted Boileau and Narcejac among its writers, Dr. Génessier grafts the face of a female victim onto her disfigured daughter Christiane. The "eyes without a face" are Christiane's, as she is obliged by her father to wear a face-like mask that reveals only her eyes; she carries it for most of the film and the final failure of the graft implies the definitive impossibility of her recovering beauty and transparency. *Les Yeux* has been rediscovered as "a masterpiece of poetic horror and tactful, tactile brutality" (Hoberman 2003). "Brutal and lyrical in equal part, it is one of the most memorable entries in French *fantastique* cinema" (Sélavy 2018), one that is profoundly related to major themes of the post–World War II philosophical context (Geroulanos 2013). It is revealing of the way *Les Yeux* was initially perceived that, in the USA, it was released under the title *The Horror Chamber of Dr. Faustus* and as a double feature with *The Manster* (1959), a sci-fi/body-horror production involving a man mutating into a murderous two-headed monster (shot in English in Japan, it is now appreciated by camp aficionados and feels like a forerunner of David Cronenberg's "body horror"; Lucas 2008).

Les Yeux can be connected not only to several low-budget 1960s horror pictures, but also to Pedro Almodóvar's 2011 *La piel que habito* (*The Skin I Live In*), which repeatedly pays homage to it while adding transgender change to the significance of faces as marks of identity. In a completely different genre, John Woo's *Face/Off* (1997) enacts a face swap between FBI special agent Sean Archer and assassin and terrorist Castor Troy. This provides the occasion for spectacular action scenes, pursuits and fights between John Travolta (Archer's original appearance) and Nicolas Cage (Troy's). The swap, however, was accidental. The goal of temporarily giving Troy's face to Archer is to help him fight crime and restore order. But after Troy unexpectedly wakes up from postoperative coma and discovers what has happened, he forces the surgeon to give him Archer's face. In a clear tribute to a classic motif, the special agent's face is preserved in a glass vessel identical to the usual ectobrain container. Behind appearances and temporarily adopted social roles, each man remains totally himself, constantly disgusted by having to inhabit a body that looks like the enemy's and to adopt the persona of the other. Emphasizing how convincingly each character plays the other, Žižek (2001) argues that *Face/Off* demonstrates the symbolic efficiency of the mask, and enacts the incompatibility between Jacques Lacan and Emmanuel Levinas; yet he does not take into account the bland, family-friendly happy end that comes about when Archer recovers his face after Troy's death.

Finally, in *body* or *biological horror*, bodies are threatened and reshaped into extreme abjection. They can be invaded from the outside by creatures that try to dominate them; possessed by intruders from within that manifest themselves by and through bodily features; attacked by parasites and other beings who exploit them, maim them or consume them; or become transgressive freaks, anthropomorphic monsters that defy the supposedly natural boundaries of gender and humanity (Tudor 1995). Through disease and decay, deformity and mutilation, mutation and excrescence, all manner of anatomical metamorphoses make bodies fundamentally unreliable. They no longer function as trustworthy foundations of identity, and therein lies one of the "more horrifying flavors," the essence of the terror the genre produces (Lopez Cruz 2012, 167). However, the transmogrifications enacted in biological horror do not visibly concern the brain.

In the cinema of David Cronenberg, undisputed master of the genre, the "New Flesh" emerges as a mode of existence that physically does away with the barriers between mind and body, the natural and the artificial, the real and the virtual, the human and the technological (Papenburg 2011). The brain can be part of the transformations, but remains unseen inside the head, and what happens to it is not shown directly on the screen. *Videodrome* (1983, extensively discussed in Beard [2006], Chap. 7) is the best example of this. Videodrome, a torture-and-murder television show, broadcasts signals that cause cancerous brain tumors. For Professor Brian O'Blivion, who lives only as a face on TV and helped create the show, "the television screen is part of the physical structure of the brain." He therefore considers the tumors as a "new organ" or "new outgrowth" of the human brain; yet these are not displayed.

To sum up: in movies, as in the human and the life sciences, neither the heart nor the hand, two organs symbolically and pictorially associated with personal experience and personal identity, reach the ontological status of the brain. Similarly, radical bodily transformations may alter individuals psychologically, but do not turn them into other persons. Moreover, as we shall see, if living heads are not like other body parts, it is primarily because they enclose a brain. The rich imaginary of transplantation includes various instances of "rebellious grafts" that enjoy a certain degree of autonomy vis-à-vis the transplant recipients (St-Germain 2015, Chap. 2). But if the transplanted brain appears as the fullest case of that autonomy, it is because the transplantation makes the recipient identical with the donor. Sometimes, and for a little while, the old *body* defies its new brain, thus bearing out the idea that the surgery is a whole-body transplant. Essentially, however, since the principle that "where goes a brain there goes a person" holds, there is really nothing to rebel against.

The Donor Portion

Filmic brain transplants are mainly allografts, that is, surgeries where donor and receiver belong to the same species. In such cases, X remains X *in* or *with* Y's body. When X's brain is relocated in Y's decerebrated body, X is the receiver and Y the donor. Thus, as most commentators have concluded with regard to the brain-transplantation thought experiment, the operation must properly be seen as a *whole-body transplant*. Brain movies adhere to such an interpretation, and they do so by way of various plot and character configurations.

Some filmic scientists, descendants of H. G. Wells's Dr. Moreau, experiment with xenografts, or interspecies transplants. In *The Atomic Brain* (1964), thus entitled because radiation inexplicably enables non-surgical brain transplants (but it is also known as *Monstrosity*), a lustful female octogenarian wants her brain transplanted into an attractive young woman's body. In her mansion roam weird creatures, former humans given an animal brain. Her personal mad doctor ends up placing her brain in a cat's body. After he accidentally locks himself in the transplant machine, the smart animal presses the right button, and blows everything up.

The seemingly most preposterous operations may be the ones with best historical support. Two decades after Soviet scientist Vladimir Demikhov grafted a puppy's head to an adult dog, a surgeon in *The Incredible Two-Headed Transplant* (1971) creates two-headed snakes, rabbits, and monkeys; he then grafts a psycho-killer's head on a mentally disabled young man's body. (The two-headed dog surgery is recorded in a documentary available on YouTube; see Film list under *Demikhov*.) In *The Thing with Two Heads* (1972), a racist white physician contrives a ludicrous two-headed gorilla; the donor's head should be eventually removed to produce a one-headed hybrid. Since the doctor is dying, he wants his head grafted onto a healthy body – which, against all expectations, happens to be that of an African American convict. After thirty-eight days the original head was to be removed and the grafted one would command its new body. However, since the convict is found innocent, the doctor's head must be left to die – and it dies asking for another body. The more singular non-human interspecies brain transplant is pretext for silly fun in *Hot Cross Bunny* (1948), where a doctor plans to give Bugs Bunny a chicken's brain.

Apes

The simian motif deserves the rank of brainfilm subgenre. Why would anyone transplant an ape's brain to a human body, or vice versa? From *L'homme-singe* onward, the reason is that such transplants easily generate action. This, as we have seen, applied to the pulps; and we find it again in motion pictures. Plots are sometimes designed to be funny, and help introduce variety into a series. In *A Bird in the Head* (1946), a Three Stooges short movie (the eighty-ninth out of 190), a scientist finds Curly's brain small enough for a gorilla. This prompts the characteristic slapstick of one of the most famous comedy teams in history. At about the same time, the motif appears in two movies (the fourth and sixteenth of forty-eight) featuring The Bowery Boys, another popular team of comedians. In *Spook Busters* (1946), a mad scientist wants to take part of one of the boys' brain and put it into a gorilla; in *Master Minds* (1949), he plans to kidnap one of the boys and transfer his brain into a monstrous humanoid.

In various combinations with other elements, violence most often dictates the atmosphere and outcome of brain transplantations. Virtually omnipresent, conceited, power-hungry, or simply evil scientists are obsessed with trying out their "theories," seek personal vengeance, or use their surgical hybrids to dominate the world. The three motives are combined in the Mexican pictures *Ladrón de cadáveres* (*The Body Snatcher*, 1957) and *Las luchadoras contra el médico asesino* (*Doctor of Doom*, 1963 – literally, *The Women Wrestlers Against the Killer Doctor*), where seedy surgeons transplant gorilla brains to female wrestlers' bodies and manipulate their creatures to attack somebody on the ring.

The gland fad we observed in pulps did not circumvent filmic apes. In *Captive Wild Woman* (1943), an endocrinologist transfers to a female gorilla "glandular extractions" from a human patient with excess amounts of sex hormones. The notion made sense. Glandular xenotransplantations entered the scene in the 1920s, when the Russian-born French surgeon Serge Voronoff (1866–1951), who had transplanted thyroid glands from chimpanzees to humans with thyroid deficiencies, attempted to graft primate testicles in men. His goal was not merely to restore virility, but to rejuvenate the entire organism. By the 1930s, thousands of men, some of them rich and prominent, had been treated around the world, and Voronoff had made international headlines and entered popular culture (Berliner 2004; Rémy 2014). Voronoff had studied transplantation techniques with the French surgeon Alexis Carrel (1873–1944). Carrel received the 1912 Nobel Prize for Physiology or Medicine for developing a method of suturing blood vessels. However, he was also famous for his development (together with legendary aviator Charles Lindbergh) of the perfusion pump, which was used to preserve animal organs outside the body and eventually opened the way for open-heart surgery, as well as for keeping a culture of embryonic chicken heart alive for over three decades starting in 1912. The "permanent life of tissues outside of the organism" (as reads the title of Carrel's first article reporting his results), gave rise not only to scientific controversy, but also to various hopes and fantasies about immortality and the replacement of body parts.

In *The Man in Half Moon Street* (1945), a slow-moving picture with a noir look, the all-too-obviously named Dr. Julian Karell seems to be thirty-five, but is actually over a century old. His youth depends on undergoing a gland transplant every decade, and for that, he needs human victims. (Based on the same play, the less subtle *The Man Who Could Cheat Death* [1959] displays more violence and emphasizes the doctor's rotting face as he fails to rejuvenate one last time; produced by Hammer, a British company specializing in horror films, it included two stars of the genre, director Terence Fisher and actor Christopher Lee. See Chapter 5 on Hammer.) For the endocrinologist of *Captive Wild Woman*, however, glands were not enough: to create "a human form with animal instincts," he still needed a human "cerebrum." He finds it in his objecting female assistant. The gorilla becomes an attractive though singularly inexpressive young woman named Paula Dupree (the role was played by an actress known as Acquanetta, judged at the time to have exotic looks and nicknamed The Venezuelan Volcano). Paula assists the tamer who brought her from Africa. However, when she sees him kiss his fiancée, jealousy throws her back to a simian state. Mayhem follows as she saves him from a lion before being shot by a policeman. Although, apparently, the surgery does not fully give the gorilla the human donor's identity, the brain plays such a crucial role that the doctor complains he might need "a new brain" to keep the gorilla girl in human form.

Jungle Woman (1944), the first sequel to *Captive Wild Woman*, makes only passing remarks about glandular substances. The second and last sequel, *Jungle Captive* (1945), is more interesting in this regard: Moloch, the misshapen assistant to the unscrupulous Dr. Stendhal, who wishes "to prove or disprove [his] theory of restoring life," steals from the morgue the corpse of the "ape woman." Back in his secluded country lab, the doctor tries to revive her thanks to the blood of his unwilling collaborator Ann. He succeeds, but does not know how to give human form to the simian creature. To find out, he obtains (again by way of Moloch's murderous tactics) the records of the late Dr. Walters, the endocrinologist who performed the first experiments in *Captive Wild Woman*. Thanks to Ann's "glandular secretions," the ape woman becomes again Paula Dupree. Her behavior, however, suggests that her brain is "subnormal, in some ways subhuman." Stendhal must acknowledge, "Paula's brain is gone. Her reactions are those of an animal." That, however, is not an insurmountable obstacle: Walters had given the ape woman her female assistant's brain, and his records provide the necessary instructions for the "transplanting of the cerebrum." In the meantime, though, Moloch's tender side has stirred and he has become protective of Ann. He tries to prevent Stendhal from operating on her; the doctor guns him down and gets ready to extract Ann's brain. In the meantime, Paula has (without explanation) reverted to ape woman, strangles Stendhal, and is killed by the police when she is about to slaughter Ann.

The simian motif seems to define the oldest brain-movie variety, which could also be seen as a subgenre of the larger ape-movie category. As often with the early cinema, it began with reference to comedy and Grand Guignol. In 1909, pantomime might have been the essence of *L'homme-singe*; a decade later, *Go and Get It* (1920) featured a reporter trying to solve the murders committed by a gorilla with the brain of a dead convict seeking revenge. Over the years, the subgenre ended up blending various ingredients of the B category: the mad scientist, good looking female victims, violence, morphed or disfigured bodies, generally outdated but stereotyped science visuals and discourse – all tied together by the brain motif. By 1983, *The Man with Two Brains*, discussed below, refers to a human-brain-to-gorilla transplant as a wink to B movie fans and as a humorous tribute to a venerable filmic topic.

For all its success, the simian motif has intrinsic limits. On the one hand, from the original *King Kong* (1933) to its 2005 remake, through various lesser productions – but also Frederick Wiseman's disturbing documentary *Primate* (1974) – cinema apes, like real ones, do not need human brains for viewers to anthropomorphize their behavior or inner states. On the other hand, the human-to-monkey scenario is sometimes no more than an easy way to jump-start the action. Nevertheless, precisely because the donors are humans and the receivers, anthropoids, the relevant films must deal, no matter how perfunctorily, with the consequences of placing a human brain in a nonhuman body.

In *The Monster and the Girl* (1940), while looking for a gangster who married his sister and probably forced her into prostitution, a man is framed and sentenced to death. As he awaits in death row, a doctor obtains his consent to transplant his brain into a gorilla's body. The ape "should be proud when he wakes up with a human brain." The doctor believes that finding out whether the hybrid experiences such human qualities as love or wisdom will open "a new chapter in scientific history." The animal's outward appearance remains the same, which led the *New York Times* critic quoted above, to speak of the "anonymous – and no doubt perspiring – soul in a flea-bitten ape skin." Yet, the gorilla has remarkably human eyes, is recognized by the donor's dog, executes several mobsters (hence the movie's other title, *The Avenging Brain*), and tries to express his brotherly love before being killed. As far as intentions and emotions are concerned, he clearly is the victimized woman's brother in an ape's body.

Semigrafts

In full-brain transplantations, the persistence of personality, eventually with some features potentiated or adjusted, is to be expected. What happens, then, in semigrafts, in partial brain transplants? The continuity of personal identity is the crux of the surgery; insofar as they combine a piece of X's brain not only with Y's body, but also with Y's brain, semigrafts have the potential for more psychological complexity or at least more tortuous story lines. Thus, in *Return of the Ape Man* (1944), Professor Dexter thaws a prehistoric man and seeks to give him the capacity to describe the prehistoric world by grafting "a segment" of a modern brain. Indeed, he explains, a whole-brain transplant "would remove the entire connection with his former life" and therefore make him a totally new person. The surgery mingles personalities or, in a foolproof recipe for action, keeps them side by side.

In the thriller *Black Friday* (1940), whose screenplay was co-authored by Curt Siodmak, Dr. Ernest Sovac (Boris Karloff in one of his incarnations as brain surgeon) tries to save the life of his friend, Professor George Kingsley, by giving him part of gangster Red Cannon's brain. The same actor, Stanley Ridges, plays both parts. When Sovac discovers that Cannon has half a million dollars tucked away somewhere, he wonders if "the Cannon brain in Kingsley's head retain[s] the knowledge of the hidden money." Hoping to appropriate the booty to establish "a great laboratory and give the world the benefit of [his] scientific knowledge," he takes Kingsley to New York City, certain that the familiar surroundings will rekindle the gangster's memory. Under Sovac's suggestive influence, the professor morphs into the mobster, acquiring the latter's voice, gaze, gait, and criminal habits. The problem, as the doctor says, is that one never knows "when the murderous brain of Red Cannon may take possession of Kingsley." In the meantime, Sovac forces the gangster to give up the money by threatening to make him stay Kingsley for good. Back in Kingsley's quiet university town, Cannon's brain remains "completely dormant" until a police siren rouses it during one of the professor's lectures. The gangster reclaims his due, attacks Sovac's daughter, the doctor shoots him, and as Red Cannon lies dying, he reverts to Kingsley. As Sovac sums it up, Cannon is Kingsley, and Kingsley is partly Cannon's brain. Although the way this situation is enacted depends on tacit expectations about the power of a grafted brain portion, the person remains the brain.

Almost eight decades after *Black Friday*, *Get Out* introduces a psychic twist into how someone's personality can persist in spite of whole-brain transplantation. The African American bodies into which white brains are transplanted preserve the host's consciousness in a "sunken place" where they have been locked up via hypnosis. In the scene that gives the picture its name, at a party organized and mainly attended by white Americans, the strange behavior of a black man calls the attention of black photographer Chris Washington (Daniel Kaluuya). As he tries to photograph him, the flash goes off accidentally; the man reacts with fear, his nose begins to bleed, and he yells "Get out!" at Chris. What looks like an aggression is a friendly warning from the reawakened consciousness of the African American person whose body has been used as receptacle for a white brain. The fact that such a reaction is triggered by a flash and is reminiscent of photosensitive epilepsy shows that, aside from its political meanings (Sharf 2017), the "sunken place" is a brain location.

In their consequences, semigrafts recall split or multiple personalities, which are a particularly rich dramatic device. Semigraft brainfilms, however, shine by their quirky plots rather than by psychological complexity. The comedy *Man with the Screaming Brain* (2005), for example, is about a businessman who has part of his injured brain replaced by tissue from his murdered driver's brain. The surgeon hopes that the treated organ will "overcome the donor portion" and that the patient will "once again function as a whole." That, of course, does not happen. In the meantime, the businessman's wife has been assassinated by the seductive but deranged gypsy woman who had injured him and killed the driver (who was in turn her former lover). In the end, the businessman remains two-in-one, while, predictably, his wife's brain is transplanted into the gypsy's body. The movie highlights the organ by flashing a brain just before a memory from the temporarily dormant personality bursts into the protagonist's consciousness. Highlighting a remarkable cinematic continuity across more than six decades, the short, bursting appearance of a brain keeps reminding us that "we are" that organ.

Like science-fiction brains in vats, stories about brain parts are older than their cinematographic incarnations. The fine Soviet production *Heart of a Dog* (1988) closely follows Mikhail A. Bulgakov's witty novella of 1925, in which Professor Preobrazhensky (inspired in the real-life Dr. Voronoff) transplants human testicles and a hypophysis into stray dog Sharik. Sharik becomes a man, Sharikov, who satisfies his vestigial canine instincts as employee of the municipal department responsible for clearing the city of cats. After he turns Preobrazhensky's life into a nightmare, the professor reverses the procedure. His goal had been to establish the viability of hypophysis grafting and its effect on rejuvenation; the interspecies transplant had the unwelcome consequence of transforming identity. To the extent that the hypophysis "is the brain itself, in miniature" (Bulgakov 1968 [1925], 104), it carries its original owner's individuality. Although Bulgakov alludes to the fad for rejuvenation through monkey testicle transplantation, both the novel and the movie, which closely follows the text, emphasize the brain. In the film, the only graphic surgery scene shows Preobrazhensky placing the hypophysis into Sharik's brain.

Living Heads

In semigrafts, action results when the transplanted organ portion temporarily conflicts with or takes over the whole; in xenografts, the donor's brain transforms the receiver into a member of the donor's species. This synecdochic logic, in which parts stand for wholes and containers for the contained, also applies to living heads. Of course, not all "disembodied heads" involve brain themes. There are none, for example, in *The Thing That Couldn't Die* (1958), where the head of Gideon Drew, a devil-worshipper beheaded by order of Sir Francis Drake in 1579, remains alive in a casket; after it is exhumed, it psychically controls others until it is placed back on its body. Some ectobrains (Donovan's, for example) have the same capacity. Overall, however, in motion pictures, the main goal of keeping a head is to safeguard a brain, and thereby a person whose continuing existence is a crucial ingredient of the plot and the visuals. (This was the essence of the *Amazing Stories* pieces of 1926 and 1928, "The Talking Brain" and "The Head.)

In *They Saved Hitler's Brain* (1968), a notoriously crude production, Nazi officials maintain the Führer's head alive in the South American republic of Mandoras, and plan to conquer the world under its leadership. Unchanged since the end of the war, the head is kept under a glass bell in a perfusion device (Brainfilms 3.16). The same happens in *The Frozen Dead* (1967), where a scientist cryogenically preserves the heads of Nazi criminals. *The Man Without a Body* (1957) starts out adhering to the usual logic of head preservation, only to turn weirdly around. As millionaire Karl Brussard (George Coulouris) is shown the X-ray that reveals his fatal brain tumor, he relishes in his organ: "I built an empire out of nothing – and this is the brain that did it." It must therefore be saved. Brussard places his hopes in Dr. Merritt (Robert Hutton), who has revived a monkey's brain and transplanted it into another monkey's body. The rationale of the experiment, however, goes awry without anybody remarking it. For what Brussard wants is to get a *new brain* for himself. Oblivious to the fact that without *his own* brain he would no longer be himself, he steals Nostradamus's well-preserved head from the tomb of the legendary sixteenth-century astrologer, and has it revived by Dr. Merritt (Brainfilms 3.17). Wreckage happens before any surgery is attempted. (As is often the case, the most nonsensical fantasies can end up making sense. A 2019 article in *Nature* described "the restoration and maintenance of microcirculation and molecular and cellular functions of the intact pig brain under ex vivo normothermic conditions up to four hours post-mortem" thanks to an extracorporeal pulsatile-perfusion system [Vrselja et al. 2019]. This result is of course a world apart from Merritt's, who hoarded vats full of upsetting organs stereotypically sustained by throbbing pumps and bubbling flasks – but both raise the question of whether brains can be revived.)

As we saw with Donovan, ectobrains can be driven by a desire to be masters of the world. However, the expressive features of a talking head bring about comical, grotesque, or pathetic effects that do not arise from a naked brain. Hitler's head is the most outlandish instance of the frenetic drive to dominate at the expense of surviving without a full body. However (as the pulps also illustrate), living heads differ from brains in vats in that they usually do not wish to survive, especially not when they are kept alive in order to be exploited. I say "usually," since heads such as Hitler's or Dr. Hill's (in *Re-Animator*) want to live to satisfy their evil impulses. In *The Brain That Wouldn't Die* (1959), which displays one of the best living heads of all cinema (Brainfilms 3.18), Jan (Virginia Leith) "dies" in a car accident. Her boyfriend, Dr. Cortner (Jason Evers), saves her head, and looks for an appropriately attractive body to make her "complete again." She, however, wants to die – the movie opens with her voice moaning that wish – and, since her brain is "still untouched," plans to use it to get her way. Encouraged by Jan, a monster made up of failed grafts that Cortner keeps in his lab kills the doctor; as a fire destroys the facilities, it carries away the girl whose body was to receive Jan's head. This film is also known as *The Head that Wouldn't Die*, a suitable title that mistakenly appears at the end. "Nothing you can be," Jan tells the monster, "is more terrible than I am. A head without a body!" (The heads kept alive in jars in *Futurama*'s thirty-first-century Head Museum do not suffer to that point, but do not really enjoy their life either; Brainfilms 3.19.)

In the 1959 German production *Die Nackte und der Satan* (*The Head*, literally *The Naked and the Devil*), Dr. Abel, played by celebrated French actor Michel Simon, has invented a serum that keeps organs alive after the rest of the body has died. Abel suffers from a cardiac condition; crafty Dr. Ood (Horst Frank) is entrusted with transplanting his heart, but he instead preserves Abel's "disembodied" head (Brainfilms 3.20). The surgeon opposes the head's insistence on being let to die, citing irrefutable reasons: "Your brain made you great, the rest doesn't count. I kept your brain alive; you will live. … I saved your brain for mankind, Professor." Evoking *Frankenstein*, Abel accuses him of having "a criminal brain" (see Chapter 5). In all its wonderful Z-class absurdity, the dialogue could not be a clearer expression of the brainhood ideology on screen.

The BBC art television miniseries *Cold Lazarus* (1996) offers a more intellectually refined version of the trope. In the year 2368, humans live in an ultra-technologized dystopic world, dominated by the interests of corporate media. The rebel movement RON (Reality or Nothing) wants to overturn the situation by violent means. The head of twentieth-century writer Daniel Feeld (Albert Finney) has been cryogenically preserved (Brainfilms 3.21). Dr. Emma Porlock (Frances de la Tour) and her colleagues activate Feeld's memories, together with the associated emotions, by pumping neurochemical substances into different parts of the brain; this provides the opportunity for a lot of scientific-sounding *neuro*-talk. Feeld's memories take form as projections on a screen; media mogul Daniel Siltz (Henry Goodman), who plans, with Porlock's complicity, to broadcast them for profit, is able to see them from his mansion thanks to a brain-shaped headgear (Brainfilms 3.22). A question discussed in Porlock's team, and which leads her colleague and RON member Dr. Fyodor Glazunov (Ciarán Hinds) to destroy the head, is whether Feeld, though merely a wired-up head floating in liquid nitrogen, is aware of his condition. He is – "We are his torturers," says Glazunov – and has been begging the scientists to let him die (Potter 1996, 377). For all the technological distance that separates Abel and Feeld, there is little phenomenological and no ethical difference between Merritt and Porlock. The pulps had rehearsed all this in similar ways. In "Fortitude" (1968), Kurt Vonnegut, a pulp reader in his youth, combined the figures of Frankenstein and the cyborg in the story of a woman's living head connected to a roomful of machines that function as an artificial body (instead of killing herself, as she wishes, she kills the doctor, whose head ends up preserved alive alongside hers); the story became an episode of the TV series *Kurt Vonnegut's Monkey House*.

These fictions have real-life counterparts (Lamba, Holsgrove, and Broekman 2016; more generally on head transplantation, see St-Germain 2017, which focuses on Canavero, mentioned below). The horror that head transplants inspire is patent in the reactions to the late Cleveland neurosurgeon Robert J. White's "cephalic exchange transplantation," that is, the grafting, first performed in 1970, of one monkey's head onto another monkey's beheaded body. Successful with the tabloids, it inspired scorn from scientists, and was associated with "Frankenstein fears" and "medical technology run completely mad" (Anon. 2001). White believed most people would agree to give physicist Stephen Hawking, who died in 2018, a new body (Jungblut 2001). Decades later, the Italian neurologist Sergio Canavero announced his project for "cephalosomatic anastomosis" (i.e., "head transplantation with spinal linkage"): "First human head transplant could happen in two years" (Thomson 2015; Canavero 2015). In the commercial realm, realizing that "it makes no sense to preserve ten times more tissue than necessary," most members of the Alcor Life Extension Foundation opt for "neuropreservation" (https://www.alcor.org/FAQs/faq02.html#neuropreservation). The company claims that its goal is not to preserve heads, but brains, which it protects against freezing injury by means of "neuroseparation" and "vitrification." While recognizing that successful neuropreservation depends on future nervous-tissue-repair technology, Alcor foresees that "virtually any injury that left the brain intact [sic] would be reversible by programmed tissue regeneration," and expects that the extra-cerebral body *may* be replaced during revival. This must reassure the neuropreserved, who presumably would not like to revive as impaired brains in vats.

Living heads under perfusion were also a mid-twentieth-century scientific reality. The Russian documentary *Experiments in the Revival of Organisms* (1940) shows Sergei Sergejewitsch Brychonenko's team at the Moscow Institute of Experimental Physiology and Therapy reviving dogs thanks to an "autojector" that functions as artificial heart and lungs. The device kept the animal's heart beating outside its body, and maintained its head alive for up to three and a half hours. The film's "scientific audience" at the 1943 American-Soviet Friendship congress in New York, "thought this work might move many supposed biological impossibilities into the realm of the possible" (Anon. 1943). Although the experiments took place – and were so well known that Dr. Abel mentions them in *The Head* – the movie itself gives the impressions of a restaging, and the dog's severed but living head looks as fake as any fabricated with the basic special effects of the era. (On Brychonenko see Böttcher and Alexi-Meskishvili 2003.)

By the 1950s, then, heads like Abel's in *The Head* or Jan's in *The Brain that Wouldn't Die* (alive in a shallow pan, sometimes under a glass bell jar, bathing in a solution and with multiple pipes connecting it to a pump) were not an alien sight. Pulps had textually and graphically depicted them way before, and (alongside non-pulp literature) had explored the appalling relationship between unscrupulous scientists and a disembodied head. In the above-mentioned 1925 novel *Professor Dowell's Head*, Dr. Manfred Kern, who assisted Dowell in experiments on keeping separate body parts alive, kills him and stores his head alive to exploit for his benefit the knowledge it contains. The professor laments that he has lost the world, and equates the sense of his body with himself. Kern's assistant Marie Laurent, who has discovered his boss's scheme, wants to avenge "those miserable heads he resurrected for the hell of a bodiless existence" (Beliaev 1980 [1925], 146). In both the book and its screen adaptation (*Professor Dowell's Testament*, 1984; Brainfilms 3.23), Dowell and Kern are said to work on "resurrection." A resurrection in which persons are portions of their bodies is utterly unchristian; historically, however, the movies are on target, for in the medieval iconography of hell, the fragmented body stood for eternal punishment (Bynum 1991).

Maintaining heads alive is either a way of keeping a person under punitive or utilitarian control (as in the case of Abel and Dowell), or a stepping-stone toward grafting, as in the case of Jan or of a woman called Irene in *The Head*. The latter case is perhaps the only instance of a relatively happy end in a picture of this subgenre: Irene is a young hunchbacked nurse with a beautiful face; Dr. Ood (the "Satan" of the film's original German title) wants to give her "a perfectly formed body, a new body." For this purpose, he kills strip-tease dancer Lilly (the title's "Naked"), and grafts Irene's head onto her body. He later notes that while Irene is still "ruled by her head," by which he means her brain, her body is making new demands. Having learned the truth, Irene herself wonders, "Which is my past, which isn't? The past of Lilly's body, or that of my head?" We return below to the post-surgical existential tensions that these questions encapsulate in movies where the resulting hybrid of A's headbrain and B's body is treated as a "freak." Here, the words of Irene's friend Paul reassuring her throw crude light on the conditions of a happy existence, on the strength of societal expectations, on normativity, and on the road traveled since the 1950s: "Don't be afraid. Now you have a normal body. You can fall in love, you can be like everyone else."

Some Filmic Allografts

The tensions inherent in the notion of an incarnate eternal life come to the fore when personal immortality depends on the persistence of a human ectobrain (Chapter 4). In *Donovan's Brain*, if the cerebrum lives, the person does; when Jan insists that "Donovan is dead and cremated," Pat retorts he "is still alive and kicking" (Siodmak 1942, 112). Donovan extends his agency as pure ectobrain by telepathically possessing Pat. More commonly, however, personal identity and individual immortality realize themselves in a heteroembodied brain, an organ grafted on a body different from the original one. The *Frankenstein* series sets this out systematically. After the initial two classics of the 1930s, Frankenstein pictures abandon the theme of the creation of life, and turn the brain transplantation fantasy into the core of their plots. While they do so in the modes of horror, gore, or parody, it is always a phrase from the Monster to his creator in one of the movies that best summarizes the crucial event: "Your father gave me life, and you gave me a brain." Chapter 5 deals with this in detail.

Basic brainhood questions – Is the combination of A's brain with B's body still A? If my non-cerebral body is also myself, how can I be my brain transplanted into another body? Does a fragment of my body suffice for me to be me? And will it be enough to make me immortal? – are an endless source of inspiration for filmic fantasy. Ageing or fatally ill individuals, not only mad scientists, but also millionaires such as Brussard, are so convinced of their intellect's worth that they believe it deserves to live on forever. "My genius," declares the racist surgeon in *The Thing With Two Heads*, "must be allowed to continue." The fluctuation between cerebral and psychological criteria for personal identity, a central philosophical and bioethical topic, is often dramatized as the scientist's quest for brain-based immortality. However, unlike real-life doctors, for whom "brain transplantation" consists of grafting small portions of localized tissue (Boyer and Bakay 1995; Lee 2007; Morrison 1987), movie surgeons handle entire organs.

Even when surgery itself is not displayed, full-organ transplantation allows for the visualization of brains inside (and sometimes outside) vats, and literally gives flesh to what would otherwise remain a mind transfer. This can be accomplished in various cinematographic styles. In *Brain of Blood* (1972), a cheap gore film, the brain of Amir (Reed Hadley), benevolent ruler of an Islamic nation, is placed, due to the temporary lack of better options, in the head of a horrible freak; the surgery scene includes close-ups of a gaudy, blood-soaked brain on a glass platter (Brainfilms 3.24). The hybrid goes berserk and is killed in spite of explaining that he is actually Amir. After the brain is transplanted again into a body identical to the original, Amir appoints the scheming surgeon as head of a mega-ministry of science. Generally, however, the performance value of brain transplantation derives from the fact that the resulting creature looks *different* from the original, and from the individual and interpersonal puzzles, emotions and behaviors that arise as a consequence.

Who is Julia? (1986) illustrates this in the TV-soap-operatic mode. Two young women die at the same moment. One, the lower-class, plain-looking, dark-eyed brunette Mary Frances (Mare Winningham), drops brain-dead just at the moment when Julia (Judith Ledford), a rich, blue-eyed, blonde fashion model, saves Mary's son from being killed by a huge cement truck – which, predictably, crushes her. In a fairly realistic scene, surgeons then graft

Julia's intact brain onto Mary's intact body. The rest of the story revolves around Julia's distress and the challenges of being trapped in a body that corresponds neither to her life-story and self-perception, nor to her circle of wealthy socialites. Emotional complications naturally arise with both husbands, but in the end Julia remains Julia in Mary Frances's body. This television melodrama stands out among comparable clichéd productions in that it remains focused on the transpersonal issue.

Memory Run (1996) illustrates the futuristic-dystopic-action approach. In 2015, society is controlled by the Life Corporation, which is opposed by a resistance movement; gangs try to steal from the elite and sell to the rebels. The Corporation's aged leaders want their brains grafted to younger bodies. Josette is assassinated while making love with a male gang leader, whose brain is subsequently placed in her head. The outcome is a transsexual hybrid called Celeste Montgomery (Karen Duffy). After Celeste disrupts the reception where she is presented as a brain-transplant success, she is thrown in prison, escapes, and joins the resistance. The movie treats the "trans" experience superficially, but comes up with a fascinating case of self-pregnancy: as a consequence of her fatal one-night stand, Josette's body is now expecting a child. In the meantime, the Corporation chairman's brain has been transplanted into the head of Josette's lover. Celeste kills him, accepts the loss of her original male body, assumes her femininity, and contemplates the sunset with her child and a male partner. Happy ends, especially if romantic, corroborate the viability of brain transplants.

Renewing a relationship or finding a partner can even be the surgery's original goal. In *Magdalena's Brain* (2006), surgeon Magdalena Welling (Amy Shelton-White) plans to inject into a muscular young man's brain part of the fluid in which her physically disabled husband's memory is grown. Once the material is "integrated," the recipient's badly located brain tumor will be removed, he will become one of the smartest persons in the world, and she will benefit from her husband's brainmind in a sexy body (Brainfilms 3.25). For all its computer talk, brain imagery, and sleek photography, the movie shares crucial premises with considerably less ambitious pictures, such as the semi-erotic horror movie *Lady Frankenstein* (1971), in which the doctor's nymphomaniac daughter grafts the brain of Frankenstein's brilliant ageing assistant into a dim-witted stud.

Brains in jars, a pulp and movie staple, can be philosophically suggestive. They can also embody horrific crime. They are visually prominent in *Gray Matter*, Joe Berlinger's documentary about the killing, as part of the Nazi euthanasia plan, of over seven hundred disabled children in a Viennese clinic (their brains were kept in jars until buried in 2002). Preserved brains, however, may also have a comic potential. In *The Man With Two Brains* (1983), the best of brain-transplantation comedies, Steve Martin plays Dr. Hfuhruhurr, whose favorite movie is *Donovan's Brain* and falls in love with Anne's brain. After calling her an "object," he must break to her the truth that she is "a disembodied brain kept alive by a scientist." Anne's ectobrain is frightened, but he reassures her: "Oh, don't be! Things are never as bad as they seem. You still have your… brain." He steals the brain (thus saving it from transplantation into a gorilla), and becomes involved with "the most complete woman I've ever known." After his nasty wife is murdered (Kathleen Turner as the gorgeous vamp Dolores), he transplants Anne's brain into her body. Anne, however, is a compulsive eater who immediately becomes obese. He doesn't love her any less for that, and in the end we see him, newly wed, barely carrying her over their house's threshold. (Warner Bros. denied permission to reproduce an image from the picture. As a precaution, I have not included any in Brainfilms, but many can be found in Internet.) In its silly way, *The Man With Two Brains* touches on many themes of earlier brain movies (and some of its gags rely on having seen them), while reducing the brainhood ideology to its simplest expression: Anne's brain in Dolores's body is to such an extent Anne herself that her bulimia instantly takes over. The movie not only humorously explores a scientific fantasy, but also evokes with a light touch the connections between physical beauty, sexual desire, love, personhood, and the uneasy relations between *being* and *having* a brain and a body. The purpose, of course, is comedy, and the issues are exploited accordingly.

Paradox of the Naked Brain

With regard to real ectobrains, the pinnacle of fragmentation was reached by Albert Einstein's brain. After the physicist's death in 1955, pathologist Thomas Harvey extracted the brain, fixated it, photographed it from all angles, and cut part of it into 240 small cubes, which he preserved, together with bigger pieces, in formaldehyde-filled hermetic glass storage jars. Microscopic slides were prepared and distributed. Would they help explain Einstein's genius? Neuroscientists since the 1980s have claimed that the left inferior parietal area contains more glial cells per neuron than the average, that the cortex is thinner and more densely populated with neurons than control brains, or that in the posterior end of the Sylvian fissure, the organ is 15% wider than controls. In the meantime, as part of its "Relics" series, the BBC produced *Einstein's Brain* (1994), a brilliantly funny movie about Japanese Einstein admirer Kenji Sugimoto's odyssey in search of the organ. Sugimoto, a real character, author of a "photographic biography" of his hero with almost five hundred images, is disappointed by scientists who show him photographs or slides. He is satisfied only when Dr. Harvey, after opening with goofy difficulty one of his jars, grabs a piece of the brain, places it on a cutting board, chops off a piece with a kitchen knife, puts it in a used pill box with some fluid ladled from the jar, and offers it to the ecstatic scholar. The entire sequence turns the finally visible fragments into the central protagonist, and suspensefully moves from showing the floating pieces in medium shot to an extreme close-up of the chosen morsel. Overjoyed, Sugimoto flies back home with the plastic reliquary sitting in front of him on the folding table.

By the time the film was released, the relic status of "elite brains" was far from new (Hagner 2004). Enshrined as incarnations of extraordinary minds, brain relics differ from those of Christian saints in that they lack the thaumaturgic powers at work in a universe that allowed for supernatural intervention and attributed to a fragment the intercessory *virtus* of the whole. Strictly speaking, therefore, brainfilm brains are not relics at all: dead or (mostly) alive, their role is to stand for persons. Such ontological function accounts for Sugimoto's intense emotional and intellectual relationship with Einstein's pathetically chopped up brain. For Sugimoto, finding Einstein's brain meant meeting the genius in the flesh, or at least encountering the essence of his being. For the most part, however, brainfilms handle ectobrains in ways, from nutty humor to shocking gore, which, rather than furthering love, empathy, projection, or identification with the organs, introduce a distance between viewers and the organs. This distance is sometimes abolished for comic effect, as in the above-mentioned *The Man With Two Brains* or the Brazilian musical *Apolônio Brasil, Campeão da Alegría* (2003), where a doctor wants to clone for commercial purposes the brain of the abnormally cheerful musician the film title calls "champion of happiness." The brain, which carries 254 *alegrones*, way over the normal average of 52, sits on a metal rod within a glass cylinder; Apolônio's friends come over in turns to observe it and have with it lively one-sided conversations (Brainfilms 3.25).

The dichotomy brain-body is a different dimension of this paradox. Expressions like "disembodied brain" or "brain without a body," often used to describe naked brains that are at the same time consubstantial with a particular person, really mean "outside a body." Yet, as already noted, they also imply that brain is not body. This is not unique to the pulps and motion pictures: for what else is meant by announcing that "Brain not body makes athletes feel tired" (*New Scientist*, July 29, 2004), or maintaining that "autism is neither a physical (bodily) disability, nor a mental illness; it is a neurological disability"? (Dekker 1999). The difference between living heads and ectobrains highlights the fact that the brain has taken over *functions* formerly attributed to the soul. And not only functions, since (as we shall see in the next chapter) stories about eternal youth make the brain operate as if it also had *features* of the soul. To that extent, it makes sense to see ectobrains as "disembodied" wholes instead of as bodily fragments. Heads are in this respect profoundly different. They possess the expressive and communicative powers that usually make persons recognizable, and that is perhaps connected to their refusal to subsist "without a body." Ectobrains, on the contrary, usually do not suffer from their "disembodiment," and wish to go on living and even extend their powers. The visual and conceptual irony is that these brains, like the superintelligent ones illustrated in the pulps, are formidably concrete, often hideously or ludicrously anatomical objects.

Evil-brain movies take this phenomenon to the extreme. In *The Brain from Planet Arous* (1957), the extraterrestrial entities are balloon-like devices whose outer surface exhibits thick convolutions and one eye on each hemisphere close to the medial longitudinal fissure (Brainfilms 3.26). As good brain Vol explains, evil brain Gor can be killed by "a heavy blow on the point known to your surgeons as the fissure of Rolando," a fold on the lateral surface of each hemisphere, which the movie foregrounds in a close-up on the *Encyclopaedia Britannica*. Gor controls other brains, and uses human beings (here, a nuclear scientist) to pursue its goals. In medieval and early modern demonology, demons possessed their victims by acting on their imaginations via the humors and "animal spirits"; brain movies extend that logic by having one brain take possession of another by way of paranormal processes that sometimes require rays and beams to operate. It has been claimed that *The Hidden* (1987) reproduces the argument of *The Brain from Planet Arous* (Dufour 2011). However, while both films indeed stage the mortal war between good and bad extraterrestrials that operate by taking over living human bodies, the evil alien of *The Hidden* is a slimy slug-like creature that enters human bodies through the mouth.

Fiend Without a Face (1958), a psychogenic variation of the brain-invasion theme, may offer the ultimate in murderous brains. In a town next to a military nuclear installation, people's brains and spinal cords are "sucked like an egg" through two small holes in the occipital region (brain leeches again). What has happened? While trying to create something like a human brain, "but without the limitations of the human body," the local mad scientist has materialized his thoughts. These remain invisible, and attack people, feeding on their brains and bone marrow. The crimes, accompanied by creepy sound effects, cannot be attributed to anyone, except to "fiends without a face." One day, an excess of atmospheric radiation reveals their form: brains with antennae and a snake-like piece of spinal cord they use as a tail to crawl and spring (Brainfilms 3.27). At the end, there is a memorable battle, which anticipates the final scene of *Night of the Living Dead*, between people barricaded in a farmhouse and hordes of effectively realized stop-motion animated brains. When the nuclear plant control explodes, the fiends melt down disgustingly.

The fact that thinking generates the "fiends without a face" and that these are ectobrains performs the relationship between mind and brain. A mind can only become incarnate as a cerebrum; thoughts become physical as an entity that look like the organ that produce them – and that is why they must feed on brains. (This does not rule out the possibility that thoughts materialize in other ways. In October 1933, twenty-five years before *Fiend*, *Astounding Stories* published Paul Ernst's "From the Wells of the Brain," a short story in which a professor turns his thoughts into matter, by way of electricity rather than atomic energy; he thus engenders a violent ape-like creature that kills him and destroys his lab; Bleiler 1998, no. 378.)

There is no evidence that the fiends' feeding on brains has purposes other than criminal and physiological. In other cases, the brain diet results in a sort of personality transfer. In *Attack of the Crab Monsters* (1957), a hugely successful B movie by a master of the category, Roger Corman, scientists travel to a remote Pacific island to look for a team of colleagues that evaporated, and pursue research on the environmental effects of radiation from nuclear tests. They start hearing voices from the vanished individuals; then one of them disappears, and his voice is also heard, guiding them toward a cave in the island. The voices turn out to be telepathically mediated messages from the title creatures (two of them in total), which, when visible and not killing, tend to fill the entire screen and advance toward the spectators in menacing low-angle shots. Their purpose is to lure the humans, which they will devour and assimilate. What has happened? The remaining scientists explore a possible explanation:

> Dr. Karl Weigand [nuclear scientist]: Apparently we have one of those biological freaks, resulting from an overdose of radiation poisoning. … Any matter therefore that the crab eats will be assimilated in its body as solid energy, becoming part of the crab.
> Martha Hunter [marine biologist]: Like the bodies of the dead men?
> Weigand: Yes; and their brain tissue, which after all is nothing more than a storage-house for electrical impulses.

> DALE DREWER [marine biologist]: That means that the crab can eat his victim's brain, absorbing his mind intact and working.
> WEIGAND: That's as good a theory as any other to explain what's happened.
> MARTHA: But, doctor, that theory doesn't explain why [slain scientists] Jules' and Carson's minds have turned against us.
> DALE: Preservation of the species. Once they were men, now they are land crabs.

Implausible as it is, the theory does account for such crucial features of the action as the crabs' ability to "speak" with their victim's voices: eat a brain, and you assimilate its owner's mind.

Finally, oversize brains (another pulp favorite) are a class in themselves. They virtually always signal danger and menace. Offering various combinations of superior force, an inclination to violence, and a superhuman intelligence in the service of wicked purposes, they have been said to reflect a postwar mistrust of experts and scientists. In the Japanese movie *Evil Brain from Outer Space* (1964), the omnipotent Balazar has been killed. His genius, however, was so powerful, "that as he lay dying, his brain ordered built a mechanism which would keep it alive even though his body was destroyed. And now Balazar's Brain seeks universal conquest!" No brain as such is shown, but the giant saurian monster that comes to devastate the Earth has two filigreed crests that vaguely resemble thickened cortical capillaries and are prolonged along part of its back by a spine-like tail.

As in pulp science fiction illustrations, alien invaders in mid-twentieth-century film almost always have overgrown braincases. The origin of this feature is perhaps to be found in H. G. Wells's 1901 novel *The First Men in the Moon*. Chapter XXIV, "The natural history of the selenites," remarks that, of the various distortions that characterize them, one "was particularly conspicuous," namely "brain cases distended like bladders to a huge size, with the face mask reduced to quite small proportions" (Wells 2017 [1901], 153). The head of a certain Phi-oo, for example,

> is distended into a huge globe, and the chitinous leathery cuticle of the mooncalf herds thins out to a mere membrane, through which the pulsating brain movements are distinctly visible. He is a creature, indeed, with a tremendously hypertrophied brain, and with the rest of his organism both relatively and absolutely dwarfed. (ib., 154)

Such hypertrophy affects different cerebral regions and results in variously formed heads. This phrenologically inspired feature reflects a strict social organization. If a Selenite is destined to be a mathematician, "the mathematical faculties of his brain grow, and the rest of him only so much as is necessary to sustain this essential part of him. ... His brain grows continually larger, at least so far as the portions engaging in mathematics are concerned; they bulge ever larger and seem to suck all life and vigour from the rest of his frame" (ib., 157). The unparalleled mental development of an intellectual aristocracy is enabled "by the absence of any bony skull in the lunar anatomy" (ib., 158). Thus,

> the unlimited growth of the lunar brain has rendered unnecessary the invention of all those mechanical aids to brain work which have distinguished the career of man. There are no books, no records of any sort, no libraries or inscriptions. All knowledge is stored in distended brains much as the honey-ants of Texas store honey in their distended abdomens. The lunar Somerset House and the lunar British Museum Library are collections of living brains. (ib., 158)

In contrast to the Selenites, who are five-foot (c. 150 cm) "men-insects," in large-brained movie extraterrestrials, the size of the cerebrum and skull tends to correlate with its owner's physical power, which usually, though not always, serves nefarious purposes.

Bulging brains, a staple of aliens on paper and screen, provide some of the best examples. The tall bug-eyed Mutants in *This Island Earth* (1955), which the humanoid Metalunans breed to do slave work, combine an insect exoskeleton with an unprotected oversized brain (Brainfilms 3.28). Even though they are dwarves, the visually similar creatures of *Invasion of the Saucer Men* (1957), which boast "the most exaggerated eye-brain hypertrophy of all" (Skal 1993, 252), can easily overpower humans (Brainfilms 3.29). (They are also sensitive to light, to which they react with pathetic squeaks, and are literally pulverized by it beyond a certain intensity.) In *To Serve Man*, a 1962 episode of the TV series *The Twilight Zone* (1959–1964), the extraterrestrial Kanamits, almost three meters tall and boasting a proportionally tall cranium, land on our planet as self-proclaimed friends of humanity. Humans have been plagued by natural and unnatural catastrophes; coming as they do from a "far more developed" planet, Kanamits have decided to help. They convince humans to trust them, but, as revealed in a stupendous final twist, what they actually want is "to serve man"...for their own dinner.

Four decades later, the invaders of *Mars Attacks!* (1996), Tim Burton's spoofy homage to 1950s alien-invasion films, have skulls with eyeballs and a large exposed brain that reproduce those of the homonymous trading cards of 1962 (Topps 2012; Brainfilms 3.30). In *The Brain* (1988), an evil doctor keeps a huge brain in a vat, fed by "brain wave transmission" from his patients. The massive organ actually encloses an anthropophagous monster with dark bulging eyes, threatening fangs, and projecting long intestine-like tentacles with which it catches its victims. The tagline on the movie's VHS cover, "Mind Over Matter," seems absurd given the creature's unmistakable physicality (Brainfilms 3.31). It nevertheless captures the paradox of "disembodied" brains: while their strength resides in mental capacities, they would be nothing without their imposing materiality (see Danzey 1999 for an illustrated interview with the movie's special effects technician).

The paradox of the naked brain is further illustrated in Paul Verhoeven's *Starship Troopers* (1997). During one of their interstellar colonizing campaigns, twenty-third-century humans encounter a fierce species of arachnoid bugs that kill a hundred thousand soldiers in a single battle. After such a devastating defeat, the newly appointed "sky marshal" declares, "To fight the bug, we need to understand the bug." Now, who controls it? As humans find at great cost, the answer is: a monstrous wobbling hybrid of an arachnoid and a cerebrum that occasionally sucks up human brains with its huge proboscis. Heroic troopers capture it and, after pulling it out of its cave in a net, hand it over to scientists. A military intelligence officer explains, "We've got one of their brains now, and pretty soon we'll know how they think, and then we'll know how to beat them." Back on earth, a newsreel shows the trapped creature in a lab, surrounded by personnel in red chemical protection suits: "What mysteries will the bug reveal? Federal scientists are working around the clock to probe its secrets." Probing here consists of puncturing the suffering animal with a jumbo repeat syringe, presumably to extract and analyze its cerebral substance. The film, with cinematography that is sometimes reminiscent of 1950s historical epics like *The Robe* or *Ben Hur*, was trashed when it came out. Later on, however, one commentator went as far as considering it "one of the most misunderstood movies ever," and described it as a "self-aware satire" against "the military-industrial complex, the jingoism of American foreign policy, and a culture that privileges reactionary violence" (Marsh 2013). It is significant in such a perspective that the chief of the resistance against humanity's colonizing enterprise is a *brain* bug. Such creatures tend to be inherently evil, their potent brains serving malevolent, destructive purposes. Here, however, they nobly defend themselves against terrestrial attacks.

Beyond the basic constraints of having to *show* something and use actors, movies insist on persons' corporality. In *Spock's Brain* (1968), a humanoid female breaks into the starship Enterprise, and leaves Spock "worse than dead: his brain is gone." Unbeknownst to the victim, his cerebrum is used to run an advanced civilization:

> SPOCK: I seem to have a body that stretches to infinity.
> CAPTAIN KIRK: Body? You have none!
> SPOCK: What am I?
> CAPTAIN KIRK: You're a disembodied brain.

Spock's ectobrain should live for ten thousand years. "But Spock will be dead," the Captain says. "His body is dying away this very minute." Spock's survival as a full person requires putting brain and body together again. Once more, brainfilms problematize the ideology they seem at first to proclaim: Magdalena, Lady Frankenstein, and Dr. Hfuhruhurr don't want to sleep with ectobrains, and naked encephalons can rarely dominate the world merely by themselves.

Source Code (2011) is perhaps the most poignant instance of how, if it is to work cinematographically, the brain motif forces full corporality back. Source Code is a computer program that enables an individual to "cross over" into someone else's identity. Captain Colter Steven (Jake Gyllenhaal) is a US Army pilot who died in a mission in Afghanistan. His brain, however, is kept alive. Via Source Code and a "time reassignment" procedure, it is used to search for the terrorist behind a train bombing that has already taken place, and thereby to prevent further attacks. To achieve this mission, Colter's mind (i.e., his brain's contents) is made to occupy a male victim's body. The operation is repeated several times, and in the end succeeds. The control room includes computer screens that display the pilot's brain as neuroimages (Brainfilms 3.32). Along the way, Colter finds out that he is in fact dead, that his body is seriously maimed, and that he has been placed on life support so that "part of [his] brain remains activated." Toward the end of the movie, Captain Colleen Goodwin (Vera Farmiga) disobeys her superior's orders, and, honoring her deal with Colter, lets him die. Only then are we shown his frightfully mutilated body: a thorax with an intact head and beautiful, peaceful countenance, lying in a metal box, and hooked (but only lightly) to the machinery. Only then, with the revelation of soldier's embodied form, does the full pathos of his predicament explode.

A final dimension of the ectobrain paradox concerns immortality. The brain turns out to be everything. It is preeminently matter, and the self's body, yet at the same time, as we shall see in the next chapter, it has the traditional qualities of the immaterial soul. Personal immortality can be obtained by recurrently grafting one's brain to younger bodies. Brains mature psychologically, but do not age or decay. This fantasy sustains cryogenists' hopes. But the role of transplantation underlines the fact that brains (like souls in the Christian perspective) only realize themselves when joined to a body. In movies as in medieval theology, nobody desires to live forever as an ectobrain: a brain in a vat might enable eternal life, but being an immortal person demands a full body. Film has laid out this situation and the conundrums of the "disembodied brain" more fully than any other medium.

4. Personal Survival

Abstract
This chapter discusses pictures that enact brain transplantation as means for realizing personal immortality, and addresses such questions as: To what extent do brains sustain personal continuity? Which challenges await A's brain in B's body? What happens with these transgenerational (and occasionally interracial) brains? Given the closeness of some filmic, mythical, and literary materials with regard to fantasies of longevity and immortality, the chapter includes a small sample of the latter since antiquity. It nonetheless focuses on the filmic performance of the paradox inherent in the desire to transcend the body by retaining one's brain through consecutive re-embodiments. Case studies include *The Man Who Changed His Mind* (1936), *Change of Mind* (1969), and *The Man With the Transplanted Brain* (1971).

Keywords: brain transplantation, immortality, longevity, myth, race relations, transgenerational brain

The global increase in life expectancy has turned the deterioration of the brain into a health problem of epidemic proportions (WHO 2012). The challenge is both collective and individual. At the collective level, it is anticipated that the number of people with dementia and Alzheimer's will increase to 135 million by 2050, with over 70% of them living in low- or middle-income countries, and with costs escalating proportionately, especially for those countries, beyond the annual US$ 604 billion recorded in 2010 (ADI 2013). Part of the drama of dementias is that they affect both personal identity and the conditions of personhood. Beyond a certain point, the persons whom we knew are "no longer there" and the signs they produce seem reduced to signifiers of the disease. Using a chemical metaphor, the French philosopher Michel Malherbe (2015, 225) speaks of the "ontological denaturation" Alzheimer's operates: it ceases to be an "accident of life," which is what illness usually are, even when chronic, and becomes the person's essence. That is why, for him, the question Alzheimer's raises is not the

Vidal, F., *Performing Brains on Screen*. Taylor & Francis Group, 2022
DOI 10.5117/9789462989146_CH04

usual and superficial one, whether a loved one with the illness recognizes us, but a more fundamental one: whether and how we recognize her – not as she was before, but in her current manner of being in the world (ib., 9).

Though these questions are globalized, in the sense that they may be posed anywhere and by anyone, they are rooted in Western modernity. As we have seen, according to the view that has prevailed in Western cultures since the late seventeenth century, personhood (the status of being a person) and personal identity (one's persistence and sameness over time) are constituted by memory and self-consciousness. It is their continuity that determines and supports a person's continuity, and their particular contents make each of us as who we are rather than someone else. Now, if the brain insures the functions usually said to define personhood, then we are essentially our brains, and this organ is the only part of our body we absolutely need to be persons and have a personal identity. Since the 1990s, as never before, the brain has been depicted as humanity's most important scientific frontier; largely driven by brain research, and especially by neuroimaging-based claims about the societal impact of the neurosciences, "neuroessentialism" has been on the rise (Reiner 2011). It has also been resisted (see Smith 2019 for a recent example). Yet the brain's role is obvious and indisputable, and precisely because of its basal function, neurological diseases constitute a trauma like no other in the vast spectrum of human suffering.

The appeal of brains as foundation for modern fantasies of personal survival and immortality predates both late twentieth-century neuroessentialism and the twenty-first-century "dementia plague" (Hall 2012). It can be traced to the early days of brainhood during the Enlightenment, when Charles Bonnet asserted that if a savage inherited Montesquieu's brain, "Montesquieu would still create." In 1777, knowing his death was approaching, the physiologist Albrecht von Haller wrote to Bonnet lamenting that his brain would soon be nothing but a clod of earth, and saying that he could hardly tolerate the loss of so many ideas accumulated over a lifetime. This kind of feeling sustained, in Bonnet and others, speculations about the role of a brain-like organ as basis for the continuity of the person at the time of the general resurrection (Vidal 2002 and 2011, Chap. 9). Transplantation fantasies emerged later, with the advances of surgery and brain localization, and were well established by the time science fiction pulps started to proliferate in the 1920s.

The relation between the brain and high intelligence, which often drives those fantasies, is such a basic assumption that it is hardly ever explained. Making it explicit need only be done for humor or for children. Witness the animated television series *Pinky and the Brain* (1995–1998), starring two genetically enhanced laboratory mice – the dim-witted Pinky and the arrogant Brain. The latter's schemes to take over the world always fail, yet his supposedly superior genius is proclaimed not only in his name, but also in the organ's prominent visual presence in the introduction to the series (Brainfilms 4.1). The pair's adventures are perfectly innocent compared to how mad scientists seek to preserve genius, theirs or others'. The pulps offered examples, and on screen we have already met the surgeon of *The Thing With Two Heads*, who justifies his criminal enterprise by asserting that his genius must be allowed to continue. The theme is so commonplace that it even made it into the exuberant masked-hero Mexican film industry of the 1960s. Dr. Caronete, the evil scientist of *Los autómatas de la muerte* (1962), literally *The Automatons of Death*, boasts that he has merged three prominent scientists' brains into one, "which submissively obeys me, and I have managed to get hold of all their ideas." The combined brain talks from under a glass bell (Brainfilms 4.2). Caronete's goal is to obtain the formula for a neutron bomb, but he is defeated by Neutron, the masked "atomic superman." In *Blue Demon contra cerebros infernales* (*Blue Demon vs. the Infernal Brains*), the masked wrestler-hero of the title fights an evil scientist who, assisted by several miniskirted raygun-carrying automaton-like beauties, kidnaps eminent colleagues in order to extract and replace their brains, and appropriate their knowledge. In both cases, animal brains are prominently displayed; shot in bright hues, *Blue Demon* includes the most unreal brain transplantation in movie history, carried out by simply pressing a brain into the patient's forehead. (Brainfilms 4.3)

The Colossus of New York (1958) provides an interesting variation on the genius-brain transplantation nexus. Jeremy Spensser, a brilliant young scientist who has discovered the means for ending food shortage around the world, is accidentally killed by a truck on the eve of receiving the "International Peace Prize" at the United Nations. His father, famous neurosurgeon William Spensser, decides that Jeremy's work must continue for the benefit of humanity, and transplants his brain into the body of the huge robotic creature that gives the film its name (Brainfilms 4.4). It is not clear why Jeremy's brain has to be placed in a robot-like entity. Perhaps the idea was to make it a recognizable descendant of earlier characters, such as the *Maschinenmensch* of Fritz Lang's 1927 *Metropolis*, or (for a different public) of Professor Jameson in "The Jameson Satellite," published in 1931 in the pulp magazine *Amazing Stories*. (Viewers of *RoboCop* [1987] will recognize in the colossus an anticipation of the title cyborg – a massive metal body into which the brain of a good human cop has been implanted.)

For Dr. Spensser senior (Otto Kruger), "[i]n the brain, and in the brain alone, lies the glory of man." He asks the best friend of his dead son Jeremy to imagine the "advance in civilization" that could take place if genius' brains were "allowed to continue their work, unhampered by their bodies" – to which the friend responds by emphasizing the union of body and mind achieved through the soul, and asserting that a brain cut from human experience would become "dehumanized to the point of monstrousness." Jeremy's brother Henry (John Baragrey), an expert in automation, initially refuses to help his father:

> HENRY SPENSSER: No, it's inhuman!
> WILLIAM SPENSSER: Inhuman? It would've been inhuman to deny the world of his genius.

He nonetheless ends up collaborating. After having asked to be destroyed, Jeremy-in-the-robot agrees to continue his experiments. However, as expected, the Colossus (who has somehow acquired extrasensory perception and the capacity to kill people by means of rays emitted from his eyes) indeed gets out of control and wreaks havoc in the UN building where a ceremony in Jeremy's honor is about to take place. He calms down only when his young son confronts him; he then asks the boy to turn the switch that will terminate him, thus realizing his initial wish.

The promise of immortality through the brain has been rightly identified as a transhumanist fraud (Tritsch and Mariani 2018). But we are here interested in self-admitted fantasies where brain transplantation allows aging persons to inhabit younger bodies. A first operation extends their life; successive ones may insure their immortality. The most chimerical aspect of such fiction is not the surgery, but the fact that it makes the brain operate like the soul, maturing psychologically, but not deteriorating as organic substance. The brain's birth date marks it as belonging to a certain generation, which is increasingly left behind by the repeated renewal of its bodily receptacles. The difference between the brain and the soul, of course, is that the former *is* material, and must remain connected to something that nourishes it (a natural body or an artificial machine) to carry on.

What happens with these transgenerational brains? To what extent do they sustain the persistence of the older person? How, if at all, is personality changed through the new body? What are the internal and external challenges the surgical hybrid must face? Which "lesson," if any, is to be drawn from the paradoxical desire to transcend the body by keeping one's brain through consecutive re-embodiments? Given the affinity of some filmic and literary materials with regard to fantasies of longevity and immortality, this chapter will include a tiny sample of the latter (for more, see Ferreira 2012).

Immortality and the Brain

Ambivalence is perhaps inherent to issues of longevity and immortality. We can be afraid of aging and death without, nonetheless, wanting to live forever. Throughout history, immortality has been strongly associated with everlasting torment (Prometheus, Sisyphus, the damned in the Christian Hell). Moreover, as movingly demonstrated by Dante's *Paradiso* and Botticelli's illustrations for it, beatitude of the sort Christianity postulates as humans' ultimate reward – an intense but static *visio Dei* – does not lend itself well to vivid narrative and pictorial depiction. In Christian art, the harrowed bodies of the damned offer a colorful and varied contrast to the luminous, yet more abstract and visually less interesting tranquility of the blessed. Similarly, modern fictions tend to associate immortality, if not perforce with punishment and suffering, at least with situations that make everlasting life a problematic and not altogether rewarding state of being.

Where does human immortality come from? In the Greco-Roman and Judeo-Christian traditions, it does not result directly from deliberate choices and actions of the beneficiary, but is usually granted by divinities as a condition for the realization of an individual final destiny (e.g., Hell or Heaven), as a sort of reward for heroic deeds (e.g., Hercules), or as a form of compensation (e.g., Tithonus, discussed below). Neither in those cases, nor in old or cutting-edge versions of filmic reincarnation (e.g., the "regeneration" that Time Lords undergo in the British TV series *Dr. Who*, a process used twelve times since 1969 to introduce a new actor into the main role) are body parts or their transformation designated as the specific vehicles of immortality. The same applies to rejuvenation legends. For example, in a famous painting by Lucas Cranach the Elder in Berlin's *Gemäldegalerie* (c. 1546), decrepit women enter the Fountain of Youth and emerge as immodest maidens. Here, external form is transformed for the better, but there are no hints about personal identity, which presumably persists with the affordances of a younger body. This would be consistent with the fates of bodies according to the Christian doctrine of the resurrection, which will rise perfect, and with the same age as the crucified and resurrected Christ. In some cases, therefore, resurrecting will involve getting older, in others younger. Yet it will always entail the inability to age and die. In contrast, the indefinite life extensions that are the object of filmic and literary fictions do not happen once and for all.

Brain fictions involve bodily and psychological rejuvenation, both in partial form. On the one hand, the transplanted brain that insures the person's continuity in a new body does not become younger. Only the non-cerebral body does. On the other hand, although the surgical hybrids have the same personalities as the original individuals, their new bodies affect them. Brain transplantation thus works like a bath in the Fountain of Youth. If indefinitely repeated, both may give an indefinite lifespan to a fully embodied individual. The difference lies in the sui generis nature of fictional brains. They can be destroyed, and might require technological assistance to survive outside a body. However, in an absolute reversal of the causes giving rise to current anxieties about dementia, they are depicted as having the benefit of anatomo-physiological immutability and potentially endless endurance. Under such circumstances, life ends because of destructive human actions rather than as a consequence of natural biological processes.

The imaginary brain's indefinite lifespan differentiates fiction from various real-world techno-scientific attempts to conquer death via rejuvenation or organ preservation. In the experiments with severed animal heads carried out in post-revolutionary Russia (Krementsov 2009, 2013), brain transplantation was to provide a new but limited lease of life. In more recent contexts, the brain must become the object of manipulations that improve on its immediate post-mortem condition, that is, on its state at the time of its removal from the patient's cranium. Indeed, cryogenic "neuropreservation" is "primarily a tool for preventing bodily decay until new techniques for molecular level repair and enhancement, such as nanotechnology and cloning, mature. It is envisaged that these technologies may then be employed not only to renovate, but also to augment the existing faculties of the subject, completing the project of age-reversal and life extension" (Parry, 2004, 394). In contrast, literature and film assume that, even if it occasionally calls for repair, an undisturbed brain can go on living forever.

Adam and Tithonus

Hanif Kureishi's (2002) short novel *The Body* reiterates the classical fiction of one's brain in someone else's body (Krüger-Fürhoff 2012, 2.2). One of its main virtues is that it stages the thought experiment in its purest form, with no cyberpunk gimmicks or scientific jargon, and refrains from turning the philosophical and phenomenological issues it raises into theoretical discourse. John Updike (2004) noted that *The Body* "has the terse speed and casual logic of a screenplay and might make a good movie." In fact, it had *already* been filmed by the time Kureishi wrote it, and the author admitted that movies inspired him:

> I watch late-night TV – trash TV – and there are lots of programs about people having bits cut out of their bodies or other bits added and so on. I thought, why go to all the trouble to have a bit done here and there? Why not just get a whole new body? I became interested in what people thought having a new body would do for them. And I was really interested in the philosophical questions about identity: Who would you be? What makes you who you are? (Kureishi 2004)

Clearly, the writer's thinking about "a whole new body" betrays not only his movie-watching habits, but also his university education in philosophy. On the one hand, as we have seen, philosophical thought experiments about personal identity tend to concern various forms of preserving and transplanting brains, which are routinely interpreted as whole-body transplants. On the other hand, there are many more "trash" productions about entire bodies or total personality transfers than about body parts.

The protagonist and first-person narrator of *The Body* is Adam, a playwright in his mid-sixties. During a party, he meets Ralph. This young actor is actually a seventy-year-old man whose brain has been transplanted into the body of a thirty-year-old. He is what is technically known as a Newbody. Ralph convinces Adam to go through the same procedure, which takes place in a run-down warehouse outside London. Adam, however, is hesitant and prefers to see the operation as a "short-term body rental." When given the choice of bodies of both genders and various skin colors, he settles for a "classically handsome," Italian-looking man with "a fine, thick penis and heavy balls" (Kureishi 2002, 27).

In what a nurse describes as his new "facility," Adam becomes the fashion model Leo Raphael Adams, and devotes himself to a life of sex and drugs. As he eventually discovers, most of his young companions are in fact Newbodies. One of them, the evil millionaire Matte, wants Adam's body for his dying brother. Adam refuses to sell it and returns to the warehouse in the hope of getting back his old facility. When he arrives there, Matte and his men are waiting, with a surgeon on standby, prepared to get Adam's body – and, of course, discard his brain. Adam manages to run away, but with no hope of ever escaping his incarnation as a Newbody.

What are the connections between Kureishi's story and academic philosophy? In his 1969 article "Brain Transplantation and Personal Identity," Roland Puccetti (1969, 67, 70) referred to then recent neuroanatomy and neurophysiology to conclude, "there are no permanent barriers to successful brain transplantation, though by present standards it is scientifically visionary." Three decades later, again on the basis of scientific information, Eric Steinhart (2001) argued that Puccetti had been wrong, since, he explained, the psychological features and functions of persons are in fact "realized" by "parallel distributed processing networks dispersed throughout the whole body" at the nervous, endocrine, immune and genetic levels. Like most fiction, *The Body* seems to hold both claims before our eyes, as reconcilable alternatives, or perhaps as a figure–ground phenomenon. Which personhood configuration stands out (is perceived as figural) depends on a focus determined by momentary interests, context, and various internal and external conditions. Kureishi indeed makes the continuity of personal identity depend on the presence of the same brain in a different body. At the same time, Adam's brain lives on in a young body that prevents Leo Raphael from being the older person he wants to be. The story enacts the double validity of brainhood and of fully embodied personhood. Although we are our brains in some essential ways, the brain is not alone in bringing about and performing the self, which, as Adam's fate highlights, emerges from interlocked organic, relational, and social processes. Kureishi thus joins dimensions that academic analysis sometimes keeps separate: the brain as seat of selfhood, the person as fully embodied entity, and the phenomenological self.

In addition to narrativizing phenomenological and ontological questions, Kureishi's story revitalizes deep and ancient connections between immortality and desire. To retain Ulysses, Calypso offers to make him "immortal and ageless" (*Odyssey* 7.259). He declines, his yearning for Ithaca being stronger than his lust for the nymph. Others were not so fortunate. One of the most heartrending renditions of the link between desire and immortality is provided by the story of the Trojan prince Tithonus. Eos, the goddess of dawn, abducts him and Ganymede to be her lovers. When Zeus steals Ganymede, she asks in compensation that Tithonus be made immortal. But since she forgets to ask for eternal youth, Tithonus is condemned to live forever – in a forever-aging body. In one of the Homeric hymns to Aphrodite, the goddess of love tells Anchises (her mortal lover and father of her son Aeneas) of "foolish Dawn" who neglected to ask Zeus "for youth, to erase [from Tithonus] deadly old age." So, continues the hymn, "when the gray hairs first rained down / on his handsome head and noble chin, / then Dawn completely avoided his bed." And later, "when hateful old age weighed him down, and he could not move his limbs or raise up, /... / she set him in a chamber and closed the shining doors. / His voice flows on without ceasing / and the strength in his supple limbs is gone" (Raynor 2004, 82–83).

After first refusing to sleep with the aging Tithonus, cruel Eos locks him up in a beautiful room where he wretchedly laments over himself for eternity. In some versions of the legend, as Tithonus's body shrivels, the goddess takes pity on him and transforms him into the interminably singing cicada. Contrary to the Sybil of Cumae in a similar story, the miserable Tithonus could not even look forward to dying. The Sybil obtains from Phoebus her wish to live as many years as there are grains in the handful of dust she holds; however, when she rejects the god's advances, he denies her eternal youth. As the centuries go by, her body withers, she becomes reduced to her prophetic voice – *vocem mihi fata relinquent*, writes Ovid in the *Metamorphoses* (XIV, 153) – and desires only to die.

Kureishi retains the essential bond between immortality and sexual desire, but with a twist. In the polytheistic regime, the immortality of a human being depended on satisfying gods or goddesses; in post-monotheistic modernity, humans themselves seek (or try to give) immortality for their own pleasure. In addition, the predicaments of Adam and Tithonus are related. Tithonus's misery comes from the persistence of his being in a perpetually aging body. In Alfred Tennyson's *Tithonus*, the hero speaks of "happy men that have the power to die," and begs, "Release me, and restore me to the ground." The anguish of Kureishi's Adam is not rooted in the same sense of lasting obsolescence, yet also derives from his having or being in a body that does not correspond to the chronological age of his brainmind. Both stories depend on the dichotomy and antagonism between one's brain-seated self and one's non-cerebral body. In both narratives, the organ that is responsible for personhood and insures the continuity of personal identity matures and evolves; however, it neither ages nor advances toward death.

In the myth, it is presumably the soul that insures the person's continuity. In the modern story, it is the brain, and re-embodiment takes place in an operating room. The modern surgeon has replaced the ancient gods, and the whims and power of the deities have been displaced by the skill and hubris of the scientist. In Kureishi and other literary and filmic fictions, the brain takes on the long-standing functions of the immortal and immaterial soul. The union between a soul and a body, which was long the ontological foundation of living beings, has been replaced by the link between a body and a brain. What Newbody are and feel as persons is shaped by the interaction of the two, especially by their individual attitude toward the "facility" into which their brains have been transplanted. From Tithonus to Adam, this attitude and the entire Newbody experience are rooted in a dual generational affiliation: the apparent one of the body, and the hidden one of the brain. The body plays the role of a chosen disguise or an imposed iron mask.

For fictional immortals, facing younger generations is particularly trying. Tennyson's Tithonus revolts against the way

> ... strong Hours indignant work'd their wills,
> And beat me down and marr'd and wasted me,
> And tho' they could not end me, left me maim'd
> To dwell in presence of immortal youth,
> Immortal age beside immortal youth,
> And all I was, in ashes.

Although the youth of others is not everlasting, indefinitely facing younger generations only deepens the agony of the perpetually aging. Adam suffers less, since while he enjoys being part of the younger generation, he knows his rejuvenation is in principle reversible, and takes advantage of his youthful body while maintaining the psychological distance of a wiser sixty-year-old.

Commenting on the sexual and drug-consumption mores of his body-age peers, Adam says, "I knew I was not of them, because I couldn't help wondering what their parents would have thought" (Kureishi 2002, 68). He shares their dissolute habits. Yet in the end, he cannot bridge the generational gap that separates his body and his person. He must endure being himself (i.e., having his own original brain) in a body that, he feels, is completely at odds with who he actually is. Before becoming a Newbody, he had felt a similar discomfort, but in reverse, as an awareness of being outdated, as the uneasiness of no longer fully belonging to the world. Before going, out of boredom and dreariness, to the fateful party where he met Ralph, Adam reflected on how out of touch he was with the surrounding culture, and concluded: "I imagine that to participate in the world with curiosity and pleasure, to see the point of what is going on, you have to be young and uninformed. Do I want to participate?" (ib., 4). Thus, like the heroes of classical mythology, Adam was ready for Ralph's proposal – though, like them, not for its ultimate consequences.

In a Platonic move for the neurochemical age, Kureishi depicts the body as a prison for that which makes the person. This ontological constituent is no longer the soul, but the brain. Yet, if it is a prison, the body is a paradoxical one: in its capacity as the brain's tool (as in earlier worldviews it was the instrument of the soul), it allows the brain/soul to realize and manifest itself, interact with the world, and avoid total solipsism. Saying that the self *inhabits* a body here amounts to saying that there is a particular brain in that body, and implies attributing a person's features to his or her brain – as when Dr. Cory says that Donovan's brain thinks. No art form has exploited this psycho-anatomical metonymy more than film; in many cases, it is what turns the brain into a full-fledged protagonist. The philosophical pendant of such cinematographic role is the "mereological fallacy" (from the Greek *meros*, "part"), which cognitive neuroscience has been accused of committing systematically, and which consists of ascribing consciousness, understanding and other mental functions to the brain itself (Bennett and Hacker 2003). Yet when neuroscience perpetrates the fallacy, it reifies the brain and encounters a methodological, empirical, and theoretical pitfall; when film performs it, it does not generate incoherence, but rather images and plots that problematize neuroessentialism.

Before the 1980s and the replacement of bloody, surgical-knife procedures with computer-like operations, digital imagery, or discreetly implanted microchips, many motion pictures displayed brains in vats, ectobrains floating in nourishing solutions, maintained alive waiting to be transplanted into new bodies. As we saw in Chapter 3, these ectobrains are the functional equivalents of Christian souls, which remain active but disembodied in the long interval between death and the general resurrection. The person's full restoration is accomplished through brain transplantation. Plots are driven by the search for an appropriate body and by postoperative consequences, usually catastrophic, sometimes just foolish. The primary goal and significance of the surgery, namely to perpetuate persons beyond their original embodiment and thereby demonstrate the power and hubris of science, tend to be obvious. In many pictures, though, some teachy dialogue makes them explicit. Some of the situations that ensue from brain transplants are found in films where personality transfers happen by other means. For instance, in *All of Me* (1984), the soul of a dying millionaire woman ends up in her male lawyer's body, and in *Freaky Friday* (2003), a mother and a daughter switch bodies. These movies, however, belong above all in the venerable "comedy of errors" genre, where mistaken identity (here through body swaps) is used as a comedic device, and where the mechanisms for transposing persons are secondary to the narrative and involve no particular visual resources – least of all images of the brain, research laboratories, or surgical equipment.

Staying the Same, Becoming Someone Else

Among the many movies that perform brain transplantation, three stand out in the extent to which they earnestly take the surgery as a thought experiment: *The Man Who Changed His Mind* (1936), *Change of Mind* (1969), and *L'homme au cerveau greffé* (*The Man With the Transplanted Brain*, 1971). In contrast to many other productions, these pictures use the problematic assumption that humans are cerebral subjects as the element that gives their scenario continuity, rather than as an ad hoc action trigger. They incorporate it as a constitutive element of the narrative and the filmic texture, consider it as the main trope to be dramatized, and tackle with serious intent and a sober style the transformations that result from a person's survival *in* and *with* an extra-cerebral body different from their original one.

In the early twentieth century, French writer Maurice Renard, whose *Les Mains d'Orlac* was discussed in Chapter 3, developed many of the themes that later gained filmic form. His 1908 novel, *Le Docteur Lerne, sous-dieu* (*Dr. Lerne, Undergod*), is dedicated it to H. G. Wells, whose mad scientist in *The Island of Dr. Moreau* (1896) pieces together chimeras by means of vivisection. Lerne instead operates by swapping animals' heads and, later, by transplanting brains (the narrator, victim of such surgery, finds himself in a bull's body). He also switches the brains of his two assistants Wilhelm and Karl:

> Ah! The good fellows!... Who would think their entire bodies have been amputated? And yet each, since that day, has been living in his friend's carnal house. Look!
>
> He called in his assistants and, lifting their hair, revealed the purplish scar. The two Germans smiled at each other. (Renard 1908, 214)

Lerne's original ambition, however, was to give persons a new, younger body, thereby securing their immortality. He considered the self as identical to the brain, but wished to attain his goal without having to perform cerebral transplantations. That objective fails, and Lerne's outlandish surgical activity is in part the consequence of such failure. Brains turn out to be indispensable.

The Man Who Changed His Mind (1936)

The English film *The Man Who Changed His Mind* was directed by Robert Stevenson (1905–1986), who moved to Hollywood in the 1940s, and between the 1950s and the 1970s directed nineteen films for the Walt Disney Company, including the popular musical *Mary Poppins* (1964). It shares with the classic *Frankenstein* of 1931, discussed here in Chapter 5, a screenwriter (John L. Balderston) and a principal actor (Boris Karloff); and like James Whale's classic, it is subtler than its usual categorization as science-fiction horror would suggest.

A black-and-white production with lots of scientific-sounding dialogue, *The Man Who Changed His Mind* effectively begins when the beautiful Dr. Clare Wyatt (Anna Lee) decides to work with the aged chain-smoker Dr. Laurience (Boris Karloff), a once-respectable scientist who now carries out experiments in his somber manor. In a manner typical of the era, his home laboratory combines apparatuses evoking electricity, physiology and chemistry: microscopes and dynamos; high voltage electric converter wire equipment; Voltaic piles; a galvanometer; liquids bubbling in and flowing among Schlenk tubes and flat- and round-bottomed flasks suspended by clamps; and the less common brain in a glass vat – perhaps the first brain kept alive in a vat ever shown in a movie (Brainfilms 4.5). As one of Clare's senior colleagues puts it, she "is going into the wilds, to work for the mad brain specialist."

Laurience has come up with a technology for transferring mental contents from one brain to another. "Until now," he explains to an increasingly worried Clare while showing her a preserved brain, "it's never been possible to, as it were, extract the thought content from a living brain, and leave it alive but empty. I can do it; I can take the thought contents of the mind of a living animal, and store it, as you would store electricity." The trope of transferring or commuting minds is far from new; in the pulps, and in film since at least *The Man Who Changed His Mind*, it has generally involved explicit brain manipulations. During the transfer, the animals sit side by side, wearing wired helmets through which brain contents will pass from one to the other in the form of current (Brainfilms 4.6). The swap begins by inverting the position of plugs on an apparatus similar to a telephone switchboard, and the process is displayed in the form of a crackling electric arc. When it is finished, each animal has acquired the other's personality.

From *The Man Who Changed His Mind* in the mid-1930s to *Flash Gordon and the Brain Machine* (discussed below) in the mid 1950s, and from *The Fiend With the Electronic Brain* (1969) to *Johnny Mnemonic* (1995), *Eternal Sunshine of the Spotless Mind* (2004), *The Final Cut* (2004) and beyond, helmets – silly-looking if old, and, if new, graced with a vintage touch or stylized as futuristic headphones (as for example in *Identity Crisis* and *Second Thoughts*, the late-1990s *Outer Limits* episodes mentioned above) – have been a major cue to brain-altering technologies, as well as metonymic signs that cerebral contents are being moved, remade, or erased. Used in the same ways and for the same purposes, helmets were mainstream in pulp science fiction, and in Stapledon's 1937 novel *Star Maker* (mentioned in Chapter 2), people have their brain centers radio-stimulated via a "specially constructed skull-cap."

The important element, though, is the function, not the technology itself. Thus, the scene in James Cameron's blockbuster *Avatar* (2009) where the personal identity of Jake Sully, a paraplegic former Marine, is transferred to the genetically engineered body of a Na'vi (the humanoid inhabitants of a planet humans wish to conquer) includes the fMRI-like scanner where he is placed, as well as futuristic see-through screens (the year is 2154) colorfully displaying the process in 3-D functional neuroimages. *Mutatis mutandis*, this is no different from Dr. Laurience demonstrating with two chimps that he can transfer mental contents from one living animal's brain to another.

When Clare realizes that Laurience plans to try this out with humans, she is appalled and refuses to help him further. The doctor, who is infatuated with Clare, seeks to convince her (and here the motivation is different from anything in *Avatar*): "I can take a young body, and keep my own brain ... Think of it: I offer you eternal youth, eternal loveliness!" In the meantime, Clare has met the journalist Dick Haslewood (John Loder), son of press magnate Lord Haslewood (Frank Cellier). Although Laurience is discredited in the scientific community, the pompous lord offers him a laboratory in his London "Haslewood Institute of Modern Science." After the doctor is ridiculed at a prestigious conference, his patron fires him. But Laurience manages to tie Haslewood to the cerebral transfer chair, and replaces the lord's mind with that of his crippled assistant Clayton (Donald Calthrop). (The swap between humans does not require helmets; the subjects sit in separate rooms, and the exchange is signaled by alternating bright light flashes visible through translucent doors.) Haslewood (i.e., Haslewood's mind in Clayton's body), dies immediately after the transfer, while Clayton's brain survives in the nobleman's body. In the meantime, Clare has become engaged to Dick Haslewood. Driven by jealousy, Laurience is determined to take possession of Dick's body. For that, he obviously needs Clayton's help. Clayton, however, has discovered that Haslewood's body suffers from a fatal heart disease, and claims Dick's body for himself. Laurience kills him, and when Dick arrives at the Institute, the scientist forces the mind exchange. Clare later manages to put Dick's and Laurience's minds back into their original brains. The doctor dies asking for forgiveness and makes her promise to destroy all his equipment.

The Man Who Changed His Mind conflates brain and mind in interesting ways. Although Laurience claims that he can take a young body and keep his own brain, he does not plan to transplant brains, but to transfer without surgery their contents, that is, "the thoughts, the personality, the mind" that define an individual. These are localized in the brain, but "brain" sometimes stands for "mind." When Laurience tells Clare that he can keep his own *brain* in a new young body, he means his *self.* Thus, in spite of the brain's proclaimed role, the criteria for defining personal identity are purely psychological. Contrary to what happens in many other fictions, the eternal youth and loveliness Laurience promises Clare do not *depend* on brain transplants. Yet the doctor is characterized as a "mad brain specialist," and professes that he can keep his own brain in a younger body. Not for nothing is the film also known as *The Brainsnatcher*, and in French and German as *Cerveaux de rechange* and *Der Mann, der sein Gehirn austauschte*.

Both the conflict and the empirical or logical dependence that characterize the relationship of cerebral and psychological criteria for personhood are performed here in the context of a scientist's quest for brain-based immortality. About three decades before professional philosophers systematically began using brain fictions to discuss personal identity and its physical vs. psychological criteria, a motion picture explored the same issues while simultaneously assuming and relativizing the idea that humans are cerebral subjects. The movie alternately tells us that we are our minds and that we are our brains. While the juxtaposition of the two possibilities suggests their identity, the floating vocabulary denotes difficulties and challenges that are inherent to the "mind-body" problem as it has evolved since the seventeenth century.

Two later pictures move the brain transplantation drama into the social realm, as well as into a different scientific and filmic era. They replace the character of the mad brain scientist by less histrionic doctors in white coats, the time-honored gothic lab by clean modern operating rooms with normal-looking assistants in scrubs, and the magical electricity-driven extraction and transference of a living brain's "thought content" by explanations with some more apparent scientific verisimilitude. For all its sci-fi character, brain transplantation not only could be accepted as plausible in principle, but also as a procedure raising questions that belonged to the realms of professional science and philosophy. Indeed, in the three and a half decades between *The Man Who Changed His Mind* and the pictures we shall discuss next, organ transplantation had become a reality, and "brain death" had been defined.

The first successful kidney transplant was performed in 1954 between identical twins; various immunosuppressive drugs were developed in the 1960s and prolonged the survival of experimental kidney transplants; the first clinical liver and heart transplants took place in 1963 and 1967 (Barker and Markmann 2013). The latter in particular, performed by the charismatic

Cape Town surgeon Christiaan Barnard, received worldwide media attention and could hardly be unfamiliar to anyone who watched TV, flipped through magazines, or read newspapers. While ethical questions related to human transplantation had been raised before, the case of the heart made them especially urgent:

> Removal of a kidney from a living donor was partially justified by the fact that kidneys are paired organs; a person can live with only one. But removal of a viable heart definitely ends the life of its source. So the debate over the definition of death was revived: is it possible to assert that a person whose brain has ceased functioning is dead? (Jonsen 2012, 264)

In 1968, the Harvard Medical School ad hoc committee "to examine the definition of brain death" provided an affirmative answer. One of its motivations was precisely to replace "obsolete criteria for definition of death," which could "lead to controversy in obtaining organs for transplantation" (Beecher et al. 1968, 337). The committee did not "redefine" death; rather, it detailed neurological signs of irreversible coma. Although "brain death," that is, death defined as the irreversible loss of brainstem or (more commonly) whole-brain function, predominates in clinical practice everywhere, there are considerable differences in diagnostic procedures, and controversies regularly arise in the case of patients who would enter the brain-dead state if supportive measures were withdrawn. The following movies do not question the fact that the body donors are dead or seek to explain the criteria of death; neither do they raise questions about the ethics of the surgery. But the way they dramatize the consequences of having one's brain in a different body belongs in a larger context in which the brain was moving center stage.

Change of Mind (1969)

Robert Stevens's *Change of Mind* (1969), a picture that remains subdued in spite of the energetic original score by Duke Ellington and His Orchestra, uses the brain transplantation fiction to explore race relations in 1960s USA. Stevens was one of the directors and producers of the early-1950s TV series *Suspense*, and directed many episodes of the TV program *Alfred Hitchcock Presents* and *The Alfred Hitchcock Hour*, which ran between 1955 and 1965.

The movie opens on close-ups of an open-skull operation, an intensely reddish brain, an EEG chart. White district attorney David Rowe has terminal cancer; Dr. Bornear (Anthony Kramreither) is saving his life *in extremis* by transplanting his brain into the body of Ralph Dickson, a black man ran over by a car. The result is a white lawyer in a black man's body. The ads and posters suggest a predominantly romantic plot (Brainfilms 4.7), but the story is more interesting. For it is in his new black persona that Rowe (Raymond St. Jacques) must prosecute a white racist sheriff for the murder of a young black woman. The scenario, heavy-handed on both sides of the racial divide, is both obvious and contrived, and perhaps suffers from not being more fully focused either on the legal case, or on the surgery's social and psychological consequences. Yet it combines both in a skillful way.

Every commentator misses something that others consider significant. For the late Roger Ebert, famous film critic at the *Chicago Sun-Times* and first member of his profession to win a Pulitzer Prize for Criticism, the plot of *Change of Mind*

> hardly inspires enthusiasm. The brain of a white district attorney is transplanted into a black man's body, and the movie is about how he adjusts to his new color and almost wins the big case. This sounds like one of Hollywood's common ploys: trying to make a movie twice as successful by employing not one but two contemporary themes. People are interested in transplants and race relations, right? So why don't we...
>
> Well, strangely enough, *Change of Mind* is never as bad or tasteless as it could have been. It concerns itself mostly with the hero's emotional and ethical problems, and becomes a sort of fictional *Black Like Me*. But we still can't forget the absurdity of the premise. A BRAIN transplant?
>
> And so, instead of appreciating Raymond St. Jacques' fine performance as the district attorney, we are distracted (a) by the reminder that the DA is really the brain inside the body and (b) by thoughts of how St. Jacques must feel, as a black man, playing a white man playing a black man. The implications are interesting, yes, but the distractions get in the way of the performance. We're forever figuring out the angles.
>
> The other problem is that the movie turns out to be about a controversial murder trial, instead of about the experience of becoming Negro. (Ebert 1969)

What Ebert considered absurd and distracting is for us a significant way of making the movie's point; and pushing spectators to "figure out the angles" certainly was one of the picture's virtues. In 1959, the Texan white journalist John Howard Griffin underwent a dermatological treatment to temporarily darken his skin. Passing as a black man, he embarked on a six-week trip through the racially segregated southern states of the USA. He recounted the experience in *Black Like Me*, published in 1961. The cover of the first edition announced, "A white man learns what it is like to live the life of a Negro by becoming one!" So Ebert was right when he spoke of a "fictional *Black Like Me*." In the movie, however, the "absurd" brain transplant is precisely what makes the transracial experience possible, and determines its form in a particular time and place.

The surgery places *Change of Mind* in a specifically pulp and B-movie lineage, into which it introduces several features that play a considerable role in the story: the change in skin color is involuntary and not done for a particular purpose related to race; the transformed protagonist is not an unknown visitor in a new place, but a well-known public figure who must continue to interact with family and colleagues; his metamorphosis into a black man is not cosmetic; the new body he inhabits is not originally his; people, both black and white, know that he is a white individual "in" a black body. The plot's "distracting" aspects largely follow from these features; they crucially contribute to the psychological and social texture of the story, and shape many of the film's visual details.

For instance, the Washington, DC, mayor finds the looks of the postoperative Rowe "a little shocking"; Rowe's visitors and co-workers act with visible embarrassment; his wife Margaret (Susan Oliver) won't let him touch her; his mother feels she can't ask Margaret to love David when she can no longer accept him as son ("It's me, mother. – How can you look so different without being different?"); Dickson's widow Elizabeth (Janet MacLachlan) interrupts their lovemaking to comment "Ralph is dead"; in the nightclub where Elizabeth sings, an attractive black woman recognizes Rowe but treats him as black, while a black man taunts him, "Oh... It's the brother with the new brain. ... You know what's stitched inside this freak's head? A white politician's brain." Political opportunism also plays a role. At first, Rowe's political party no longer wants him to run for district attorney. As party head and Senate majority leader Bill Chambers (Jack Creley) tells him, "To a white man, you're black. To a black man, you're a freak. You couldn't get elected as dog-catcher here in Dorene county." Predictably, after Rowe wins over black voters thanks to his vigorous pursuit of the case against the white sheriff, the party considers asking him run for attorney general. Yet, when Rowe discovers that the murder was actually committed by a black man and asks for the case to be dismissed, black citizens are furious.

These situations define the social drama of the movie and contribute to bring about the "change of mind" the title refers to. How does this drama relate to brainhood? The film proclaims the cerebral subject ideology. Thus, a journalist asks Dr. Bornear, "What is he now, doctor: a white man with a black body, or a black man with a white brain?" The surgeon does not reply, but, at first sight, the film's answer is unambiguous. Several times Rowe asserts the continuity of his personal identity under a different appearance ("It's me, mother"), and remains himself to the point of dismissing a case against his own political interests and his reputation as civil rights defender. In a rare romantic moment, when he still believes in his marriage, he tells his wife, "The brain is a wonderful thing. It's really everything: David in me, Margaret in you." Science seemed to confirm such assertions. Bornear's associate, Dr. Kelman (Ron Hartmann), explains that the country's top authority on forensic medicine concluded "that since the brain of David Rowe survives, the brain that reasons, has compassion, personality, loyalties and love, which has memory, instinct and sensation, then David Rowe, district attorney of Dorene county, survives medically *and* legally."

Yet Rowe's medical and legal permanence conflicts with the historical conditions of his social existence. Rowe grows increasingly disappointed and estranged from Margaret. When she is appalled at his cynical depiction of politics, he is angered by her "white morality." In a country that had only recently passed civil rights laws, Rowe's re-embodiment transforms not only his mind and body, but also his position in society, the attitudes toward him, and his own sense of self. His pre-operative defense of racial desegregation takes on an existential significance that was completely absent when he was still a white district attorney.

The movie offers no resolution and finishes with Rowe's taking leave of Margaret and flying toward an unknown destination to "think things over." Such open, interrogative ending corresponds to the film's ambivalence regarding the conditions of personal identity. We are cerebral subjects – all the protagonists *say* it. At the same time, what they *do* demonstrates the inadequacy of the brainhood ideology to account for Rowe's transformation. His change of mind is not a consequence of physiological changes ensuing from the brain transplantation. Rather, it is mediated by historical circumstances and interpersonal relations. In the end, only the composite of a "white brain" and a "black body" is able to experience, realize, and confront the transformative impact of a new skin color.

From the point of view of how the black experience of race is explored in US films at the time of the civil rights movement, *Change of Mind* is similar to Melvin Van Peebles's *Watermelon Man*, launched the following year. In this successful 1970 comedy, Jeff Gerber (played at the beginning of the movie by black actor Godfrey Cambridge in whiteface), a risibly racist white insurance salesman wakes up one morning to discover he has become black. Like Rowe, he experiences bigotry and discrimination; police arrest him without reason, neighbors threat him with anonymous calls ("Move out, nigger"), he loses his family, and gives up his job. Here too, the new circumstances bring about a change of mind that completely reorients the protagonist's life and political outlook (Jeff militantly accepts his new identity and opens an insurance company for black people). Both the overnight change in skin color and the white man's brain being transplanted into a black man's body can be seen as little more than devices to prompt plots about the experience of being black in a racist environment. They are in that respect perfectly equivalent. This, of course, does not rule out specific features and different perceptions. For example, whereas *Change of Mind* is a rare example of the theme of race involving scientific fiction (or fictional science), Jeff's transformation in *Watermelon Man* is pure unmotivated magic. As for critical reception, largely by virtue of the directors' different careers and identity (Van Peebles, who is black, pioneered black-focused films and became an important figure in "black cinema"), *Watermelon Man* has seemed critically subversive in a way Stevens's film has not (Gates 2014). Nevertheless, interrogating the seemingly trivial brain-switch artifice brings up questions that do not appear when the focus is placed on the racial issue, and underlines the need to ultimately integrate the themes performed and the devices used into a single object of filmic analysis.

The Man With the Transplanted Brain (1971)

The French movie *L'homme au cerveau greffé* (*The Man With the Transplanted* Brain, 1971) was directed by Jacques Doniol-Valcroze, who was also actor, screenwriter, and producer, as well as co-founder and first editor (1951–1957) of the influential *Cahiers du Cinéma*. Like the homonymous novel by Alain Franck and Victor Vicas on which it is based, the film tells the story of a surgical hybrid: "With the intelligence of one man and the flesh of another, he [the surgeon] has made a new being" (Franck and Vicas 1969, 229). While "flesh" here refers to the non-cerebral body, "intelligence" designates the function or contents of the transplanted organ. This synecdoche is the basis of the plot, and once again enacts Puccetti's dictum, "Where goes a brain, there goes a person."

The novel opens with a lengthy preface outlining the history of organ transplantation, and situates the fiction in the framework of questions about life, death and the future of medical science as they could reasonably be raised in the late 1960s:

> Legal death is thus defined by brain death.
>
> But what if it is precisely the brain that one wishes to take from one body to graft it on another body?

> The dilemma is clear: either the brain is dead, harvesting is possible – but what would be the use of a dead brain? Or it is still alive, and in that case...
>
> Therein resides the entire drama: *a brain transplantation is possible only if the brain is removed from a person who is still alive.*
>
> Should we conclude that a brain transplantation will never be done?
>
> Of course not. ... What was impossible yesterday is often possible today. As to what tomorrow will be like... (ib., 13–14)

The film, like the novel itself, explores these questions from the perspective of a future where brain transplantation has become possible.

The premises of the plot remain well within the genre. Middle-aged surgeon Jean Marcilly (Jean-Pierre Aumont) and his collaborator Robert Desagnac (Michael Duchausoy) have been experimenting with brain transplantation in animals and waiting for the opportunity to try it out with humans. When the body of the young Franz Eckerman (Mathieu Carrière), fatally injured in a car crash, arrives at Marcilly's clinic, the surgeon, who knows he is fatally ill, asks Desagnac to graft his brain onto the victim's body. In the end, the resulting individual (let's call him Franz2) voluntarily assumes Franz's persona to lead a new life with Elena (Nicoletta Machiavelli), the beautiful Italian who was about to divorce Franz at the time of the deathly accident.

In *Change of Mind*, the grafted brain completely dominated the rest of the body, and the transformations of the self derived from the hybrid's encounter with his social environment. In contrast, *The Man With the Transplanted Brain* stages the re-emergence of Franz's personality, accompanied by certain antagonisms of brain and body, as crucial elements in Franz2's metamorphosis into a self-declared new individual. Right after the operation, Franz2 introduces himself as Professor Marcilly and Desagnac calls him "Jean." He speaks with a slight accent, but his demeanor is Marcilly's. To a colleague who asks him if he is used to his new form, Franz2 replies that he still finds it strange to hear his new voice, have an accent, and experience difficulty finding some words. Such practical challenges, he says, are small yet striking. "And the rest?" she asks. "The rest," Franz2 replies, "is terrifying." Desagnac discusses with him the complexities of the situation given that, officially, Marcilly is dead and Franz hospitalized. They decide to present the experiment publicly seven weeks later at a scientific conference.

In the meantime, Franz2 meets Franz's wife, discovers they are about to divorce, and moves into Franz's apartment. He must undergo a medical check every two days; during one of them, an increasingly worried

Desagnac emphasizes, "We must *invent* a human being. After all, you live in someone else's body." They opt for leaving Franz2 at Franz's home so as to continue the experiment outside the laboratory. Franz2 and Elena revive their relationship, and little by little, some of Franz's usual behaviors reappear. Franz was a racing pilot; Franz2 drives a car at top speed and barely avoids an accident. Franz2 handles a cat affectionately, and then suddenly drops it with violence; a rapid alternation of Marcilly's and Franz2's faces highlights the conflict of the two personalities. Franz2 is puzzled; Elena tells him he loved dogs, but hated cats. Franz had a penchant for alcohol; Franz2 drinks a bottle of rum without realizing it; when Elena scolds him, he denies having drank. As Franz2 explains in his medical persona, "the subject seems to have abruptly become prisoner of the body's drives, as if the cerebral element had suddenly ceased to govern." (I use "drives" to translate *pulsions*, the French word usually employed for Freud's *Triebe* and rendered in English as "instincts"; the psychoanalytic overtones would have been obvious to any French even mildly conversant with psychoanalysis.)

The remark about the power of Franz's body is followed by a succession of scenes whose juxtaposition demonstrates the coexistence of two persons in Franz2, as well as the collision between their different social worlds. The first one shows Franz2 visiting Marcilly's widow Elisabeth (Monique Mélinand) in her vast bourgeois apartment. When Desagnac arrives, he is surprised to find Franz2. They move to Marcilly's study, where Franz2 explains that he wished to see his family and environment – which nevertheless, he tells Desagnac, he does not miss. In the following scene, Franz2 returns late to his flat, quarrels with Elena, fills a glass with alcohol; as he is about to drink, he sees himself in a mirror, and throws the glass on the floor. Back at Marcilly's, Elisabeth finds on her husband's desk a piece of paper with a doodle he was in the habit of making, and which was not there before Franz2's visit.

Later on, the automatisms and conflicts are superseded by Franz2's conscious choice of a new life. There remain some identity slips, as when Franz2 introduces Elena and Marcilly's daughter Marianne (Marianne Eggerickx) to each other as, respectively "my wife" and "my daughter." But awareness and emotion predominate. When Desagnac objects, "You are not Franz Eckerman," Franz2 responds, "I know, Robert, I know Eckerman is dead; but the truth is that I, Jean Marcilly, love this woman [Elena]." While the dialogues reproduce enduring associations of the brain with reason, and of the body with passions and emotions, Franz2 evolves toward a reconciliation of the two in a new individual.

Marcilly's radical existential decision to impersonate Eckerman is catalyzed by the beautiful Marianne, who falls in love with Franz2, and tries to seduce him. "You love your wife, but you desire me." Franz2 denies it, they kiss, and while she is fixing him a drink, he escapes from her apartment. Back home, he phones Desagnac, introduces himself as Franz Eckerman, calls him "doctor," addresses him as *vous*, and asks him to tell Marianne no longer to follow Franz. While phoning, however, he automatically makes the surgeon's idiosyncratic scribble. When Marcilly deliberately takes on Eckerman's civil identity, which had until then been a mere cover for the surgeon's brain and personal identity, he turns the doctor's death and the patient's survival into public and irreversible social realities.

Distressed, Desagnac argues with Franz2 that the traces of Eckerman's personality are only a temporary phenomenon, and that he *is* Marcilly. Desagnac admits to not knowing if Franz2 has the right to enact the surgeon's choice, or if he should interfere with it; but the essential thing, for him, is that the experiment has succeeded and could be repeated. The essential thing, Franz2 retorts, is the right to be happy. Alluding to the scribble she found on Jean's desk, Elisabeth Marcilly suspects Desagnac hid something from her; he admits it, adding that "it was... it is" Jean's will. In the meantime, Franz2 and Elena happily drive away into the forest. The German title of the novel adequately summarizes it all: *Morgen bist du ein anderer* (*Tomorrow You Are Someone Else*). The choice to become the other into whose body one's identity has been transferred generally involves the brain, but not always surgery. For example, in *Avatar*, Jake's choice to fully become a Na'vi entails a brain manipulation presupposing that the self is a unitary entity that can be transferred as a whole (Wolpe 2010).

Moreover, such a choice always requires a body that might have a problematic relationship with its new brainmind. In *The Man With the Transplanted Brain*, contrary to the doctors' expectations, the brain does not fully dominate the body. In this respect, the novel is more audacious and tragic than the film. The hybrid of surgeon Daniel Berson and the young Pierre Lizio actually becomes the lover of Berson's daughter, who is, in the book, Desagnac's fiancée. Adding insult to incest, and following Pierre's impulses, Berson/Lizio cheats on her; she dies in a car accident while running away from him, and he commits suicide by throwing himself under a car. The novel's tragic ending conveys a lesson about the dangers of scientific hubris and of meddling with the essence of humanity; it may also be the moral of a fable in which the drives and passions of the body end up dominating the purported seat of reason. In contrast, the film, by way of cinematic means and a happy ending, highlights not only the return of Franz's bodily impulses and the contradictions experienced by the composite of A's body and B's brain, but also the final balance of brain and body through a deliberate choice that gives definitive social existence to the result of an unprecedented organ transplantation.

In spite of the surgery and the connections the film makes between the brain and the non-cerebral body, the brain is presumed to be to a certain extent distinct from the body, rather than an integral part of it. The issue is not histocompatibility, but the ancient question of the union of two essentially different substances. The brain takes on the functions of the soul as substantial foundation of self, and even as that which assures its persistence beyond bodily decay. Marcilly is supposed to survive in Franz's body; as in other fictions, successive transplants of an individual's brain into younger bodies could insure that individual's immortality. In these fictions, however, brains are always older than bodies (about two decades in *L'homme au cerveau greffé*), and we are not told if after being grafted they will rejuvenate, simply not age, or deteriorate. Brains just are, and we are they.

***

Beyond the individual dilemmas of a brain trapped in an unfamiliar body, the outcomes of the movies we have just sketched point to the intrinsically relational nature of personhood. In Marcilly's story, as in Julia's (who stays with her husband) and in David Rowe's (who takes leave, perhaps temporarily, of his wife), the final act always concerns relationships and how the protagonists' new embodiments reconfigure their place in a community and society. What these characters become is not merely a sequel to "where their brains go," but involves emotions and desires deeply engaged in social and interpersonal dynamics. Other pictures convey the same message.

In John Frankenheimer's disturbing *Seconds* (1966), with which Kureishi's *The Body* has considerable unnoticed affinities, middle-aged banker Arthur Hamilton (John Randolph), who leads a boring life with his wife in the suburbs of New York City, is first lured and then coerced into undergoing an operation that will turn him into a young man. The procedure is plastic surgery; in a scene including shots of an actual rhinoplasty, we see doctors working on Hamilton's face. The operation visibly affects the entire body, and the result is an impressive "Reborn" with the body of Rock Hudson. As is the case with many other Reborns, Hamilton's "adjustment" to life as a younger man fails, fatally in his case. The ultimate reason is that the whole-body renewal has left him with his original brain. The affective issues he would still have to settle from his past life have become unsolvable; moreover, although his new identity as the painter Antiochus "Tony" Wilson in a hedonistic California beach community is pleasant, he is shocked to discover that the other members are all Reborns. Like Adam in Kureishi's *The Body*, he wants to reverse the procedure, but is not allowed to do so. In the end, Tony is released for "cadaver use" and his body will serve as "catalyst" for a new Reborn. The film closes with a POV shot of what he would see were he still conscious: a surgical light above him, and a drill about to be pushed into his head. (A POV or "point of view shot," one of the forms of the so-called subjective camera, shows what the character sees; Kuhn 2009.)

In Tarsem Singh's *Self/less* (2015), tycoon Damian Hale (Ben Kingsley) decides to "shed" his terminally ill body and have his mind transferred into the "empty vessel" of a body that, he is told, was "genetically engineered for perfection." As in *The Man Who Changed His Mind* eighty years earlier, the procedure does not involve brain transplantation. The transfer of someone's mind into a new body takes place in a machine vaguely reminiscent of a CT scanner, surrounded by displays of brain scans on computer screens. Such *mise en abîme* – displaying brains on small screens as the means of performing them on the large one – refreshes the scientific façade of the operation, and underlines the continuity across decades of the brain motif and the neurocentric ideology (Brainfilms 4.8). What makes *Self/less* more complex than *The Brainsnatcher* (the older movie's alternative title) is that the mind transfer functions like a semigraft of the sort discussed in Chapter 3 in connection with *Black Friday* (1940), where the grafted portion of a gangster's brain periodically takes over a professor's entire personality (we also saw how, almost eighty years later, *Get Out* [2017] complicates the situation by letting part of the host's consciousness remain in spite of total brain transplant).

In *Self/less*, Damian's new body (played by Ryan Reynolds) had belonged to someone else, a man called Mark, who had sold it in exchange for an insurance that would save his daughter's life. So Damian has been cheated: "you thought you were buying a new car, and it turns out it has a few miles on it." Mark's mind invades Damian's in the form of flashbulb memories of a woman and child. Damian looks for them. In the end, he chooses to suspend the medication that would irreversibly suppress Mark's identity from his brain; by allowing this identity to take over, Damian lets himself die, and Mark can return to his beloved family. As in all other movies, personhood is embrained. Yet, contrary to what happens in brain-transplantation stories, Damian may freely decide to let go of his person precisely because his identity has been transferred to a brain that is not his, and is precariously stored as information, rather than being consubstantial to his own physical brain.

As in *Self/less*, what lends existential depth to the transgenerational rejuvenation plot of *L'homme au cerveau greffé* is that, contrary to the doctors' expectations, the brain does *not* fully dominate the body. That allows the films to conclude with a balance of brain and body, performed through the main protagonists' final choice in favor of a healthy body and a younger look. The choices nevertheless lead to opposite outcomes. While Damian gives himself up entirely in favor of his host body, Marcilly – firmly anchored in his brain and not only his mind – prefers to remain himself and enjoy his new embodiment.

Such a situation dramatizes the union of two essentially different entities, and again makes the brain assume the soul's function as substantial foundation of the self. It nonetheless avoids substance dualism. Like other movies based on the transgenerational plot, it gives the brain a crucial ontological function as the organ of personhood. At the same time, it enacts the self as made up of social and interpersonal processes and experiences. In short, through their depiction of an extreme existential situation, motion pictures visually and performatively reassert that being ourselves of course requires a brain – yet is not predicated upon neurobiological states alone, but also upon extra-cerebral circumstances. The same can be said about literary fiction. The late 1990s saw the emergence of a literary subgenre, sometimes labeled "neuronovel," which uses neuroscientific discourse as a means of expression within the narrative (Roth 2009). Characters are not simply explained in neurochemical terms. Rather, it is by way of these terms they are created and exist in the text. Neuronovels seem committed to a reductionist neurocentric ideology. In closer reading, however, the neuroscientific idiom is less a conceptual statement than a literary device that opens up room for ambivalence and criticism vis-à-vis that ideology (Holland 2019, Chap. 3; Ortega and Vidal 2013).

Similarly, Kureishi's *The Body* endorses Puccetti's dictum, "Where goes a brain, there goes a person" – but only to problematize it. The brain remains a crucial condition of selfhood, yet the depiction of Adam's physical, psychological and social plight as a Newbody turns personhood into an embodied and relational phenomenon. The younger body is not merely a practical tool or a burdensome privilege, but that which mediates Adam's being-in-the-world. In short, as already noted, rather than committing the mereological fallacy, literature and film push to the limit the synecdoche of the brain that thinks and acts. Their treatment of brainhood performs and brings to awareness ordinary attitudes. Sociological studies show that people assimilate neuroscientific ideas pragmatically and for their immediate relevance, and mainly when those ideas substantiate existing beliefs and modes of understanding (O'Connor and Joffe 2013). Even persons diagnosed with brain-based conditions do not attribute to neuroscience an absolute capacity to define or explain subjectivity. In general, as the social sciences abundantly document, one's experience of age and self depends not only on physical condition and appearance, but also on one's "embeddedness" in a social world.

As illustrated by the tensions between the age of the body and the age of the brain in Kureishi's Adam and several movie characters, transgenerational brains fictions amplify the challenges ensuing from that sociological fact. The struggles involved in moving one's brain from body to body turn out to be essentially relational, and to concern in fundamental ways an individual's place in the social world. By narrating and enacting them, fiction helps sharpen our gaze with regard to the neurologization of persons, and directs our attention to the intersubjective dimension of personhood. This dimension is comparatively little explored in philosophical discussion, which tends to focus on self-consciousness, first-person perspectives and individual autonomy at the expense of how relating to oneself and to others may be intertwined (Ikäheimo and Laitinen 2007). It is, after all, because there are other humans that Tithonus's voice can be heard as he slowly withers in the arms of "cruel immortality … at the quiet limit of the world."

5. Frankenstein's Brains

Abstract
This chapter documents how, in the long history of Frankenstein productions, the original theme of the creation of life was replaced by brain transplantation, and explores various forms of that radical transformation. It discusses the origins of the brain subplot and the relation of motion pictures to Mary Shelley's novel (1818). It also examines the entire Frankenstein film industry since 1910, with emphasis on the series produced by Universal (1931–1948, including James Whale's foundational classic) and Hammer (1957–1973). In contrast to the tendency to find in the Frankenstein motif all sort of societal "anxieties," this chapter demonstrates the significance of factors internal to the film industry in the formation of a narrative and visual tradition.

Keywords: brain transplantation, Frankenstein, James Whale, Hammer Film Productions, Mary Shelley, Universal Pictures

We have so far explored how the cinema performs the relationship between personhood and the body by means of fictions concerning the brain and its contents. From the "mad brain specialist" of *The Man Who Changed His Mind* (1936) and the crude disembodied brains of 1950s B movies, to *The Matrix* (1999), which offers a version of the philosophical fable of the brain in a vat (Chalmers 2005), and further on to the dying tycoon and the ailing elderly whites of *Self/less* (2015) and *Get Out* (2017), motion pictures have localized individuality essentially in the brain, and have imagined ways for personal identity to transcend the body's demise by transplanting the brain or its contents into other, typically younger and healthier bodies. Drawing credibility from both science and philosophy, they implicitly follow Roland Puccetti's 1969 conclusion, "Where goes a brain, there goes a person." At the outset, movies assume that the brain is the somatic limit of the self and consider that the noncerebral physical body is secondary to personal identity. However, the body's role as repository of the brain

Vidal, F., *Performing Brains on Screen*. Taylor & Francis Group, 2022
DOI 10.5117/9789462989146_CH05

and as the recipient's interface with the world shapes the hybrid subject's experience, and generates the motives and imbroglios that drive action.

Frankenstein films deserve a special place in the history of such fictions. At a general level, this is because "Frankenstein" designates "an authentic modern cultural myth" (Marcus 2002, 190). Though most frequently associated with the potential dangers of transgressing limits in the life sciences, the story has resonated much more widely "through its extraordinary resistance to simple resolutions and its almost inexhaustible possibilities of significance" (Levine 1979, 18). Film has been a major medium for performing the myth in its myriad facets and ramifications. Of relevance here is whether the responsibility for the enacted catastrophes is direct or indirect. As Andrew Tudor observes,

> With growing public concern about atomic energy during the fifties, the idea of science *unwittingly* causing disaster becomes more common, a pattern that is repeated in the late seventies and eighties, where scientific "side-effects" give rise to pollution and ecological imbalance. A similar shift is apparent in the relative proportions of different kinds of monsters in different periods. When mad scientists are in the ascendant, and individuals are thus responsible for the threat through their own actions, monsters are mainly medical creations more or less directly descended from the Frankenstein prototype. During periods of indirect scientific responsibility, however, accidental mutations become much more common, as a consequence first of radiation and, later of pollution. (Tudor 1989, 134, and more generally Chap. 7)

By virtue of its basic structure, the Frankenstein myth retains its power in spite of the decline in the popularity of the mad scientist it usually portrays (Frayling 2005; Haynes 2014). The same applies to brain transplantation movies: the surgeon remains a key character because someone has to plan and carry out the brain transplant.

Yet the special place of the cinematic Frankenstein among brain fictions arises from its internal evolution. It has been often observed that in the 1940s, protagonism shifted from creature to creator. A different, but intrinsically related and crucial change has hardly been noticed: Frankenstein pictures abandon the original theme of the creation of life, and place a brain transplantation subplot at the core of their narrative. We shall here examine such transformation with a focus on the two "classic" Frankenstein series, released by Universal Pictures and Hammer Film Productions between 1931 and 1973.

Shelley's Novel and Frankenstein Films

The Frankenstein story has been a steady source of theatrical and filmic inspiration. A chronological list of most major feature movies between 1910 and 1994 comprises seventy-one items (*A List*); other movies have been released since then, and many more have a tangential relationship to elements of the original story and its derivatives (Glut 1984; Jones 1994; Rohrmoser n.d.). Not all of these pictures involve brain transplantation. The cerebral subplot, however, is common to almost all of the "classics" making up the Universal and Hammer film series that shaped the twentieth-century image of Dr. Frankenstein and his creature, and it persists until today both in film and other media, such as comics, games, and children picture books and graphic novels (Alder 2018; Bukatman 2018; Krzywinska 2018).

Universal Pictures, whose original name was Universal Film Manufacturing Company and is also known as Universal Studios or just Universal, was founded in New York in 1912, with production studios in Hollywood. In the 1920s, it shot several horror and monster movies; the success of *Dracula* (1931) encouraged it to stay in the horror-monster business, and its first *Frankenstein* (1931), directed by James Whale and featuring Boris Karloff's epochal appearance as "The Monster," was released in the same year (Mank 1981). Whale's *Frankenstein* introduced the brain motif, but only later did transplantation replace the original theme of the creation of life. The second series was produced between the mid-1950s and the mid-1970s by Hammer, a British company founded in 1934 and best known for its horror movies (Hearn and Barnes 2007; McKay 2007; Meikle 2009). The brain subplot provides central visual motifs and a narrative trigger throughout the series. Most later Frankenstein movies cite and pay homage to the Universal and Hammer productions; the most famous one including the brain motif is Mel Brooks's *Young Frankenstein* (1974), which is rich in self-reflexive humor and dependent, for full enjoyment, on familiarity with the Universal pictures.

How does the brain subplot relate to the movies' *prima facie* inspiration, Mary Shelley's 1818 *Frankenstein; or, The Modern Prometheus*? The novel gives no information on how Dr. Victor Frankenstein put his creature together (Sutherland 1998), or on how he gave it life. Moreover, the two processes must be distinguished. In the 1831 Introduction to the novel, Shelley wrote, "Perhaps a corpse would be re-animated; galvanism had given token of such things: perhaps the component parts of a creature might be manufactured, brought together, and endured with vital warmth"; and Victor described himself as "not unacquainted with the more obvious laws of electricity" (Shelley 1831, x, 28). These allusions opened the way for the spectacular use of electricity as animating medium in Universal's first *Frankenstein*. (Electricity became thereafter a standard element of many Frankenstein movies. Sometimes its presence does not go beyond a few sparks emanating from a lab machine, but it also gives life, and it eventually kills, as when the creature in the Frankenstein episode of the anthology series *Tales of Tomorrow* [1952] is accidentally electrocuted.)

As for the creature's body, Victor admits that he "dabbled among the unhallowed damps of the grave," that he "collected bones from charnel houses," and that the "dissecting room and the slaughter-house furnished many of [his] materials" (ib., 40, 41). The narrative includes no such later movie staples as nightly forays into cemeteries or morgues, no organ removal from corpses, no stitching together of bodily parts, no scars on the creature's skin, and not even a hint of the brain's significance for his identity. All these elements, which have become integral to the Frankenstein imaginary, amplify the novel's reference to "the grave" and the rest, but, like electricity, come directly from Universal's 1931 production. There are of course numerous other differences between the novel and the movie series. Yet as horror cinema specialist Peter Hutchings (2008, 123) points out, "judging any Frankenstein film in terms of its adherence to the novel is a futile activity. The films exist instead in relation to a series of cultural transformations of various fragments of the Frankenstein story."

By the time Frankenstein and his monster emerged as cinematic entities, even the idea of "fragments of the story" had ceased to be relevant. Representing or performing the doctor or his creature no longer required referring to anything in Shelley's novel. Although the credits usually make some claim about their source, for example "Based on the characters created by Mary Shelley" in *The Horror of Frankenstein* (1970), most movies routinely revisualize various elements, such as the Monster's aspect, which belong to specifically filmic canons. If we nonetheless ask how the brain plot transforms the story, we see that it does not affect just "fragments," but, to use Mary Shelley's words in her Preface to the novel's first edition of 1818, the very "event on which this fiction is founded." Shelley judged that event "impossible as a physical fact"; however, since some scientists considered it "as not of impossible occurrence," she claimed that she was not "merely weaving a series of supernatural terrors," and that "[t]he event on which the interest of the story depends is exempt from the disadvantages of a mere tale of spectres or enchantment" (Shelley 1831, 1). That event is what Victor Frankenstein describes as "bestowing animation upon lifeless matter," "the creation of a human being," "infusing life into an inanimate body" (ib., 38, 40, 43).

The result was horrifying: "A mummy," deplores Frankenstein, "again endued with animation could not be so hideous as that wretch" (ib., 44). Films have exploited this to the full, and frequently over the top; even in the rare productions where the creature is initially good-looking, such as *The Revenge of Frankenstein* (1958) and *Frankenstein, the True Story* (1973), he becomes monstrous as the story progresses. (An exception is the handsome athletic creature of the 2004 TV miniseries *Frankenstein*, who looks like the 1980s pop singer the actor used to be. Several features of this series, including the Monster's sad, articulate and sensitive personality, have led some commentators to see in it the most faithful adaptation of Shelley's novel.) The creature's repulsive facial scars and deformities evince Dr. Frankenstein's surgical method. With time, stitches on the forehead become prominent; sometimes they are the only trace of surgery at all (Brainfilms 5.1; see also the portrait gallery of the creature from 1826 to 1994 in Skal 1998, 44-45). They signal that the "event on which this fiction is founded" has ceased to be the making of an inanimate body and the infusion of life into it, and has instead become the persistence of an individual's identity thanks to the transplantation of his brain into the Monster's body. The continuity of someone's personal identity replaces the making of a new person; transplantation takes over creation. The foundational event of the fiction is thus thoroughly redefined. What motivated such a change, and what does it mean?

The Final Touch: *Frankenstein* (1931)

The first Frankenstein movie (c. fifteen minutes long, silent, black-and-white, but tinted) was made in 1910 by Thomas Alva Edison's production company. The doctor here proceeds by dropping a potion into a large cauldron from which a disheveled, grimacing, shambling creature with messy long hair and stringy, elongated hands and feet gradually emerges from the flames, flapping a skeletal arm up and down. The effect, praised at the time as "the most remarkable [scene] ever committed to a film" (quoted in Wiebel 1997, 25), was obtained by burning a papier mâché dummy and then reversing the film (see also Drees 2005). Its creation involves no bandages, no scars, no surgery, no assembling of odd bodily parts – in short, none of the features that became standard after the film James Whale directed for Universal in 1931.

Five minutes into that classic, Dr. Henry Frankenstein (Colin Clive) and his hunchbacked assistant Fritz (Dwight Frye) reach a gallows in the dead of night. Fritz cuts the rope from which a man hangs; the body thumps to the ground. (The assistant does not exist in the novel, but immediately became a movie staple.) After checking it, Henry reacts angrily: "The neck is broken. The brain is useless. We *must* find another brain." The following scene shows Henry's former professor Dr. Waldman (Edward Van Sloan), who in the novel is Frankenstein's kind mentor and a chemist rather than an anatomist, explaining to an auditorium the differences between two preserved brains. One is labeled "normal," the other "dysfunctional" and "abnormal." "Observe," Waldman tells the students as a close-up of his moving pencil points to areas on the brain surface, "the scarcity of convolutions on the frontal lobe ... and the distinct degeneration of the middle frontal lobe. All of these general characteristics," he remarks, "check amazingly with the case history of the dead man before us, whose life was one of brutality, violence, and murder" (Brainfilms 5.2). Brains floating in a preservative solution in a glass jar were common in the pathological collections established in nineteenth-century hospitals and medical schools (see, e.g., Alberti 2011); they were not uncommon in pulp illustrations and became a major filmic motif in the wake of Whale's *Frankenstein*.

After Waldman's lesson, Fritz breaks into the empty lecture hall to steal a brain. He drops the jar with the normal one, and hurries away with the other. In spite of his anatomical expertise, Henry does not notice the organ's supposedly obvious criminal features, and the abnormal brain ends up in his creature's body. As the completed being lies inert, Henry reassures Fritz:

> There's nothing to fear. Look: no blood, no decay. Just a few stitches. And look: here's the final touch. [He uncovers the creature's bandaged head.] The brain you stole, Fritz. Think of it! The brain of a dead man waiting to live again in a body I made with my own hands – with my own hands...

The scene highlights the ontological function of the brain. Shortly thereafter, once the creature receives the electrical discharges that give him life, begins the sequence leading to Frankenstein's sensational fit of hysterical enthusiasm:

> HENRY [Colin Clive, speaking with rising speed and volume]: Look! It's moving. It's alive. It's alive... It's alive, it's moving, it's alive, it's alive, it's alive, it's alive, it's alive!!!
> VICTOR MORITZ [Henry's friend, restraining him with Waldman's help]: Henry, in the name of God!
> HENRY: Oh, in the name of God! Now I know what it feels like to be God!

In spite of the creature's size and monstrous materiality, his personhood and personality reside in the brain, the "final touch" without which a body is an organism but not a person. This is reasserted with the revelation of the organ's abnormality:

> WALDMAN [speaking with a clipped "German" accent]: ... Wake up and look facts in the face! Here we have a fiend whose brain...
> HENRY: The brain must be given time to develop. It's a perfectly good brain, doctor. You ought to know: it came from your own laboratory.
> WALDMAN: The brain that was stolen from my laboratory was a criminal brain!
> HENRY [playing down his visible consternation]: Oh well, after all, it's only a piece of dead tissue.

The scene ends with the memorable first screen appearance of the Monster, walking slowly backward into the room before turning toward the breathless audience.

Henry Frankenstein's distress indicates that he does not entirely reject the idea that brain morphology is destiny. His dismissing the organ as "a piece of dead tissue," a defensive move, is inconsistent with the role he assigned it in the creature's making when he proudly told Fritz about the "last touch." Nothing, however, suggests that his developmental considerations are insincere. Moreover, the events that drive the action toward their conclusion, in which an angry mob burn the creature alive, question brain determinism further. In the spirit of Shelley's novel, the film shows an innocent being who becomes aggressive only in response to human maltreatment, first inflicted when Fritz frightens him with a torch.

The origins of the brain subplot remain unclear. To begin with, it is not in the play that is credited, together with Shelley's novel, as providing the film's source material. British writer Peggy Webling's theater piece *Frankenstein* (the first instance of naming the creature "Frankenstein") was first produced in 1927 (Webling 1927). As in the novel, the play's Victor has dabbled in chemistry and alchemy; he has also studied "physiology and anatomy"; and he has "handled the newly dead," spending "nights and days in vaults and charnel-houses." The creature's body is formed from materials he collects in those places. However, instead of employing electricity as animating force, Victor uses an "elixir to animate the senseless body." An electric storm provides a Gothic atmosphere; however, instead of giving life to the creature, lightning kills him instantly at the end of the play. The American John Balderston, whose adaptation of a stage version of *Dracula* had been used for the screenplay of Universal's eponymous blockbuster of 1931, was asked to do the same job with Webling's play. His version, which was never produced on stage, would become the basis for the screenplay of Whale's film (Balderston and Webling 1930). In Balderston's version, the creature comes to life by a combination of electricity and an "Elixir of Life." Dr. Frankenstein (now called Henry) attaches his creation's inert body to "wires of galvanic battery," to a machine that "fizzes and gives off queer lights, and sends out sparks." While this happens, he takes a small bottle from a cupboard, and pours its contents down the body's throat. The brain appears as only one part of the creature's anatomical makeup. Henry explains:

> I had found ways of slowing up corruption but I had to work fast. I knew my way about the graveyard. I stole the key of the dissecting room – I took what I needed as I dared – a leg or a lung or some complicated nerve tissue. I am a sculptor; I moulded a figure and a face. (To Dr. Waldman) Do you remember ten days ago when you were dissecting a brain? I took that – some of it! From odds and ends – from charnel house and burying ground, I fashioned a body – I made a man!

Elements of Webling and Balderston's version appear in the film, but a brain motif with the significance it would gain in Whale's film is nowhere to be found. (A volume published in 2010 as *Frankenstein. A Play in Three Acts* [Balderston 1930] misleadingly suggests that the text is the film script, while it in fact is the play by Balderston and Webling.)

In his memoir *Hollywood d'hier et d'aujourd'hui* (1948), the director and screenwriter Robert Florey, who was initially in charge of the movie and contributed to the final script, claims to have invented "l'épisode de la substitution des cerveaux et de la création du monstre" (quoted in Forry, 1990, 105, n. 28). While in his history of Frankenstein dramatizations, Steven Forry (ib., 92) writes that Whale "incorporated Florey's ideas, including the substitution of a criminal brain for the Creature," medical historian Susan Lederer (2002, 39) maintains that "[s]creenwriter John Russell introduced the plot device of using a criminal brain rather than a normal brain to explain the monster's urge to kill." Be that as it may, the brain subplot began as a specifically filmic twist to the Frankenstein story, and became one of the central conventions of later Frankenstein pictures. Science writer Philip Ball (2011, 87) aptly summed up its significance for the Frankensteinian heritage:

> The hardest blow to the psychological core of Shelley's tale comes from the crude way in which the monster's pathological nature is rationalized.

> There is no longer the bitter tumult of the rejecting father and abandoned progeny; Fritz simply bungles his assignment to steal the "perfect brain" from Waldman's medical school. ... Needless to say, this all rather undermines the moral purported at the outset: Frankenstein's attempt to make a human is abortive not because it defies God and nature, but because he couldn't get the stuff.

As we have seen, Shelley's Frankenstein felt that he had also botched his creation's appearance: a mummy "could not be so hideous as that wretch." In film, the turn to the brain is incorporated into the creature's appearance via the forehead scars, and gives him his most visible sign of identity.

A 1933 article on the "make up secrets" of horror pictures aptly observed, "When you shudder at the sight of frightful characters in horror movies, it is usually the makeup man who is responsible for your thrills" (Bowles 1933). The testimony of Jack P. Pierce, Universal's chief make-up artist, shows the extent to which the brain subplot was both a constraint and a source of inspiration:

> My anatomical studies taught me that there are six ways a surgeon can cut the skull in order to take out or put in a brain. I figured that Frankenstein, who was a scientist but no practicing surgeon, would take the simplest surgical way. He would cut the top of the skull off straight across like a pot lid, hinge it, pop the brain in, and then clamp it on tight. That's the reason I decided to make the Monster's head square and flat like a shoe box and dig that big scar across his forehead with the metal clamps holding it together. (Quoted in Jones 1994, 36)

The Monster's characteristic square-shaped skull was, according to Pierce, built to give the impression of "a man whose brain had been taken from the head of another man" (ib., 37).

While these visual elements are perfectly in tune with the brain subplot they serve, the subplot itself plays at best an ambivalent role as motive for the creature's behavior. Such ambivalence, brought about in the dialogues and even more clearly in the action, was rapidly expunged. It completely disappeared from later Frankenstein films, and the brain subplot has been generally interpreted as providing the obvious cause for the creature's alleged killing urges. While an early *New York Times* reviewer correctly stated that the reason *the film gave* for the creature's "murderous onslaughts" was that Fritz "stole an abnormal brain" (Hall 1931), later commentators adopted that explanation *as their own* (but see exceptions in Hauskeller

2013, 8; Horton 2014, 52–55; Mendelsohn 2013, 210–202). For Lederer (2002, 39), "the Universal film emphasizes that the monster's evil results from his criminal brain." Caroline Picart (2002, 31) contrasts Shelley's original creature, "initially as innocent as a child," and the filmic rendition who, "having been given a 'criminal brain' (admittedly by accident), is implied to be inherently evil"; his "biological criminality and lack of speech sentence him to a life of guilt, condemnation, and social impotence." In an otherwise illuminating analysis, Paul O'Flinn (1986 [1983], 204) too affirms that the film "deletes" Shelley's view about the role of social circumstances "through its insistence that the monster's behavior is not a reaction to its experience but biologically determined, a result of nature, not nurture." Though Bruce Kawin (2012, 57) seems more nuanced when he writes, "Harsh treatment and the criminal brain combine to make the Monster a destroyer," there are no elements proving that the brain effectively plays such a role other than Waldman's assertion.

The lack of evidence for the role that commentators attribute to the brain becomes clear if we look at the creature's behavior. Sure enough, he kills Fritz and Waldman – but defending himself from their attempts to wound and destroy him. The most egregious of his apparent crimes happens in what some consider as the film's most famous scene, where he tenderly accepts the invitation to play with the little Maria. Far from being afraid, she holds his hand and asks him, "Will you play with me?" They toss flowers into a pond; the beauty of the floating flowers moves the creature, and when they run out of them, he innocently throws Maria in the water, obviously trusting that she will float as gracefully as the flowers; scared and bewildered, he frantically looks for her when she drowns. In 1937, the scene (restored only in the 1980s) was truncated, no longer showing the Monster's reaching for Maria, and cutting directly to the child's father carrying her corpse. The omission suggested a heinous crime and justified the ensuing pursuit and killing of the creature by a mob of angry villagers. Perhaps under such circumstances can one be justified to give the "criminal brain" a causal role – but the authors quoted above refer to the restored version of the movie. (A number of scholars have discussed the scene with Maria from other perspectives; see for a recent example Towlson 2014, 39–41.)

In short, reproducing Waldman's views about the "criminal brain" contradicts both the spirit and the letter of the film. Although Whale's *Frankenstein* was consistent with contemporaneous beliefs about the brain and cerebral determinism, it did not present "a monster whose evil results from the lobes of his brain rather than his experiences or character" (Lederer 2002, 46). Audiences of 1931 were surely not surprised to hear Waldman speak of a "criminal brain" and account for individual inclinations by looking at the cortical surface: it was common at the time to locate criminality and genius in brain morphology. Still, if that commonplace played such an important role in the film's economy, it was also by virtue of its being negated in the rest of the action.

The Universal Series

It is tempting to consider the cerebralizing reading of Whale's *Frankenstein* as a reflection of the authority of the "neuro" and the brain's iconic status since the mid-twentieth century. Primarily, however, it echoes the importance the brain motif gained in later Frankenstein productions, and retrospectively projects onto Whale's masterpiece the tradition this picture contributed to initiate.

"Tradition" may be too weighty a word, but it emphasizes the continuity of the brain motif and the clichés connected with it in the Frankenstein film industry. The line of descent, however, did not begin immediately with Whale's picture. Thus, in the same director's *Bride of Frankenstein* (1935), the second movie in the Universal series, Dr. Pretorius (Ernest Thesiger) forces Henry Frankenstein (Colin Clive) to finish a female companion for the Monster. Although this does not involve brain surgery, Pretorius tells Henry: "I have created by my method a perfect human brain, already living but dormant. Everything is now ready for you and me to begin our supreme collaboration." Henry refuses, but is in the end coerced to bring the Monster's mate to life. Although there is no brain subplot or scene here, mentioning the brain provides a significant element of continuity. (Except for the Bride, played by Elsa Lanchester, Frankenstein's creatures are male. In *Frankenstein Created Woman* [1967], a Hammer production, the creature is androgynous, and the brain is not directly involved: a woman kills herself after her lover Hans is wrongly executed; the doctor revives her with Hans's soul, and the resulting entity seeks to avenge Hans's death.)

The Ghost of Frankenstein (1942) is the fourth film in the series, but the second one foregrounding a brain subplot (*Son of Frankenstein* [1939] and *Frankenstein Meets the Wolf Man* [1943] omit it altogether). It is also the first Frankenstein film without Boris Karloff, and is usually seen as marking a downturn in quality. As Tom Weaver and Michael and John Brunas (2007, 278) comment in their film-by-film discussion of the series, this production "made it plain that Universal was less interested in producing horror films than in churning out mere 'monster movies'" characterized by "grotesque making, swooning heroines and/or rip roaring action."

In *The Ghost*, both the Monster and Dr. Frankenstein's assistant Ygor have survived the destruction of the Baron's castle. Ygor (Bela Lugosi) brings the creature to the dead doctor's son Ludwig (Cedric Hardwicke), who lives in another town as an honest "diseases of the mind" specialist. When they arrive, Ludwig and his associates are about to finish an operation: "Think of it: the first time a human brain has been removed from the skull, subjected to surgery, and then replaced." Ludwig's "Think of it" are Henry's exact words to Fritz in Whale's 1931 opus; even so, whereas Henry emphasized the creation of life and spoke of "the brain of a dead man waiting to live again," Ludwig announces a medical triumph for the good of humankind. That is why he initially wishes to kill his father's evil creation. Dr. Frankenstein's ghost appears to him, and explains that the Monster is violent because, unknowingly, he gave it a "criminal brain." The solution is to replace the "malignant brain," as Ludwig describes it, by a healthy one. But whose? Ludwig wishes to use the brain of the Monster's recent victim, the good Dr. Kettering. Ygor, however, convinces Ludwig's jealous and unscrupulous colleague, Dr. Bohmer (Lionel Atwill), to transplant his (Ygor's). "My brain will be your brain!" he excitedly tells the creature.

The brain in a vat enters the operating room on a wheelcart rolled forward toward the spectators right in the middle of the screen; it is literally and figuratively center stage (Brainfilms 5.3). Ludwig wonders what Kettering will say when he finds himself in the creature's body; and he concludes the surgery observing that, while the original creature was "a homicidal maniac," Kettering's "brain is now inside the skull of the monster. I have replaced an evil brain with a good one." The new creature, who thanks his well-intentioned creator with the words, "Your father gave me life, and you gave me a brain," combines superhuman strength with Ygor's nefarious inclinations. After several violent events, the Monster becomes blind (his blood "will not feed the sensory nerves"), and when he kills Bohmer by shoving him onto the lab's electrical equipment, he also sets Ludwig's castle on fire.

Two years after *The Ghost*, *House of Frankenstein* (1944) gathered several Universal "monsters": the Wolf Man and the Frankenstein creature (whose bodies were found in Dr. Frankenstein's "house," the castle ruin left at the end of *The Ghost*), Count Dracula, and a hunchback called Daniel. Daniel (J. Carrol Neish) has helped mad doctor Gustav Niemann (Boris Karloff) escape from prison. Then, rather than keep his promise to place Daniel's brain into a perfect body, Niemann plans to take revenge on his enemies by transplanting the brain of one them "in the skull of the Frankenstein monster" and the Wolf Man's brain in the skull of another one. Daniel covets the Wolf Man's body, but Niemann wants to use it as a sort of relay: it "is the perfect place for the monster's brain that I will add to and subtract from in my experiments." In *House*, where there is no character called Dr. Frankenstein, a zany version of the brain transplantation motif is the subterfuge that precipitates a monster festival. On matters cerebral, a similar general description applies to the last film of the series, *Abbott and Costello Meet Frankenstein* (1948). With more slapstick than the customary violence, it brings together Dracula, the Wolf Man, and the Frankenstein creature with the era's most celebrated American comedy duo. The result is a farce prompted in part by a female mad scientist's plan to replace the Monster's brain by one that, as she tells Dracula, "is so simple, so pliable, he will obey you like a trained dog." Both the final title and the original one of the script, *The Brain of Frankenstein*, illustrate the fusion, by then common, of the doctor and his creation.

In *The Philosophy of Horror*, Noël Carroll (1990, 44) affirms that the Universal films "appear to uphold the unlikely hypothesis that somehow the monster has a kind of continuing identity ... in spite of the brain it has" and notes that "if we allow the fiction of brain transplants, why quibble about whether the monster is in some sense still the same monster it would have been" with a different brain? In fact, exactly the opposite happens. The Monster's persistence is purely cinematic; it does not concern his personal identity, and nobody quibbles about it. On the contrary, the series shapes the creature's filmic existence via different brains and purposefully capitalizes on such variation. This is the situation that Hammer would exploit to the full.

The Hammer Series

By the end of the Universal series, Dr. Frankenstein was gone and the brain subplot had been reduced to a formulaic gimmick. Hammer revived them both (on the mad scientist, see Kaltenbrunner 2014). *The Curse of Frankenstein* (1957), first in a series of seven films that the company released until 1974, defined the tone and the style to come. The Universal productions were all black-and-white; the early ones were characterized by expressionistic lighting and camera work, Gothic castles and ruins, big sets, and elaborate mad scientist laboratories (*Son of Frankenstein* [1939] is the last of the sort). Hammer, by contrast, favored an overall "realistic" aesthetic, used full, garish color, and placed its stories in opulent Victorian settings appropriated from the period melodramas that were popular in 1940s Britain (Harmes 2015). Laboratories remained crucial spaces, but compared to Universal's grand machineries and awesome electrical effects, often filmed in high- and low-angle shots, the Hammer labs were simpler and of more modest proportions. They were also filmed in medium shot, with the camera foregrounding normal-sized spiral wiring, glass tubes and retorts with bubbling liquids, some crackling electrical equipment, an operating table, and a vat with body parts, including brains. Surgery was here the chief laboratory event.

First screened in 1957, *The Curse of Frankenstein* was a huge international success with audiences (but not with critics), and is usually depicted as groundbreaking for the emergence of modern cinematic horror, as well as for the commercial exploitation and public acceptance of gore and graphic violence. As has often been pointed out, *The Curse* shifted emphasis from the creature to his creator. Under the label "Universal Monsters," Universal Pictures had invested in designing, operating, and merchandising brand creatures that generated public recognition and customer loyalty (Mallory 2009). Hammer inverted the strategy. In each film, the creature looks different and is played by different actors. The company's branding focused on Dr. Frankenstein. It was sustained by almost always using the British horror specialist Terence Fisher as director, and actor Peter Cushing as the cold and sinister, yet charismatic and elegant Baron Frankenstein. *The Curse* was produced under threat of lawsuits from Universal for potential copyright infringements, particularly of the Monster's aspect, and perhaps the new emphasis on brain transplantation was partly due to that circumstance. The creature's new look should in any case be seen in the framework of the several ingredients that differentiate the Universal and Hammer series. The brain plot spoke to audiences familiar with the Universal movies; its promotion helped give originality and continuity to the Hammer series, while linking it to popular Universal successes.

In *The Curse*, brain surgery is displayed on the face of "The Creature" by means of a red scar, closed with metal staples and running across his forehead just above the eyebrows. The brain inside the ghastly head is not innately "criminal." In fact, it belongs to a "genius" Dr. Victor Frankenstein killed precisely for his unique brain. Alas, the organ was spoiled when the glass jar containing it broke (a cliché since Fritz's blunder in Whale's picture). Predictably, the resulting creature is a "criminal lunatic," governed by his cerebral pathology. "I had a damaged brain," explained horror movie star Christopher Lee about his role as the Creature, "and so I walked slightly lopsidedly. ... Everything I did, I did as if it was forced out of me; as I was rather unwilling to do it, controlled by a brain that was not my own" (quoted in Hitchcock 2007, 215). Dr. Frankenstein claims that he can "repair the brain." This, of course, does not happen. It is while waiting to be guillotined that he tells a prison minister the story which, in flashback, makes up the film.

The Curse of Frankenstein launched the aesthetic and narrative pattern of the entire Hammer series. Parallel to a trend that began in the USA in the early 1960s, but without reaching the splatter level, subsequent productions tended to display increasing amounts of violence, blood, and gore. In *The Revenge of Frankenstein* (1958), which explicitly follows from *The Curse*, the brain plays an even more important role. The Baron has somehow escaped death and has established a successful medical practice as Dr. Victor Stein (Peter Cushing). Young doctor Hans Kleve (Francis Matthews) discovers him and joins him in his quest to transplant a brain. Frankenstein will thus take revenge: the previous creature, he explains, "should've been perfect. I made it to be perfect. If the brain hadn't been damaged, my work would've been hailed as a scientific achievement. The greatest of all time. Frankenstein would've been accepted as a genius of science." By the time Hans shows up, the doctor has assembled a new creature and is ready for the final touch: "All I need is a brain and then I can give it life." A "brain simulator" he has manufactured demonstrates that "the brain must be a living one. Unlike the limbs, life cannot be restored [to the brain] once life has gone. The brain is life, so a living brain must be used." The donor is to be Karl (Oscar Quitak), Frankenstein's lame assistant; spectators are gratified with a view of his brain being dropped in a jar. The transplantation succeeds. That notwithstanding, after killing a few people, the new Karl (Michael Gwynn), who is at first tall and good-looking, redevelops his deformities, and publicly uncovers Dr. Stein's true identity as Frankenstein. An angry mob then attacks the doctor and leaves him for dead. Hans transplants his brain into a look-alike body that Frankenstein had already prepared. The end of the movie shows "Dr. Franck" and his associate Hans welcoming patients at a new practice in another city.

In *The Evil of Frankenstein* (1964), new arrangements between Universal and Hammer enabled the creature to recover some of its original looks, and Dr. Frankenstein's laboratory to include some machinery reminiscent of Whale's; the makeup, though, is crude, and the lab lacks the original's expressionistic sumptuousness. Returning from exile, Victor Frankenstein (Peter Cushing) recovers his creature from a glacier, where it had been preserved frozen. He notices that the creature's brain is "good," but cannot make contact with it. He therefore enlists a stage hypnotist to "accelerate a reaction" in the Monster's brain. The creature, however, obeys the hypnotist alone – and this leads to death and destruction. Although physical brains are not displayed, the brain subplot is mediated through dialogue, and opens the way for the hypnotist's role, which is crucial for the action.

Frankenstein Must Be Destroyed (1969), which in Spain was distributed with the apt title of *El cerebro de Frankenstein*, is the fifth film in the series, and the third where the brain plays a key role. While Peter Cushing plays a particularly truculent Baron, the creature is little more than a forlorn character: Frankenstein's former associate Dr. Frederick Brandt, whose brain is transplanted into Professor Richter's body. Lasting over three minutes, the surgery sequence is particularly long; as in most films of the series, it happens below the sightline. We are shown various preparations, but during the surgical act the camera focuses on the doctors' faces; the nature of the act is indicated by blood prominently displayed on hands, aprons and instruments. We also see Brandt's excessively large, slimy, and dripping brain being taken out of the vat where it waits while Frankenstein noisily saws Richter's skullcap. The Baron's assistant in the surgery considers the success "utterly fantastic." "Not fantastic," Frankenstein replies, "advanced. The transplanting of all human organs is a logical branch of surgery. But you and your pigheaded contemporaries refuse to recognize that fact." Brandt (George Pravda), who looks completely normal except for the long scar left by skullcap removal, feels desperate about his new state: "My brain," he sadly tells his shocked and incredulous wife, "is in someone else's body" (Brainfilms 5.4). She rejects him: "I'm your husband. – You're not. You're not anything human!" Such scenes and dialogues illustrate a recurrent pattern.

In *The Horror of Frankenstein* (1970), directed by Jimmy Sangster, who authored its script as well as those of *The Curse* and *The Revenge*, "The Monster" again receives a brilliant (though oddly bluish-grayish) professor's brain. Mute and violent yet obedient, he has a bald, tall and flat head that recalls Pierce's design. However, rather than a scar across the forehead, the visible traces of the operation look like the sutures of the skull's temporal, parietal and occipital bones, held together by the usual metal staples (Brainfilms 5.5). As in *The Curse*, from which *The Horror* borrows several other elements, when the jar that contains it once again breaks, a glass shard harms the tissue. "Can't you talk?" Frankenstein (Ralph Bates) asks his grunting creature. "It must be that piece of glass." In the lab, a life-size outline of a human body with numbers indicating the members and organs to be found and grafted highlights brain transplantation as the crowning surgical act (Brainfilms 5.6).

Frankenstein and the Monster from Hell (1973) closes the series with an extraordinarily long surgery sequence. Baron Victor Frankenstein (Peter

Cushing again) has taken control of an insane asylum. With the hulking hairy body of one inmate (grafted, however, with a sculptor's graceful hands), he has created an imposing monster. Early in the movie, we learn, "All he needs is another brain, preferably the brain of a genius." Such a brain is obtained from one Professor Darundel, whom Frankenstein has driven to suicide. A first scene, almost four minutes long, shows the doctor's disciple Simon Helder (Shane Briant) sawing Darundel's skullcap; Frankenstein removes it and extracts an excessively firm brain, which he places in a vat (Brainfilms 5.7). In a second scene, about one minute long, the Monster's brain is removed. The transplant itself is not shown, but we do see a small, dark, dried-up brain landing in a white enameled metal basin; the basin is on the floor, and when Frankenstein moves toward the vat containing Darundel's brain, he kicks it accidentally, and the brain is thrust with comical elasticity against a leg of the stand that holds the vat. The head scar is stitched rather than stapled. In the end, in a scene that recalls the *Night of the Living Dead*, the other inmates rip the Monster apart. As usual, achieving the "final touch" of life and personhood is the first of several steps leading to destruction and death.

One recent production highlights the remarkable presence of the filmic Frankenstein. In *Get Out* (2017), where (as already explained) white individuals have their brains transplanted into the healthier, younger bodies of African American men and women, the surgery practically replicates, over forty years later, impactful visual elements of the scene just summarized from *Frankenstein and the Monster from Hell*: the Victorian-era surgical toolbox, the shot of the skullcap about to be opened, the brain thrown into a bucket. The screens displaying neuroimages in the background locate the plot and the surgical space in the late twentieth century. However, as in *Self/less*, the *mise en abîme* limits itself to updating the scene's appearance in a clichéd manner, introducing clues, mainly in the form of brain scans on computer screens, which would be familiar (if only as a visual motif) to anyone even vaguely motivated to see the movie (Brainfilms 5.8). At the same time that it fulfills a central narrative function, the brain subplot situates *Get Out* in visual and ideological continuity with a recognizable and popular cinematographic tradition.

Beyond Universal and Hammer

Several Frankenstein movies were made during the same period as the Universal and Hammer series, and quite a few after them. Frankenstein became a transnational filmic figure early on, with an Italian version predating the Universal series, several Mexican productions starting in the 1950s, and pictures coming out of Japan, Spain, Portugal, Italy, France, Turkey, Sweden, Canada, and Lichtenstein until the 1980s (Lieberman 2018). Most are low-budget productions, with various degrees of violence, gore and nudity; some adopt ingredients of form or content from the novel that had not been previously used, but as a rule they also allude to earlier films; some exploit the brain motif, and often, even when they do not, the Monster displays a skullcap scar.

The blond muscular creature of *The Rocky Horror Picture Show* (1975), a major cult classic, has a perfectly smooth body. Everywhere else, however, scars operate as metonymic signifiers of a Frankensteinian creation. In the US-British TV series *Penny Dreadful* (2014–2016), which revives several time-honored characters from nineteenth-century Gothic literature, Victor Frankenstein's "Creature" looks more like Victor's depiction in Shelley's novel than a Universal or Hammer monster:

> His yellow skin scarcely covered the work of muscles and arteries beneath; his hair was of a lustrous black, and flowing; his teeth of a pearly whiteness; but these luxuriances only formed a more horrid contrast with his watery eyes, that seemed almost of the same colour as the dun-white sockets in which they were set, his shrivelled complexion and straight black lips. (Shelley 1831, 43)

And yet, in the TV series, The Creature, also formed from body parts stitched together, features the obligatory forehead scar, which looks more like crackled earth than a surgical suture (Brainfilms 5.9). His brother Proteus is made from the corpse of only one man; it nevertheless displays a similar scar. Such a scar is the most obvious way to label a creature as Frankensteinian. The scar as sign is so established that even the endearing dog Sparky of Tim Burton's stop-animation film *Frankenweenie* (2012) is all stitched up, although it is not composed of alien body parts, but was revived whole, thanks to electricity, after being killed by a car (Brainfilms 5.10). Extended arms, an inexpressive face and a rigid gait can be combined with the scar to evoke the Frankenstein creature; but only the scar signifies the crucial "final touch."

That is exactly the look of the re-animated dead in *Creature With the Atom Brain* (1955), by the director who, two years later, would release *Invasion of the Saucer Men*. Made of corpses, the sturdy creatures (for there are several of them) are the work of an ex-Nazi mad scientist, now at the service of a gangster seeking revenge. They have been considered zombies (Kay 2008, 25–26), but they do not rise by themselves from the grave; neither does their existence involve a Frankensteinian type of surgery. Powered by atomic energy, they are remote-controlled via a brain implant consisting of a "packet" of electrodes connected to the amygdala (Brainfilms 5.11). The movie, with screenplay by Curt Siodmak (author of the novel *Donovan's Brain*), not only combines most of the psychological, political and scientific themes of 1950s brainfilms (Sconce 1995), but also, via the forehead scar, visually places the title entity in the Frankenstein lineage.

Beyond scars, the brain kept its role after the Universal and Hammer series. A few examples follow. In *Frankenstein's Daughter* (1958), Oliver Frank (Donald Murphy), grandson of the original doctor, obtains his creature's brain from an inviting blonde, played by the February 1957 Playboy Playmate (Sally Todd). His assistant Elsu (Wolfe Barzell), who worked for his ancestors, enthuses: "Your grandfather and father never used a female brain! ... Frankenstein's daughter!" They both note that the resulting "female being" (who does not look like a woman at all) will be "more responsive to command" than previous creatures; and when Oliver orders Elsu to tie her up, the assistant protests, "she's nicer than the males your grandfather and father made." In *Frankenstein 1970* (released in the same year by Allied Artists, the low budget film studio that a few years later produced *Hands of a Stranger*), the brain still propels part of the action: "Yours," the doctor tells his butler, "is not the brain I would've chosen, but at least you're obedient." In *Lady Frankenstein* (1971), the doctor's voluptuous daughter transplants the brain of her father's brilliant but crippled assistant into the athletic body of a dull-witted servant capable of satisfying her sexual desire; as the movie makes clear, such a situation stimulates her at least as much as her commitment to science. That does not prevent the brain from having its own screen presence (Brainfilms 5.12).

In the 1970s, Italy had a large trashy cinema industry that exploited Frankenstein, though sometimes in name only. In *Frankenstein '80* (1972), set in the twentieth century, even though there is no brain scene, the hideous monster (a violent rapist) displays two thick scars running from the superciliary arches to the back of the head. In *Terror! Il castello delle donne maledette* (1974), known in English as *Frankenstein's Castle of Freaks* and almost as sleazy as the previous one, but set in the familiar Victorian-Gothic castle, the Baron incises the Monster's forehead for surgery, and later explains that injuries to the original organ justified a transplantation. The brain is mentioned several times in *Flesh for Frankenstein* (better known as *Andy Warhol's Frankenstein*, 1970); at the time of its release, the film was described as "a coy binge in degradation" (Sayre 1974), but many now see it as a masterpiece of camp. A late avatar of so-called "Italo-sleaze" is *Frankenstein 2000: Ritorno dalla morte* (1991), where the only thing that justifies the doctor's name in the title is that the man who "returns from death" exhibits a deep raw scar across his forehead, held with the customary metal staples – suggestive, but misleading, since the scar is due to autopsy rather than to brain transplantation.

In many of these pictures, obtaining a brain and transplanting it motivates some of the action, but the brain itself does not play any real role. An exception is the sexploitation film *Mistress Frankenstein* (2000), in which the doctor gives his wife the brain of a lesbian nymphomaniac. After Mrs. Frankenstein dies in a ludicrous accident while riding a pantomime horse, the desolate husband wants to revive her. He somehow pops from behind her head a plastic brain, auscultates it, and finds it defective. Frankenstein's tuxedoed assistant (predictably called Ygor) goes to "Clive's Body Shop," buys a replacement brain and takes it away in a paper bag; the doctor simply puts it into his wife's skull. This particularly inane script, executed with singular ineptitude, may be mainly an excuse for scenes of lesbian softcore porn; it nevertheless attests to the persistence of the brain subplot and of the physical brain's filmic function (Brainfilms 5.13).

The brain subplot is present even in more aesthetically ambitious films that claim fidelity to Shelley's original and use previously unexploited aspects of the novel. Thus, in *Frankenstein, the True Story* (a TV production of 1973), Victor Frankenstein (Leonard Whiting) gives his creature the brain of his friend Henry Clerval (David McCallum): "Whatever may come of this [and nothing good does], forgive me Henry, no longer will your Adam have the brain of a peasant." Similarly, in Kenneth Branagh's *Mary Shelley's Frankenstein* (1994), Professor Waldman (John Cleese) is shown, as in Whale's film, giving a lesson about brain anatomy. After one of his patients kills him, Victor Frankenstein (Kenneth Branagh) keeps his brain in ice ("The very finest brain," he says) before transplanting it into his creature, played by a heavily stitched up Robert de Niro. Several later scenes allude to the brain.

As in many brainmind-themed movies since the 1980s, the brain itself as organ of flesh does not have to be displayed for brainhood to be performed. Thus, in *Frankenstein 90* (1984), the only purely French Frankenstein film, Victor, a twentieth-century descendant of the Baron played by the very popular Jean Rochefort, steals body parts from a national human biology center. His creature (called Frank and played by the celebrated 1960s pop singer Eddy Mitchell) has a brain of unknown origin. In a scene showing a sagittal head CT scan on a computer screen, Victor deletes part of Frank's memory to make room for instructions. This he does by inserting a chip in Frank's head, and then typing in his commands from a computer. "La difficulté," he explains, "c'était le cerveau; je l'ai résolue grâce à un microprocesseur." Technology thus helps him enflesh *un cerveau desincarné*, a "disembodied brain" (Brainfilms 5.14).

In 1910, Edison's film demonstrated once and for all that cinematic Frankensteins can do without surgery and brain transplants. There are later examples of that. In the British cable TV movie *Frankenstein* (1992), set in the early nineteenth century, the creature is formed by a sort of embryological process inside a large glass vat. In 2007, another TV Frankenstein moves the story to the twenty first century. Victoria Frankenstein (Helen McCrory) works at the Universal Xenograft Project, which artificially grows organs in a metal tank similar to an iron lung. Desperate to further organ growth for her fatally ill son William, she introduces some of his blood into the tank. An entire creature, baptized UX, develops and escapes from the tank during a power failure due to a storm (the meteorological cliché since Whale). After killing a small girl, UX is caught, and bolts are placed on two sides of his head to control him via brain stimulation. This of course recalls the Monster in Whale's film. Seeing beyond UX's frightening face (a waxy, glabrous, bony cross between E.T. and the character Gollum from the *Lord of the Rings* film series), Victoria compares it to an intellectually disabled child and wants to prove "its humanity." She had already exclaimed, "It's alive!" and now she rejoices, discovering William's typical facial expressions when she talks to him: "It thinks!" At the end of the movie, UX has grown inordinately tall, and he and Victoria have been permanently locked up in an unidentified facility to be observed as they interact. There is no classic "Frankenstein" in this case, since UX was an accident rather than a chosen goal. The movie nonetheless illustrates the widespread association of the name with experimenting with life and "playing God," especially in connection with GMOs ("Frankenfood"), synthetic biology, stem cells, cloning, reproductive technologies, and embryo research (Mulkay 1996; Turney 1998).

***

With few exceptions since Universal's *Frankenstein* of 1931, transplanting a brain has been the "final touch," the last action in creating the Monster, the gesture that, just before bringing it to life, seals the accomplishment of mad doctors' projects, embodies their supreme surgical skills, and confirms (in their own eyes) the legitimacy of their ambition. That brain is Frankenstein's because it incarnates the scientist's ultimate goal, and decisively contributes to make up the Monster (who, following a long-lasting convention, is often identified as "Frankenstein"). Its presence has inspired discussions in the philosophy of personhood and brainmind (e.g., Hess 2013; Petrounakos 2013). Such discussions can be interesting in themselves, and help perpetuate Frankenstein's value as a resource for thinking on a range of issues. However, as a cinematic entity, Frankenstein's brain is rooted above all in developments internal to the moving picture industry, and is best understood as an element of cinematic rhetoric and aesthetic. The case of brain transplantation films more generally reinforces that point. The subgenre, including many *Frankensteins*, involves for the most part human-to-human transplantations, and violence rather than comedy or a sober mise-en-scène of issues germane to the dynamics and ethics of science or personhood. As already pointed out, by the early 1960s, when brain manipulations became one of Anglo-American philosophers' favorite thought experiments, the fiction had already spawned multifold pulp stories and B movies.

Dr. Frankenstein tends to see brain transplants as the cutting edge of an established scientific practice. In 1931, however, when he urges Fritz to "think of it," he speaks of a dead man's brain "waiting to live again" in a body he made. Ten years later, the emphasis has shifted, and when the doctor of *Ghost of Frankenstein* (1942) asks his assistant to "think of it," he means: "the first time a human brain has been removed from the skull, subjected to surgery, and then replaced." And in 1969, two years after the first human heart transplant, the Baron of *Frankenstein Must Be Destroyed* depicts brain transplantation as the "advanced" stage of "a logical branch of surgery." In 1957, the doctor of *Teenage Frankenstein* is a mid-twentieth-century American descendant of the Baron who, like his ancestor in *Frankenstein Must Be Destroyed* or Dr. Pat Cory in *Donovan's Brain*, is convinced that, in the same way sight can be restored thanks to corneal transplantations, "so also can we successfully transplant other organs and members of the body, attaching and grafting them when needed, even in cases where important arteries and nerve centers have been severed." He nevertheless performs no brain surgery, but replaces his creature's face (which, like most brains in this branch of the Frankenstein tradition, has been obtained by assassinating the "donor"). While transplantation was certainly a familiar notion in the 1950s (Hamilton 2012), the operation Dr. Frankenstein envisaged was unthinkable: although the first successful corneal transplant had been performed in 1905, working human solid organ grafts would have to wait until the early 1950s (kidney) and 1960s (lung, liver, pancreas, heart), and the first full-face transplantation was carried out in Barcelona in 2010.

The psychological background and consequences of such surgery are medically and psychologically complex and highly risky (see Laskas 2014 for an outstanding reportage). They must nonetheless pale in comparison with brain (or full body) transplantation. Through the pulps and the Bs, such operation has persisted since the early days of science fiction, and has been often framed as a realistic future possibility. Whenever it seemed to approach actual realization, it has been linked to Frankenstein. In 1999, the American surgeon Robert J. White (1999, 24), who in the 1970s transplanted the head of one rhesus monkey onto the body of another, predicted that the "Frankenstein legend," including brain transplantation, "will become a clinical reality early in the 21st century." (Were they not in a documentary on Dr. White, some scenes of *The First Head Transplant* [2006] could come straight from a B or a Hammer production; Brainfilms 5.15.) Sergio Canavero, the Italian leader of a "head transplantation with spinal linkage" project mentioned in Chapter 3, quoted him approvingly (Canavero 2013). Scientists and ethicists reacted critically, and the usual references to "Frankenstein science" immediately surfaced on the Internet. Yet Canavero finds the reference to be an honor. At an event in June 2015, he went as far as asking the Chinese surgeon who reported successful head transplants on mice "to stand and be recognized as a fellow 'Frankenstein'" (Schall 2015).

All this may seem outlandish, yet makes perfect sense in the perspective of contemporary biomedicine and the ethical, philosophical, and political questions it raises. The trope of Frankenstein's brain did not depend on or derive from those questions. It has clearly interacted with them, refracting the concepts and concerns they conveyed, and involving synergies that may be "symptomatic" of changing preoccupations in particular moments and circumstances. Yet the symptom metaphor is perhaps not the most useful. For example, when Branagh's *Mary Shelley's Frankenstein* came out, Roslynn Haynes (1995, 435) remarked that interpreting the Frankenstein releases of the mid-1990s as the expression "of Western society's deep anxieties about genetic engineering, IVF and the human genome project" does not explain the rate at which versions of the story had been appearing since 1910. Such an interpretation, however, itself contributes to the significance of cinema as agent that shapes societal attention and sensibilities. The same applies to this chapter, whose focus on a hitherto neglected aspect of Frankenstein movies fits in a larger critical exploration of the "neurobiological age."

We have seen that the persistence of a rather undifferentiated brain subplot in Frankenstein pictures is largely due to conditions of production and commercialization, and that while pictures sometimes update the knowledge and technologies they display in order to look plausible and stimulate visual interest, they generally do not seek to "represent" or actively engage with the issues of science and society that exegetes identify. The reason is perhaps that the brain subplot by itself performs well enough the long-term continuity and the apparent naturalness of the brainhood ideology. In the final analysis, it is the relative autonomy of Frankenstein's brains that allows them to keep interrogating "the final touch" of human personhood and participating in debates around its ultimate nature.

6. Memories, Lost and Regained

Abstract
This chapter examines brain-and-memory movies. While countless films deal in one way or another with memory, only a few perform it explicitly as a process that takes place in the brain. In most pictures, having memories of a "real" past functions as criterion for being one's authentic self; forgetting, memory replacement, manipulation, or erasure therefore pose radical challenges to the self. With regard to memory, the default position of the cinema embodies John Locke's theory of personal identity. This manifests itself in the filmic preference, which this chapter documents, for retrograde amnesia (i.e., the inability to recall events that preceded the onset of the disease). Case studies include *Dark City* (1998) and *Eternal Sunshine of the Spotless Mind* (2004).

Keywords: amnesia, authenticity, John Locke, memory, self, memory erasure

πολλα παθειν,
nothing matters but the quality
of the affection –
in the end – that has carved the trace in the mind
dove sta memoria
Ezra Pound, *The Pisan Cantos* 76.156–160

Philosophers of cinema, especially those receptive to the "ontological" outlook of André Bazin (1918–1958), pioneer film critic and theorist, and co-founder in 1951 of the *Cahiers du cinéma*, would argue that film is not a mimetic art, but rather, that it breaks down the opposition between an original and its "copy," and creates being in the absence of an essence to which it must correspond. As Bazin (2005 [1945], 14) claimed, the photographic image of an object is the object itself; the cinema, which he famously characterized as "objectivity in time," extends that quality into the realm of

Vidal, F., *Performing Brains on Screen.* Taylor & Francis Group, 2022
DOI 10.5117/9789462989146_CH06

duration. The ontological power and prerogative of film is realized through the fact that everything that happens on screen is always present: like a Freudian unconscious, movies know no past tense. It is still the case that motion pictures engage over and over with their characters' past, usually by embedding it in their subjective memories. As Maike Sarah Reinhert (2009) demonstrates in her study of the means by which film gives plausibility to leaps in time and makes past moments feel like the "past" in spite of happening in the present, to be credible, a character's memories have to be restricted to his or her subjective, mental perspective. That accounts for the value of memory processes and conditions as filmic resources. When those processes and conditions are understood as fundamentally cerebral, the way is open for giving the brain a significant cinematographic role. This is our focus here; but, of course, the link between memory and the cinema has been conceptualized in a variety of other ways (see, e.g., Radstone 2010 for an overview, and Kilbourn 2010, especially Chap. 2, on traumatic identity in contemporary memory film, which discusses some of the pictures examined below).

Even though medically diagnosed amnesiacs are uncommon, amnesiac characters "stumble everywhere" through literature and the cinema (Lethem 2000, xiii). Amnesia in that context is best understood as a plot resource, a "reliable narrative device," rather than a symptom of audience anxieties (Bordwell 2017). Yet, like any other trope, this one changes according to context. Of the many movies concerned with memory that have appeared over the decades, few deal directly with the brain, and most of these few concern an amnesic protagonist. Together with brain transplantation, memory loss and its circumstances and consequences thus constitute one of the main scenarios for the filmic performance of the cerebral subject.

Forgetting has served plot and action from cinema's earliest days. However, it was been mainly in the 1980s, with the convergent rise of cyberpunk and the cognitive neurosciences, that the cinema explicitly began to connect memory to the brain, and combined recent philosophy of mind with the habitual problems of radical skepticism. Philosophically speaking, these problems are the common ground of most brain-and-memory pictures; as noted before, rather than offering a clear-cut view of things, they expose tensions in the epistemological concepts at play. Pritchard (2016, Chap. 6), for example, depicts radical skepticism as a paradox entailing the conclusion that knowledge is impossible. Brain thought experiments have been integral to explorations of that paradox. The paradigmatic situation is that of X's brain in a vat connected to a device that stimulates in it experiences that are subjectively indistinguishable from the ones X would have were she fully embodied. Can X know she is merely a brain in a vat? And in what sense can those experiences be said to be both "hers" and "authentic"? The questions are the same with memories, and they also involve performing the brain.

Most of the films examined or mentioned in this chapter have been produced since the 1980s, and many were created as self-conscious philosophical fictions: *Blade Runner* (1982), *Brainstorm* (1983), *The Bourne Identity* (1988, 2002), *Total Recall* (1990), *Johnny Mnemonic* (1995), *Strange Days* (1995), *Dark City* (1998), *Memento* (2000), *I Know Who You Are* (2000), *Paycheck* (2003), *The Manchurian Candidate* (2004 remake), *Eternal Sunshine of the Spotless Mind* (2004), *Final Cut* (2004), *Magdalena's Brain* (2006), and *The Bourne Ultimatum* (2007). A central feature of these movies is that although amnesia and other alterations of memory are attributed to brain damage or manipulation, they make sense only in the light of protagonists' individual lives, personal experiences, and existential quests. Both before and after providing a cerebral diagnosis for their characters' predicament, films, like short stories, novels, and the sciences of memory, must turn toward the mind, life histories, and the vicissitudes of self-awareness.

Memory movies have been a cherished object of commentators seeking to find in them more or less correct, more or less scientific characterizations of the function and mechanisms of memory. The comparison inexorably reveals the gap that separates motion pictures from psychology, psychiatry, and the neurosciences; yet the relevant aspect of that gap is that the "distortions" that come to light express beliefs and concerns of the cultures where the movies are produced and consumed. Films often mix discredited theories (e.g., about discrete memory localizations in the brain) with others that have been accepted (e.g., about the effect of emotional arousal on encoding, storage, and retrieval). Even though that mixture is by itself interesting, the most revealing aspect for our topic is that cinematographic performances of memory, be they judged mistaken or accurate by scientific standards, tend to go hand in hand with a certain inconclusiveness regarding philosophical positions. Once again, movies do not aim at being coherent or making clear-cut theoretical choices. Performing such inconclusiveness is a positive feature if it throws viewers off balance. For example, as we shall see below, the memory erasure procedure in *Eternal Sunshine of the Spotless Mind* requires memories to be localized in circumscribed clusters of neurons. At the same time, the protagonist's "resistance" to erasure suggests that memory processes are more dynamic and distributed than such localization theory implies. This displaces the problem of memory toward the experiential and phenomenological realm, while not setting it entirely apart from brain science. In short, beyond science-related beliefs and idioms, memory movies rehearse theories, questions, dilemmas and open questions about the primordial role of memories in defining the individual self, and of the brain in constituting human persons.

A Preference for Retrograde Amnesia

We discussed in the first chapter how commentators, especially those who read science-related pictures through the lens of a scientific specialty, tend to follow the "deficit model" of analysis, which emphasizes the accuracy or inaccuracy of filmic fiction with respect to scientific fact. This outlook is problematic, but useful when it helps identify significant cinematographic features. For example, it brings to light the fact that, as far as memory disorders are concerned, "most amnesic conditions in films bear little relation to reality" (Baxendale 2004). It also turns out that the most popular memory syndrome in the movies is not the most frequent one in the clinic. Anterograde amnesia, an inability to recall events that take place after the onset of the disease, is a more frequent and incapacitating condition than retrograde amnesia, the inability to recall events that preceded the onset of the disease. Nevertheless, the cinema has overwhelmingly focused on loss of memories of the past. (The mutated Precogs of *Minority Report* [2002] "previsualize" future events. The movie, however, is akin to the pictures discussed here in that information is located in the brain. The Precogs' visions, used to prevent murders, are stored in their brains as downloadable records, fed directly into the Department of Precrime computer system, and displayed as images on a screen. In Philipp K. Dick's original story, the Precogs have, "enlarged heads and wasted bodies," a sight the pulps made familiar; one is a "hydrocephalic idiot"; and due to the fact that their extrasensory perception lobe "shrivels the balance of the frontal area," they are in any case "deformed and retarded" [Dick 1997 [1956], 339, 325].)

A notable exception to the cinematographic dominance of retrograde amnesia is *Memento* (2000), in which former insurance claims investigator Leonard "Lenny" Shelby (Guy Pearce) suffers from anterograde amnesia as a consequence of a head injury sustained while defending his wife from a robber. Her murder is the last thing Lenny remembers, and his life's goal is to take revenge. To compensate for his condition, he tattoos important information on his body, makes notes to himself, and takes Polaroid pictures. The film alternates color sequences that tell the events in reverse chronological order, and black-and-white sequences that move forward in time; events are repeated in scenes that add detail or perspective to the previous version. The effect is so labyrinthine that we never know what "actually" happened. Yet, as director Christopher Nolan pointed out, *Memento* is "an extremely linear film" in which scenes are so strongly linked to each other that they could be hardly be moved around (Kaufman 2001).

The confusion we experience as spectators is supposed to make us feel the fragility of memory. Nolan wanted to put the audience in the hero's head; as he explained, "that's why the story is told backwards, because it denies the information that he's denying" (Kaufman 2001). The movie conveys the recurrences and the immobility that characterize Lenny's existence as he goes from one short term memory to the next, with his identity frozen in a last, painful recollection. In the original story, such a situation is summarized by the unidentified narrator, who tells the protagonist, "Time is three things for most people, but for you, for us, just one. A singularity. One moment. This moment … Time moves about you but never moves you. It has lost its ability to affect you" (Nolan 2001).

Even though *Memento* "contains a few notable errors" (Pendick 2002) and offers an "unrealistic" portrayal of amnesia (Seamon 2015, 174), scientists' response to it has been overwhelmingly positive. High-profile neuroscientist Christopher Koch (2004, 196) declared *Memento* "by far the most accurate portrayal of the different memory systems in the popular media," and there seems to be consensus on that opinion. Esther M. Sternberg (2001), best-selling author on mind-body in health and wellbeing, celebrated how *Memento*'s plot, dialogue, and technique "expose the different kinds of memory that we take for granted, unless they are suddenly lost." Lenny's semantic, implicit, working, procedural, and emotional memories still function. The movie passingly informs us that his anterograde amnesia is due to hippocampal damage; like other commentators, Sternberg notes that his condition is consistent with the case of the "unforgettable" amnesiac H. M. (Carey 2008). In 1953, the twenty-seven-year-old known as H. M. underwent a bilateral temporal lobe resection, involving removal of most of the hippocampus, in the hope of alleviating uncontrollable epileptic seizures. The operation produced "a grave loss of recent memory" and partial retrograde amnesia, while leaving early memories "apparently vivid and intact" (Scoville and Milner 2000 [1957], 106). Until his death in 2008, H. M. remained one of the most thoroughly studied subjects in the history of the neurosciences.

Even though there is no evidence that, as some blogs maintain, the case inspired *Memento*, Lenny's condition is consistent not only with H. M.'s, but also with other documented cases of anterograde amnesia with hippocampal lesion. The film thus stands in stark contrast to almost all others of its kind, which stage retrograde memory loss in the absence of anterograde amnesia, a combination that is extremely rare (Poseck 2006, 127). In short, commentators have had good reasons to praise *Memento* and to underscore the psychiatric and clinical inaccuracies of most other filmic enactments of amnesia (in a completely different perspective, Hutchinson and Read 2005 analyze the picture as a Wittgensteinian "philosophical investigation").

The same commentators might be tempted to condemn the cinema's preference for retrograde amnesia as a misleading choice driven by the poignant appeal of someone's losing their entire past and having to ask "Who am I?" Yet that preference makes sense with regard to the history of memory and of notions of personal identity in Western modernity. In most movies, "memory of a 'real' past remains a defining criterion of being a 'real' person" (Marsen 2004, 144), and memory has become so much "a shorthand for identity" that, without it, "we cease to exist as who we are and become only receptors of current data" (Bowman 2004, 85, 88; see also Doniger 2005, Chap. 8). Such a perspective also dominates in both literary fiction and patients' first-person narratives (Tougaw 2012, 2016).

The idea that memory is constitutive of identity has a very long history. For Augustine (*Confessions*, Book X) in the fourth century CE, it was crucial for our relationship to the world, God and ourselves. However, only in early modernity did it become the definitory element of personhood and personal identity. Such a role of memory, which is what our movies assume and perform, largely derives from the theory John Locke proposed at the end of the seventeenth century, a theory that decisively contributed to shape the modern self. According to Locke, personal identity is purely psychological, and distinct from bodily identity. Philosophers since the eighteenth century have been responding to him, pointing out problems with the memory criterion, arguing that personal identity requires physical continuity, or defending other criteria, such as free will, interpersonal relations, or social and historical situatedness (see Perry 1975 for excerpts of essential texts). The Lockean view, however, has not ceased to frame discussions of the topic, and this applies to the movies discussed here.

As we saw in Chapter 1, Locke distinguished between the *man*, the physically embodied individual, and the *person*, who is defined by psychological features. Insofar as the continuity of memory is a constitutive feature of personal identity, the phenomenon of memory loss raises some of the most complicated challenges for the theory; in answering them, Locke gave his thinking some of its sharpest formulations. What are, for example, the consequences of irreversible amnesia? "Suppose," he wrote imagining a possible objection,

> I wholly lose the memory of some parts of my life, beyond a possibility of retrieving them, so that perhaps I shall never be conscious of them again; yet am I not the same person that did those actions, had those thoughts that I once was conscious of, though I have now forgot them? (Locke 1988 [1694], II.27.20)

To which he answered by recalling the difference between *man* and *person*. Locke explained that the word "I" in the objection should be understood as applying only to "the man"; however, because "the same man" is "presumed to be the same person, *I* is easily here supposed to stand also for the same person" (ib.,).

In the Lockean perspective, such a presumption can only be wrong. As the philosopher wrote, "if it be possible for the same man to have distinct incommunicable consciousness at different times, it is past doubt the same man would at different times make different persons." That is why human laws do not punish "the mad man for the sober man's actions, nor the sober man for what the mad man did, – thereby making them two persons" and implying that "the selfsame person was no longer in that man." In conclusion, "Absolute oblivion separates what is thus forgotten from the person, but not from the man" (ib.). It follows that, if two "incommunicable consciousnesses" acted within the same body, we would have "two persons with the same body." People, Locke noted, often forget their past actions, "and the mind many times recovers the memory of a past consciousness, which it had lost for twenty years together. Make these intervals of memory and forgetfulness to take their turns regularly by day and night, and you have two persons with the same immaterial spirit," but embodied in the same physical individual (ib., § 23).

Forgetting and the transference and manipulation of memories thus emerged in the early modern period as vital challenges to personal identity and to the continuity and authenticity of the self. Irreversible and permanent retrograde amnesia or, as Locke put it, "absolute oblivion," breaks a life in two. This rupture redefines the person. Nevertheless, since it neither deprives the subject of the general status of person nor liquidates individual personal identity, it raises the question of authenticity. Even if someone loses the feeling of ownership of their own memories, the feeling of their being continuously the same does not ipso facto vanish (Klein and Nichols 2012). Overall, psychological research has not corroborated Locke's theory, but revealed a much more complex interaction between different aspects of the self and different types of memory (Klein 2014). Contrary to what the theory seems to imply, empirical evidence about the effects of memory loss show that affected individuals retain "a first-person identity" and "a sense of self-unity and continuity" (Zahavi 2014, 60). Amnesia does not obliterate the capacity to refer to oneself. This applies even in cases of permanent retrograde amnesia, such as that of Clive Wearing, a musicologist who, struck by herpes encephalitis at age forty-seven, was left with a memory span of only seconds, and unable to remember almost anything from his past (Sacks 2007; cf. the radio documentary by Andrieu and Ciboulet 2015).

These facts about amnesia have not undermined the popularity of the Lockean theory. Film stages it in situations of retrograde amnesia, and remains loyal to the theory through the cerebralization of the memory motif that took place in the context of the late twentieth-century neuroscientific turn. A remake shows this especially well. *The Manchurian Candidate* deals with American soldiers brainwashed by their Communist captors to have false memories of their commander's behavior. In John Frankenheimer's 1962 original version, the prisoners were manipulated by means of hypnosis and behavioristic conditioning. In Jonathan Demme's 2004 remake, implanting a microchip in the brain shores up those purely psychological methods. This is in line with the technological modernization typical of remakes and revivals, which (as we noted) update the conditions of verisimilitude without necessarily adding meanings or radically modifying basic ideological assumptions or narrative lines. Miniaturized and computerized procedures give mind an unmistakably cerebral materiality. Thus, although neuro-microtechnologies and the brain fluids that some films use as memory storage are a far cry from the vivid invasive surgeries and ectobrains of earlier movies (Chapter 3), both modes of representation convey a view of the human as a cerebral subject. Underlining the centrality of memory goes hand in hand with performing it as a brain function.

Sometimes memory movies limit the presence of the brain to a passing appearance. In *Total Recall* (1990), set in the year 2084, construction worker Douglas Quaid (Arnold Schwarzenegger) has recurrent dreams about Mars, where, as far as he knows, he has never been. At a holiday agency that implants artificial memories of visits to exotic places, Quaid signs up for a vacation as a secret agent to the red planet. It turns out, however, that he actually has been a secret agent on Mars. Another personality surfaces during the procedure, and, for most of the movie, it is difficult to tell whether the events we see are "reality" or programmed memories. A video of someone identical to Quaid announces "the big surprise: you are not you, you are me."

This "me" is Hauser, an agent for Mars's dictator. They used Quaid to lead them to a rebel leader, and after the leader is killed, Hauser wants his body back. Quaid, however, manages to escape, and in the end, he contemplates the fertile landscape of a liberated Mars together with the lovely woman who also appeared in his dreams. Throughout the movie, tormented by doubts about the reality of his memories (which, a character reminds him, lie in "that black hole you call brain"), Quaid keeps looking for his "real" self without ever finding it. His leitmotif remains, "If I'm not me, who the hell am I?" Memories are definitely located in the brain; the moral message of the film is nonetheless encapsulated in the rebel leader's dictum, "A man is defined by his actions, not his memories."

Localizing Memory in the Filmic Brain

How, then, do movies localize memory in the brain? We have seen that films of the 1950s to 1970s often display garishly corporeal encephala. They can also hark back to Dr. Laurience's technology in *The Man Who Changed His Mind* (1936). Thus, in *Flash Gordon and the Brain Machine* (1955), an episode of the TV series based on the Flash Gordon comic strip, Zydereen, the evil "witch of Neptune," uses an "electronic brain recorder" to appropriate the scientific and strategic knowledge contained in the minds of two human captives from the space hero's mission. Having tied them and put in place the recording headgear, she explains, "There is an eraser ray that follows the recorder ray as it passes over every inch of your brain" (Brainfilms 6.1). As demonstrated by their responses after the procedure, the prisoners become completely amnesic.

Another way of displaying such processes involves slightly physicalized forms of mind and personality transfer. In *Magdalena's Brain* (2006), already mentioned in Chapter 3, the protagonist's husband, Arthur, is a paralyzed genius. Magdalena helps him continue his work in Artificial Intelligence with the goal of developing an artificial brain "smart enough to repair [his] mind and get [him] out of this chair." Realizing this objective involves a "memory transfer" in which Arthur's mind contents are downloaded into a bluish liquid. A small amount of the fluid is to be injected into the brain of a strong, good-looking young man who suffers from a brain tumor; once the material is "integrated," the tumor shall be removed, and Magdalena's partner will end up being a sexy body with Arthur's mind. (None of this happens, and somehow Arthur leaves his wheelchair and gets back on his feet.) Even though we are not told how the fluid encodes information, we *see* that memory is contained in a physical and ostensibly cerebral substance, and that manipulating memory amounts to handling neural matter. Doing justice to the functional complexity and the molecular or anatomo-physiological details of the neurobiology of memory would surely disrupt filmic action. Some more detail is nonetheless possible.

In *Hauser's Memory*, a 1970 TV film based on the homonymous 1968 novel by Curt Siodmak (who here rehearses a variation on his 1942 *Donovan's Brain*), Karl Helmut Hauser, a German physicist who worked for the Soviets but defected to the Americans, has been shot. As a Russian official explains, Hauser was going to give them "an intercontinental defense system years in advance of anything America has." In order to recover the information, the US government orders one Dr. Kramer (Helmut Käutner) to carry out with a human subject the "memory transfer" procedure he has been successfully developing with monkeys, and which consists in injecting an organism with another organism's brain RNA (ribonucleic acid). After Hauser dies, Kramer refuses the chosen recipient because he is a convicted criminal, and decides to inject himself. However, his faithful disciple Hillel Mondoro (David McCallum) – who carries Hauser's brain in a round tin lunch box, escorted by a CIA agent who finds it hilarious to talk about a brain "like if it was a person" – does not want his mentor to sacrifice himself. He surreptitiously injects the RNA into his left arm. Kramer notes that the knowledge therein "contained ... actually continues constructive work in the new brain." The process, however, proves painful for Hillel, who endures traumatic memories, compulsively engages in behaviors rooted in Hauser's personality, and is driven to find out all he can about the German scientist. He discovers that Hauser worked for the *Wehrmacht*, was arrested by the Gestapo for treason, and emasculated during torture. He seeks vengeance, but ends up being killed by the Nazi general who had been responsible for Hauser's mutilation.

Since injecting portions of cerebral material does not amount to transplanting the entire brain, the result is, as in the semigrafts discussed in Chapter 3, an uneasy combination of two persons. The human and filmic interest of the story lies in the performance of the protagonist's lived experience after their transformation – but this transformation itself is possible only if their entire personality is encoded in substance that can be extracted from brain tissue and passed from one organism to another. The bottom line is that persons are their memories, and memories, brain substance. Beyond its ideological import, that assertion enables elements of plot, representation and performance that go well beyond the mere claim that humans are essentially their memories in their brains, and raise other fundamental questions related to personal identity.

Personal Identity and the Authenticity of Memory

Probably the most potent of those questions, in terms of filmic action and the staging of subjectivity and intersubjectivity, concerns authenticity: What are authentic memories? Only those of events that were "really" experienced? And what does "really" here mean? How authentic would our identity be if it were constituted of invented memories? What would happen to our sense of self if we knew we were inhabited by someone else's memory? Would the very notion of "someone else" make sense? The predominant cinematographic answer to such questions makes amnesia seem more disruptive of personal identity and the sense of self than false memories. The integrity of the self largely depends on the integrity of memory; memory lost is more problematic than memory received. We shall return to this in more detail when discussing *Dark City*.

In *Blade Runner* (1982), Rachel, a genetically manufactured "replicant," is fitted with long-term implanted memories that go back to childhood. That those memories are someone else's does not make them any less significant for her sense of self. On the contrary, the psychological continuity between the alien memories and her own coalesce into one personality. In this connection, *Johnny Mnemonic* (1995), a movie that has been considered the first cyberthriller (Springer 1999), illustrates the prodigious existential significance of childhood as memory-in-the-brain. As a "mnemonic courier," Johnny Smith (Keanu Reeves) has "to dump a chunk of long-term memory" – his childhood – to make room for data he will carry in a brain implant. He later wants to recover that memory. In order to pay for the necessary surgery, he agrees to transport in his "wet-wired" implant a dangerously large amount of information about the treatment of a "nerve attenuation syndrome" that has become pandemic. In addition to the gangs who want to seize the information for profit, there are rebels who wish to make it freely available to all. However, when it turns out that the memory-retrieval surgery cannot take place, Johnny is told, "the only way left is to hack your own brain." When he finally enters the virtual reality of his implant, its contents are broadcast worldwide on screens; the information about the treatment of the pandemic is thereby made public, and joyous crowds celebrate the rebellion's victory to the tune of appropriately soaring music. Thanks to the freed brain space, Johnny relives his blissful childhood memories, and this recovery of identity opens the way for a happy end (Brainfilms 6.2). Oblivion amounts to a paradise lost; remembering, to a paradise regained.

Johnny Mnemonic presupposes that memory is a collection of fixed data items that can be stored and recovered. Such a view has been contested by cognitive neuroscience (see, e.g., Eichenbaum 2012), which investigates the mechanisms of neural plasticity that may underlie memory, explains that long-term memories do not reside in singular locations but in dynamic neural connections, and describes how different brain systems process different types of memory. At the same time, like most movies of its kind, *Johnny Mnemonic* highlights the well-established link between memory and emotion. Research has long shown that emotion may enhance memory (though emotional memories are not more accurate in their details than non-emotional ones); that emotional arousal increases the likelihood of memory consolidation (though amnesia can also occur for emotionally charged events); that autobiographical memories of events experienced as emotional are more vivid than those of experientially neutral events; and that, in short, emotion plays a crucial role in encoding and retrieval (Buchanan 2007; Kensinger and Kark 2018; Phelps and Sharot 2008).

In *Johnny Mnemonic*, existentially vital, self-constituting memories correspond to "real events." In many other movies, precisely those that most overtly evoke the problem of radical skepticism, the challenge that prompts both action and discourse boils down, as philosopher Alain Badiou (2013, 199) put it, to "finding a discriminating procedure, from within a regime of appearing ..., between what is real and what is only a semblance of the real." In *Brainstorm* (1983), for example, a company has developed a machine that records sensory and mental experiences directly from people's brains and plays them into other individuals' brains. The experiences are stored and retrieved as scenes filmed through the experiencing subject's eyes. The sensory and mental videotapes register not only good sex and other fun activities, but also fear, early trauma, nightmares, physical pain, anxiety, psychosis, and even someone's death. All these events are endured or enjoyed with the full intensity of the real. In David Cronenberg's *eXistenZ* (1999), the virtual reality game that goes by that name (an instance of Badiou's "regime of appearing") is played directly into the players' nervous system. It thus abolishes, once again, the distinction between the "virtual" and the "real." As Cronenberg himself explained, for him, "reality is neurology" and, therefore, "meditation on the brain and nervous system" is "meditation on reality" (Wallace 2014). (The movie generated considerable philosophical commentary – for example Beard 2006, Chap. 14; and Pritchard 2012 – but not as much as *The Matrix*, which was launched a few weeks earlier, and to which we return below.)

Released two decades after *Brainstorm*, *The Final Cut* (2004) does not radically innovate in its tropes and technologies, but moves the paradox of skepticism to a brainmind realm involving no games or experience swaps. The story takes place in a world where microchips called "Zoe [i.e., life] implants" record every moment of a person's life, again filmed in subjective camera. After that person's death, the Zoe footage can be "cut" as an individual "rememory" to show the best moments in the life of the deceased. The hero of *Final Cut* is the cutter Alan Hakman (Robin Williams), whose lifelong misery results from the guilt he feels for the death of a childhood playmate. One day, he recognizes his early friend as a grownup in someone's rememory and decides to track him down. After Hakman discovers that his memory of the traumatizing event was false, viewing his own recording leads to a climactic moment of catharsis.

Hakman's story raises the question of whether and how a false memory can constitute a subject's "truth." Whatever the nuances of their answers, movies tend to imply that personal identity requires a repertoire, stored in discrete brain locations, of long-term eidetic or "photographic" episodic memories of autobiographical events. This position, more evocative of the memory palaces of the late Renaissance than of the chemical pathways of modern neuroscience, has the distinct advantage of being eminently representable. A conceptualization of the mind that emphasizes experience and interaction with objects, persons, and situations is far more translatable into fiction film than a focus on the synaptic cleft (this can work briefly, as in the awesome 90-second visual-effects opening sequence of *Fight Club* [1990]). In his pioneering work *The Photoplay: A Psychological Study* (2002 [1916]), Harvard psychologist Hugo Münsterberg examined film's capacity to "objectify" the functioning of the human mind, and saw in the various ways of framing, shooting, and editing an "objectification" of mental faculties and mechanisms. Thus, in his view, the close-up objectifies attention; the flashback, remembering; the combination of flashbacks with "forward glances" (equivalent to expectation and imagination) enacts the ways past and future become mentally "intertwined" with the present. (While *flashback* denotes both a narrative technique and a psychological phenomenon, Münsterberg's term *cutback* emphasizes instead the editing procedure. The more usual term for *forward glance* is *flashforward*.) We do not need to agree with the theory according to which cinema follows the same laws as the mind to see that, if these laws are to be cinematically performed, the filmic mind must be portrayed as though consistent with the constraints and possibilities of filmmaking.

At the same time, it is obvious that psychological processes can be given many different filmic forms. We have already mentioned how *Memento* goes beyond flashbacks and flashforwards to capture the experience of time and memory. A more conventional example is offered by *Final Cut*'s displaying the past in black-and-white monochromes. The relevant sequences exhibit two contrasting versions of the traumatizing childhood episode: the first one shows Hakman's memory and how he believes things happened; the second, his Zoe implant footage, filmed in subjective camera. The fact that the *subjective* camera is meant to give us the *objective* picture of events raises the question of what exactly makes up a human memory, and what the conditions of memorial authenticity might be.

The reconstructive, malleable, and manipulable nature of memory has been the object of outstanding research since Frederick Bartlett's 1932 *Remembering*, and of virulent discussions during the "false memories" controversy of the 1990s (Loftus and Ketcham 1994). With films such as Akira Kurosawa's *Rashomon* (1950), Alain Resnais's *Hiroshima mon amour* (1959) and Chris Marker's *Sans Soleil* (1983), or with the entire œuvre of Andrei Tarkovsky – who defined the filmmaker's work as "sculpting in time," and time and memory as "the two sides of a medal" (Tarkovsky 1986, 63, 57) – cinema has explored memory in many creative and profound ways. In particular, it has shown how memory engages not only remembering, but also forgetting and transformation, not only the past, but also the present and the future. The narrator in *Sans Soleil* encapsulates a conceptual and emotional understanding that is common to many movies when she says: "I will have spent my life trying to understand the function of remembering, which is not the opposite of forgetting, but rather its lining. We do not remember. We rewrite memory much as history is rewritten. How can one remember thirst?"

Despite the ideological and filmic significance of their cerebral motifs and cerebralizing principles, brain-and-memory movies are not visually focused on the brain as organ of flesh. Rather, they display it only indirectly, for example as implants, procedures, or scans on computer screens. Though omnipresent, the brain is less an agent than a medium. In *Strange Days* (1995), which combines sci-fi, noir, and cyberpunk, the protagonist deals in illegal recordings of experiences made directly from the cerebral cortex, allowing future viewers to live those experiences as if they were their own. The resulting footage includes the entire experience as mediated by the brain and filmed as POV scenes. Since the experience is transmitted and relived as the same POV scenes, the subjective camera in effect transfers a fixed memory from cortex to cortex without distortion. *Brainstorm* stages a similar procedure; *Final Cut*'s Zoe implants are in the brain; *Johnny Mnemonic*'s protagonist recovers his childhood memory only by hacking his brain; the *Strange Days* devices record from one brain and deliver to another; and, as we shall see, in *Dark City*, memories are engineered by manipulating a cerebral fluid.

Like the neurosciences, motion pictures proclaim that memories are brain mechanisms and that experiences have neural correlates; and yet, giving meaning to those mechanisms and correlates requires placing psychological experience and subjective and intersubjective processes center stage. Thus *Memento*, though hailed as being "close to a perfect exploration of the neurobiology of memory" (Sternberg 2001), in fact reduces neurobiology to Lenny's distressing awareness that he suffers from a brain disorder. As far as Lenny's identity is concerned, it inscribes his memories in his "extended mind," that is, *outside* his damaged brain (Clark 2010), and predicates his authentic self "on a willed decision to create and incorporate only truthful representations of experience" (LaRocca 2017, 187). The movie is more of a philosophical than a neuroscientific fiction – one, it has been argued, that "tests" Locke's theory of personal identity, and "asks us to abandon the notion that personal identity is transitive [and] that our memories must be true" (Smith 2007, 38).

Erasing Memories

Neither experiences nor memories are intrinsically traumatic, or traumatic for everyone in the same way and with the same consequences. Moreover, memories are not Zoe recordings. Rather, it is likely that they are not merely consolidated *together with* a certain emotion, but also shaped by the affect itself. While finding out the truth may be a worthwhile endeavor, the fact that (in *Final Cut*) Alan's existence is marked by a false memory does not make *him* any less authentic. The veracity of memory does not coincide with the authenticity of self. Doug in *Total Recall*, the manipulated humans in *Dark City*, or even the *Blade Runner* replicants are no less authentic because they have false memories. Debates about "therapeutic forgetting" or "memory dampening" have raised this issue within the neurocultural world.

Much of the relevant research derives from animal studies. Conditioning the laboratory rat is the most commonly used experimental paradigm for studying memory. The predominant approach is that of "classical" or "respondent" conditioning, also known as "Pavlovian" after the Russian physiologist Ivan Pavlov (1849–1936). An innate, "unconditioned response" to an "unconditioned stimulus" (in Pavlov's classic experiments, a dog salivating in response to the presentation of food) becomes the "conditioned response" to an initially neutral "conditioned stimulus" (e.g., a sound). The dog involuntarily "learns" to salivate in response to the sound. Another paradigm is that of "operant" or "instrumental" conditioning, in which a behavior is followed by various forms of "reinforcement" or "punishment," thus leading to an increase or decrease in its frequency. Psychologists and neuroscientists use variations of these paradigms, especially the classical, and experimentally treat memory formation as the involuntary learning of a behavior by means of conditioning.

About 2000, neuroscientists revived a minority opinion among researchers of the 1960s and 1970s, according to which a temporally graded retrograde amnesia could be obtained in rodents for a memory that was reactivated or retrieved just before the amnestic procedure (Sara 2000). Research with laboratory rats subjected to Pavlovian fear conditioning has suggested that, when reactivated, memories become labile and must undergo "reconsolidation," a process involving protein synthesis (Nader, Schafe and LeDoux 2000). However, if protein production is inhibited immediately after the memory is reactivated, then the memory is lost (Debiec, LeDoux and Nader 2002). Thus, after memory retrieval, activating the production of a certain protein in the amygdala enhances reconsolidation and strengthens an established fearful memory, whereas inhibiting its production impairs reconsolidation (Tronson et al. 2006). The fact that disrupting reconsolidation appears to erase "initial encoded plasticity" (e.g., the association between a musical tone and an electric shock) may "lend some validity for therapeutic use of agents that disrupt reconsolidation to reduce the fear-arousing aspects of emotional memory in posttraumatic stress disorder [PTSD]" (Doyère et al. 2007). Neuroscientists at the time debated whether reconsolidation is universal, how it works, and what its clinical applications might be (Dudai 2004, 2006; Dudai and Eisenberg 2004).

The discussion took a new direction in 2007, with the discovery that inhibiting a certain enzyme in the cortex of the laboratory rat results in the erasure of long-term associative memories. Since no reactivation is needed to render the memory trace susceptible to the inhibitor, the persistence of memory seems to depend on the ongoing activity of the enzyme after the memory is regarded as consolidated into a long-term stable form (Shema, Sacktor and Dudai 2007; Shema et al. 2009). The Israeli neuroscientist Yadin Dudai, one of the authors of the discovery, remarked that the therapeutic goal "is to erase not necessarily a single complete chunk of memory but ... to blunt or erase the extremely annoying emotional burden of the traumatic experience" (Abi-Rached 2009, 85).

Medical interventions would thus aim to "dull" or "dampen," rather than to delete. This is also the case in connection with findings about extinction training in humans. When a stimulus already associated with a mild but painful electric shock is presented again to the experimental subject during the "reconsolidation window" in the absence of the shock, the "fear memory" is durably expunged (Schiller et al. 2010; Quirk and Milad 2010). The fear associated with a stimulus can thus be "edited out," but that does not eliminate the subject's recollection of the stimulus itself, or (if we were not dealing with only skin conductance response as a fear indicator) the fact of having been afraid of it at some point (for recent reviews of PTSD, especially in connection with reconsolidation mechanisms, see Abdallah et al. 2019; Pineles and Orr 2018; on reconsolidation itself, Lee, Nader and Schiller 2017).

Yet, in a telling instance of how movies become part of the technoscientific imaginary, research on reconsolidation has been often associated with *Eternal Sunshine of the Spotless Mind* (2004), where two former lovers, Joel and Clementine, have their memories of each other erased. In *Eternal Sunshine*, the magazine *Forbes* reported, "A scientist asks you to recall a memory, gives you a pill and alters your recollection. It sounds like a scene from the 2004 film *Eternal Sunshine*. … But it's exactly what McGill neuroscientist Karim Nader is doing with folks who suffer from post-traumatic stress disorder" (Eaves 2007). Nader is the first author of the *Nature* article on fear memories that revived the notion of reconsolidation (Nader, Schafe and LeDoux, 2000). In light of his research, declared the *McGill Daily*, "science fiction proves to be more science than fiction" (Aiello 2006). Similarly, in connection with the success of neurobiologist Joseph LeDoux's team in preventing the transfer of a fearful memory from short- to long-term storage in rats (Doyère et al. 2007), a neurophilosophy blog asserted, "the ability to erase memories is no longer restricted to Hollywood script-writers" (Costandi 2007). A commentary in the *Washington Post* proved more skeptical, and criticized *Eternal Sunshine* for taking the notion of therapeutic forgetting "to science fiction extremes" (Stein 2004). Indeed, as psychologist John Seamon (2015, 62) pointed out, memory loss affects "large chunks of time," not, as in *Eternal Sunshine*, only those related to a circumscribed context (in the movie, memories associated with a former lover). The attraction of film as reference point in this field remains nonetheless as strong as ever. For instance, in their 2019 research literature review "Memory editing from science fiction to clinical practice," emotion specialists Elizabeth Phelps and Stefan G. Hofmann open with *Eternal Sunshine*, allude to film throughout their article, and conclude that, although techniques to edit unique human memories are likely to be developed, "just like in the movies, we may find that if we succeed …, there will be unexpected consequence for how we think about memory and its role in defining who we are" (Phelps and Hofmann 2019, 49).

Commentators' emphasis on memory erasure may be symptomatic of neurocultural obsessions and neuroscientific wishful thinking, but overlooks one of the picture's crucial features. As we shall see below, erasure is of course essential to *Eternal Sunshine* – but chiefly because both the narrative and the filmic textures are driven by its *failure*. Joel's main resistance against having his memories erased implies the belief that they can be irreversibly deleted. In contrast, movies dealing with amnesia tend to make the opposite assumption, namely that memories are never totally lost. Thus, in *Johnny Mnemonic*, where the erasure is voluntary, the memory of the protagonist's childhood is entirely retrievable. In other cases of premeditated memory loss, traces remain operational. *Eternal Sunshine* opens with Joel impulsively taking the train to the forgotten place where he first met Clementine. In *Paycheck* (2003), inspired (like *Total Recall*) by the American science fiction writer Philip K. Dick, a reverse-engineer agrees to have erased from his memory the three years it took him to crack the design of a machine to see into the future. When he attempts to claim the millions owed him, he discovers that he has signed away the money, and in exchange receives an envelope with miscellaneous everyday objects. Presumably thanks to his work, he unknowingly knew that those things could help him escape from the killers who would chase him. Thus, even after memory erasure, unconscious traces of his past life served him well.

In *The Bourne Identity* (2002), Jason Bourne (Matt Damon) is a spy whom his bosses want to eliminate. He has no idea of who he is or why he is being hunted down. Amnesia, however, does not prevent him from putting his linguistic, lethal, and other secret-agent skills into high gear while he crisscrosses Europe evading assassination attempts and searching for his identity. The protagonist is the killing-machine avatar of David Webb, who, in the television adaptation of the original novel (*The Bourne Identity*, 1988), possessed the same skills, but had, in addition, undergone plastic surgery, remembered episodes from the days before the onset of amnesia, and hoped to "put the pieces back together, some of them at least." In the third and final Bourne movie (*The Bourne Ultimatum*, 2007), the hero, when not involved in chases and fights, experiences flashbacks that reveal the causes of his condition in the "behavior modification" program that transformed Webb into Bourne. After "three years trying to find out who I am," he remembers – and ceases, from his own point of view, to be Jason Bourne. Recovering true memories coincides with regaining true identity. In the meantime, there is often not much about their past that the amnesic heroes can put into words (declarative memory), but their implicit memory, especially procedural, is efficient enough to drive much of the action.

Whereas the pathological condition of *Memento*'s Lenny results from injuries, and Bourne's amnesia from manipulation, the protagonist of *Sé quién eres* (*I Know Who You Are*, 2000) combines two etiologies. Mario (Miguel Ángel Solá) is said to suffer since 1980 from alcohol-related Korsakoff's syndrome, an amnestic disorder. His psychiatrist, Paloma (Ana Fernández), discovers that Mario's retrograde amnesia actually began in 1977. Hypothesizing that he became an alcoholic due to a traumatic event he unconsciously "prefers to erase from his memory," she researches his past and gives him methylphenidate, a psychostimulant widely used under the trade name Ritalin for attention-deficit hyperactivity disorder. After discovering the truth, she makes Mario remember that event: hired by right-wing Spanish generals to assassinate one of their pro-democracy colleagues, he also killed the victim's small daughters, and one of them died before his eyes. In the end, Mario recovers his past and forms new memories. Thus the retrieval of repressed memories goes hand in hand with the recovery from anterograde amnesia to mend the protagonist's personal identity and reinstate possibilities for a future life. The more detailed analysis of two pictures will illustrate how, through plots and visuals dealing with memories lost, given and regained, cinema can deal with issues of authenticity, mind, body and brain as they are raised in connection with personal identity.

Eternal Sunshine of the Spotless Mind (2004)

Eternal Sunshine of the Spotless Mind (2004; Butler 2018) deserves to be singled out among the "memory, self, and brain" movies produced in the context of the global neuroscientific turn. The movie, about a man's struggle to retain the romantic memories he has initially chosen to erase, has been described as a romantic thriller, as a celebration of love and the possibilities of a second chance that uses the premises of the genre Stanley Cavell dubbed "comedy of remarriage" in order to "chart the convolutions of the human brain in the throes of breakup and reconciliation" (Edelstein 2004). It has also been analyzed as an exploration of the nature of authentic mourning (Carel 2007), of the process of losing and recovering identity (Hill-Parks 2006), or of the insufficiencies of the classical utilitarian perspective (Grau 2006; Terrone 2017 discusses the remarriage vs. utilitarianism interpretations). Various idioms and concepts have been used to elucidate its complex, dislocated aesthetic from the point of view of cinematic style and form. For example, *Eternal Sunshine* has been considered exemplary of "atemporal cinema," a filmic style characterized by narrative structures that defy linear chronology even though the diegesis does not require such manipulations. Atemporal cinema "does not distort forward-moving time simply because of the demands of story," as is sometimes the case of science fiction; rather, the warping of time emerges from the way the story is told, rather than from its contents (McGowan 2011, 8). The temporal confusion spectators feel as a result – as is potently the case with *Eternal Sunshine* – is said to introduce them to "a way of experiencing existence outside of our usual conception of time" (ib., 10, and Chap. 3 on *Eternal Sunshine*). In an interpretation that again emphasizes narrative structure and visual strategies, Gondry's picture appears as an instance of "puzzle films," that is, motion pictures that reject classical storytelling techniques, "break the boundaries of the classical, unified mimetic plot," and replace them with complex storytelling (Buckland 2009a, 5).

Within such a framework, *Eternal Sunshine*, like *Memento* and *Dark City*, appears as an instance of what Thomas Elsaesser has called the "mind-game film," which delights "in disorienting or misleading spectators" (Elsaesser 2009, 15). Such pictures proceed by potentiating a feature that is both unique to and constitutive of the cinema, namely that "film images can simultaneously happen in multiple universes or oscillate between different kinds of time frames and reality levels" (Elsaesser and Hagener 2015, 175). Despite their great diversity, mind-game stories "abandon the notion of one reliable, absolute reality, mostly by presenting a non-actual story world such as a future scenario (sci-fi) or by narrating themselves through the perception of a distorted protagonist (psychological delusion/ghost story)"; within that paradigm, "memory anxiety" constitutes a distinctive concern (Hesselberth and Schuster 2008, 96, 97). Describing the means of visually obtaining the desired mind-game effects, Ellen Kuras, *Eternal Sunshine*'s director of photography, remarks that "[m]uch of the syntax of the dramatic action leads you to believe that you're in a memory, or a memory of a memory, but the reality of where you are in time and space is not exactly clear" (Pavlus 2004). Protagonists' inner experience is thus at the center of the ontological quandaries read into the movie, which thus also appears as an exemplar of "subjective realist multiform narrative" (Campora 2014, 112, and Chap. 6 on *Eternal Sunshine*). With regard to its use of sound and its overall structure and stylistic configuration, *Eternal Sunshine* draws largely from the aesthetics of music video (Vernallis 2013).

As far as offscreen culture is concerned, *Eternal Sunshine* has been said to typify "the contemporary interest in identity, memory, trauma, and twisted or looped temporal structures" (Elsaesser and Hagener 2015, 169). Scholars have explored how *Eternal Sunshine* manifests such "interest, and explores a range of philosophical, psychological and moral issues (Grau 2009). Yet, even though the concern for memory and identity has been intimately tied to the *neuro* since at least the 1990s, the role of the brain in the movie has not been the object of specific commentary. José van Dijck (2009, 168) argues that, beyond embodying the notion that "memory is not simply triggered by objects," but happens through them – so much so that "brain, mind, technology, and materiality are inextricably intertwined in producing and revising a coherent picture of one's past" – the movie performs the idea that memories "are also mediated by the socio-cultural practices and forms through which they manifest themselves." She connects that insight to the observation that the picture appears in more than one respect "in sync with current understandings of how the brain forms memories" (ib., 162). It remains, however, to ask how *Eternal Sunshine* performs the brain. Like *Memento*, it is said to manifest such a keen awareness of recent neuroscience and memory research, as well as of "the role of the media and their input in the formation of memory discourse," that both movies "can be read as fictional realizations of scientific reconsiderations" (Nungesser 2009, 31).

This is believed to apply in particular to the unreliability of remembering and the fact that memories can be reshaped when activated. At the same time, by means of plot, dialogue, and other properly cinematic means, *Eternal Sunshine* interrogates the ascendancy of the *neuro* and the view of the human as cerebral subject to which it may seem to adhere. Indeed, as has been aptly pointed out, one of the rewarding features of the movie is that it contains "almost no dialogue that sounds like actual neuroscience" (Johnson 2004). This is consistent with the observation that, whereas earlier pictures such as *Blade Runner* (1982), *Total Recall* (1990), or *Dark City* (1998) dealt with the subjectivity of memory and issues of loss, forgetting, and nostalgia while remaining centrally interested in the technological manipulation of memory, *Eternal Sunshine* and other pictures of the early 2000s give less importance to technology, are more preoccupied with blurring the distinction between remembering and forgetting, and tend to forgo typical science fiction aesthetics (Teo 2013).

The German rendering of the cryptic original title is admirably well found. *Vergiß mein nicht!* evokes a pretty, small bright blue spring flower called *Vergissmeinnicht*. The flower is known in many languages by similar terms (e.g., in Spanish *nomeolvides*, in English *forget-me-not*); the supposedly romantic French has no equivalent, and calls it by its genus, *myosotis*. In the Middle Ages, it was thought to have the power of ensuring that those who wore it would not be forgotten by their lovers; one legend derives its name from a drowning knight's call to his lady. By breaking *Vergissmeinnicht* into separate words and giving it the form of an imploration ("Don't forget me!"), the German title refers to the core themes of the film, further evoked by the associations of *myosotis* with loss, remembrance, and the physical end and emotional continuance of love. It also underlines the connection between psychological memory acts and a concrete, if fragile, object – something that in the film will be significant. In short, while the crassly prosaic Italian *Se mi lasci ti cancello* ("If you leave me, I erase you") could be the title of a second-rate slapstick comedy, and the similar-sounding Spanish *¡Olvídate de mí!* ("Forget me!") says exactly the opposite of what it should, the title *Vergiß mein nicht!* is a perfect adaptation of the original title.

Directed by Michel Gondry, initially a successful creator of commercials and video clips, and written by Charlie Kaufman, who authored the screenplay of *Being John Malkovich* (1999), *Eternal Sunshine* illustrates the "maze cinema" style, where the narration begins at the end and meanders toward the point of departure, as well as a device close to the "mindscreen" narrative technique that displays on screen the contents of a character's mind. While the term designates a "visual (and at times aural) field that presents itself as the product of a mind" (Kawin 1978, xi), *Eternal Sunshine* uses something like it to perform psychological processes that are presented as happening inside the brain.

The story, for which Kaufman won an Oscar in the category of original screenplay, evolves fluidly in different times and reality dimensions, moving non-linearly across past, future, and present, abruptly changing perspectives and viewpoints, casting about various sequences and instants of existence, and shifting without transition between parallel "external" and "internal" realities. To tell the story, Gondry favored editing, voice-over, light, focus, and the movement of a handheld camera over special effects. He thus produced a visually compelling, though labyrinthine and sometimes redundant film.

Joel Barish (Jim Carrey) discovers that his ex-girlfriend, the temperamental Clementine "Clem" Kruczynski (Kate Winslet), has had him and their failed relationship erased from her memory. Enraged, he decides to undergo the same procedure at Lacuna Inc., the enterprise where Dr. Howard Mierzwiak (Tom Wilkinson) carries out the "focused erasure" of troubling memories. The resulting lacunas – empty memory spots – are obtained by means of a surgical procedure. The first step consists of Joel's telling Mierzwiak about Clem and their relationship in detail; the conversation is taped. The second step, crucial in the procedure, confronts Joel with memorabilia he has been asked to bring to Lacuna. With his head in a scanner, Joel is shown the objects one by one; since refraining from verbalizing produces a better "emotional readout," he is instructed to react to them only mentally. Indeed, as Dr. Mierzwiak explains, "There is an emotional core to each of our memories. As we eradicate this core, it starts its degradation process." The process enables the "mapping" of each object-related memory in the brain. In images that resemble computerized tomographies, the brain is shown as a close-up of a computer screen; memory locations appear as green spots (Brainfilms 6.3).

With the finished map stored in a computer, the awkward Lacuna technicians Stan (Mark Ruffalo) and Patrick (Elijah Wood) join Joel for the night in his apartment. They connect his head to his laptop thanks to the usual helmet, and sedate him. Working from a laptop computer, Stan targets the memories, starting with the most recent ones, and destroys the corresponding brain tissue. If all goes well, the subject wakes up having "emptied his life" of the ex-beloved. Beyond the most recent bad memories, however, Joel, who is lying inert on his bed, no longer wants to let go of Clementine. We then enter into his neuropsychological world, and see him trying to run away from the procedure. Joel even pleads, "Mierzwiak, please let me keep this memory. Just this one." Or: "I wanna call it off. ... I don't want this anymore!" Of course, since these demands are unconscious wishes staged as mindscreen, nobody can hear them.

Joel's revolt takes the form of visually striking scenes that combine episodes of the past, moments of classically cinematic action (good guys chased by bad ones) and, finally, Clem's disappearance or the memory's disintegration. For example: Joel and Clem break into an empty beach house, and as the recollection is targeted, the house collapses; or they are in a bookstore, and as the memory is deleted, the names of the book sections fade, the books turn to empty pages, and the image blurs; or they sit in a car watching a movie, rush out of the car just as it vanishes, and run past a fence, trying to go faster than the disappearing planks. Always in Joel's brainmind, Clem asks him to find a place where there are no memories of her; they end up in his childhood. In an overstated scene, Joel, dressed in a child's pajamas, hides under a giant kitchen table. Clem, as a babysitter with minidress and white boots, tells him "it's working." "Look," she says in baby talk, "we're hidden." In the end, however, the childhood house also crumbles. Before the last memory is wiped out, Clem tells Joel to meet her again at the place of their first encounter. The film actually begins with Joel's waking up after the erasure night, and impulsively going there.

Joel's attempts at escaping take place while Stan has put the computer on automatic pilot; in the meantime, he and Mierzwiak's cute assistant Mary Svevo (Kirsten Dunst) are getting drunk and stoned, dancing around and having sex. (Mary's family name is too obviously meaningful: Italo

Svevo's 1923 novel *Zeno's Conscience* consists of the life-report a man has written for his psychoanalyst, who hoped it would be a "good prelude" to the treatment.) Suddenly, however, when Joel and Clem hide in his childhood, Joel goes "off the map." While Mierzwiak is trying to find him, Mary recites "inspirational" quotations. One gives the film its title:

> How happy is the blameless vestal's lot!
> The world forgetting, by the world forgot.
> Eternal sunshine of the spotless mind!
> Each prayer accepted, and each wish resigned.

These are lines 207–210 of Alexander Pope's *Eloisa to Abelard*, written in 1716. Eloisa contrasts her own fate – a nun after having been separated from Abelard, now castrated and a monk – with that of the cloistered virgins who, lacking an earthly love to remember, do not suffer from "hopeless, lasting flames" (line 261).

Mierzwiak finds the quotation "lovely"; Mary replies, "I just thought it'd be appropriate, maybe." She then kisses him, confessing she has loved him "for a very long time," and becoming immediately upset. As Mierzwiak consoles her, his wife Hollis arrives, and informs Mary that she has "already had him." Mierzwiak is then forced to explain that he and Mary "have a history," but that it has been erased. Indeed, Mary has totally forgotten their relationship, and does not even know it was deleted from her brain. Yet, like Eloisa's lasting flames, her love persists (albeit unconsciously), and when it reawakens, she feels it has lasted a long time. Back at Lacuna, listening to the tape of her pre-erasure narrative fills Mary with sadness and indignation. She then returns to the patients the tapes of their own narratives, thus leading Joel and Clem, after their post-erasure re-encounter, to face what each had said about the other – and stay together nonetheless.

The processes that lead to the film's opening scene, in which Joel wakes up after the erasure night and automatically takes the train to the place where he had met Clem, are explicitly located in Joel's brain and involve the surgical destruction of chosen neurons. At the same time, they are unmistakably mental, and unconscious. Both the performed actions and the means of representation realize some of the features, such as exemption from mutual contradiction, timelessness or the substitution of psychic for external reality, which Sigmund Freud (1915, § V) attributed to the mechanisms of the "system Ucs," and which mind-game films often seem intent on performing.

As we saw, however, movies assume that your having memories of a "real" past tends to be the main criterion of your being "really" who you are. In *Eternal Sunshine*, filling in memory lacunae may drive characters to mend a loss. By the same token, the eliminated information can be misused. Lacuna technician Patrick (Elijah Wood), a pathetic loser who desperately wants a girlfriend, attracts Clem with Joel's mementoes and narrative. In mindscreen, Joel complains, "He's stealing my identity. He stole my stuff. He's seducing my girlfriend with my words and my things." Robbing somebody of their identity requires nothing more than appropriating their memories. For all the materiality of the objects and actions that sustain such psychic robbery, Patrick does not need to have Joel's body as long as he can use Joel's memories. This conveys, in a manipulative mode, the Lockean theory of personal identity as the default position most spectators are presumed to recognize and accept. The cinema performs this presumption as a core narrative and visual element. Nevertheless, beginning with the fact that films stage embodied characters, they perform selves as being not only memories, but also bodies. The question is: which body makes up the self?

In *Eternal Sunshine*, Patrick's stealing Joel's memories seems to declare the irrelevance of the body. Having Joel's memories is enough to lure Clem. Now, these memories can be removed only from a specific organ of the body: the brain. "Brain scan" and "brain damage" are among the film's plot keywords. Reviewers, however, have paid no attention to its brain elements beyond chuckling at the helmets Lacuna places on its clients' heads, or amusedly quoting Mierzwiak's explanation that memory erasure amounts to "brain damage" but isn't worse than a night of heavy drinking. Brain-related moments and items seem to be no more than entertaining extras, maybe a nod to the neuroscientific turn.

This is in a sense understandable. Although a few scenes of *Eternal Sunshine* include some of the customary visuals of science fiction, the film does not belong to the genre. The Lacuna procedure is perhaps futuristic, but the helmets are spoofy, the computer and imaging equipment low-tech, the company's facilities ridiculously shabby, and the erasing sequence largely farcical. The paucity of special effects and the undercutting of technology through parody belong to the spirit of the movie. Charlie Kaufmann claimed, "The idea that there is a memory-erasing machine – I'm so uninterested in that, you know. I feel like such a Hollywood screenwriter 'cause that's in there" (Feld 2004, 139). *That*, however, is not merely a gimmick. "Hollywood" must have assumed that the technology would appeal to spectators, that brain scans would be familiar to them, that they would readily accept the memory theory of personal identity, and that they would find it natural that, to erase particular memories, you must destroy the appropriate areas of brain tissue. To that extent, and in spite of the place it gives to mindscreen, *Eternal Sunshine* participates in the cerebralization of the psyche.

The movie juxtaposes the story of the two-year relationship between Joel and Clem, mainly mindscreened during the night in which the second story (the erasure and Joel's escape) takes place. The second story drives the film and provides the foundation for its structure and visual choices; and what happens in it physically takes place in the brain. Memories are localized in it on the basis of activity recorded by a scanner. Memory maps look like computerized tomographies. Erasure implies damaging the brain. Stan realizes that Joel is "off the map" by looking at brain images. As for Joel, he may be driven by will and desire, but his hiding places are brain locations, and the escape scenes are figurative performances of non-visual neuropsychological processes. Joel locates himself in there: "I'm in my bed," he says, "I know it. I'm in my brain." In short, mindscreen is brainscreen. The sequence of Joel's capture makes that perfectly clear. After closing up on Joel's brain as displayed on Mierzwiak's laptop, the camera moves to Joel on his bed, wearing the erasure helmet. It then cuts to a mindscreen scene in which Joel hides with Clem in a foam bath in the sink of his mother's kitchen. Back in Joel's room, Mierzwiak zooms on the brain image so that it shows in red the spot he is trying to locate; he presses a button, and the cluster is eliminated. The camera then cuts back to Joel's mother kitchen where, upon erasure, the happy couple literally goes down the drain. Again in Joel's room, the coordinates on Howard's laptop glide to a new target: "OK," he says, "we're back in" (Brainfilms 6.4). By rapidly juxtaposing a brain scan, with Joel, with a mindscreen scene, and again with a brain scan, *Eternal Sunshine* makes a powerful statement about neurobiological causality, merging the subject's active unconscious, as he lies in bed, with the brain that is being manipulated.

Joel's assertion "I'm in my brain" expresses his temporarily locked-in condition. Yet he is not captive of his brain as a Platonic soul is imprisoned in a body. His resistance to the procedure challenges the power of neurotechnology, and seems to question the reducibility of personhood to brainhood. At the same time, the movie does not deny the ideology of the cerebral subject outright. Many films dealing with life science technologies demonstrate a similar ambivalence. In one of the most famous, *Gattaca* (1997), the main character has been naturally conceived, and that excludes him from a society that privileges genetically engineered individuals. Instead of revolting, he doctors his body in the pursuit of goals that only those individuals may achieve. In *Eternal Sunshine*, Joel does not break with the system – though not because he does not want to, but because his escape from memory erasure is necessarily confined to his brain. His flight is a frantic race in a maze of neural networks, and only within that space can he try to renegotiate his contract with Lacuna.

How *Eternal Sunshine of the Spotless Mind* performs that ambivalence, that capacity of film to stage different viewpoints without seeking to reconcile them, turns it into a particularly subtle production in the context of films rehearsing memory, brain, and identity. On the one hand, to the extent that it adheres to a memory theory of personal identity and foregrounds the cerebral localization of memories, it admits that humans are essentially their brains. As we saw, in *Eternal Sunshine*, mindscreen is brainscreen, and happiness can be partly pursued by intervening directly on neural tissue. On the other hand, the film variously nuances the brainhood assumptions it conveys. Some details are no more than passing, and probably unintentional hints. Although the procedure assumes a narrow localizationism, some of the neuroimages that appear on Lacuna's computer screens suggest that memories are interrelated or that each each one involves the simultaneous activation of several regions. More importantly, the mapping of memories requires self-narrative, concrete objects, and an emotional response, thus subordinating technology to lived experience. Besides, in the presence of the forgotten beloved, the person's reactions show that love survives amnesia; the fact that this is a filmic cliché does not weaken its meaning or its function in the plot. Finally, there are considerable stylistic differences in the way *Eternal Sunshine* treats the erasure procedure and Joel's brainmind reality. Neurotechnology, including the scanners, computers, and helmets, as well as the Lacuna office and technicians, are depicted in a satirical mode, and the time-honored evil mad scientist has metamorphosed into the gentle Dr. Mierzwiak. The most inventive, if often overdone, use of filmic resources is reserved for mindscreening Joel's frantic flight from neurotechnology.

Insofar as both styles are employed, *Eternal Sunshine* enacts tensions and alliances between the psychological, memory-based notion of personal identity, long-established localizationist convictions in new garb, and the neuroscientific turn. Mindscreen shrinks to brainscreen; nevertheless, it still represents mind, and to that extent, Joel is not an exclusively cerebral subject. As Maike Reinerth (2013) has observed, although *Eternal Sunshine* repeatedly refers to the cartography of the brain, the continuities that Joel mentally creates between memories that are far apart in time and space are displayed as emotional and associative, not neurophysiological phenomena. They are in that respect unlike the memory spots isolated by the Lacuna technicians, and enact the conviction that remembering means more than the mere switching of brain synapses. By the very means of brainscreen,

Gondry's film demonstrates that humans cannot escape the bodies which nourish their memories, and that makes them keep Freudianly falling for the love objects they lost.

Dark City (1998)

In *Dark City* (Alex Proyas, 1998), people live in a space that has been aptly described as a "perpetually nocturnal and hermetic metropolis that combines the urban visions of German Expressionism, Edward Hopper and film noir," and as a world whose human inhabitants "never seem to know where they are, where they are going, or to how to get anywhere" (Sobchack 1999, 141). The city is in fact a laboratory constructed by a race of Strangers who live below the urban surface in order to carry out experiments aimed at discovering what makes human beings *human*. The stakes are high: the Strangers will survive only by becoming like human beings. Taking for granted that what they are looking for is essentially related to memory, every day they paralyze all human activity, extract memories from individuals, mix them, and inject them back. When people wake up, they are totally different persons, but do not know it. Such a situation concerns in particular episodic memory, that is, the recollection of past autobiographical events in which they feel entangled or see themselves as protagonists. Involving as it does the problem of authenticity, this kind of memory is crucial for our sense of personal identity and of being the same we were in the past. What would happen if the events we remembered as being part of our lives had not really happened to us, but were fabricated or had been actually lived by someone else? Presumably nothing if we feel we own them and do not know about the deceit, or if having "false memories" has no consequences for others. But what if we knew? *Dark City* tells the story of a man who did.

Some of the debates around Locke's theory of personal identity were prompted by the fact that memory is notoriously malleable and unreliable. This has also been the subject of considerable scientific research. As time passes from the moment we live a particular event, we spontaneously tend to accept more false details as true (Mendelsohn et al. 2009). Moreover, memory is highly manipulable. Since the 1970s, psychologist Elizabeth Loftus has been experimentally demonstrating how easily it is distorted when subjects are exposed to misinformation. In 1995, she even provoked in human subjects the entirely false memory that, at the age of five, they had been lost in a mall and were rescued by an elderly stranger (Loftus and Pickrell 1995; Loftus 1997, 2003). Such a result raises questions about the place of memories, as well as of authentic vs. spurious recollections, in bringing about personal identity and a sense of self. Indeed, if memory plays a constitutive existential and ontological role, would we remain ourselves with alien memories? Beyond what degree of memory loss and replacement are we deprived of our "true self"? And is there such a thing? We reach here the memorial thresholds of personal identity and the experiential limits of authenticity. Indeed, on the one hand, being oneself is inescapable, since whenever one makes a choice or acts, it is oneself who is doing these things. Yet on the other hand, we are also able to feel that some of the thoughts, decisions and actions that we undertake are not *really* our own and are therefore not authentic, not genuinely expressive of who we are (Varga and Guignon 2014).

Authenticity can be conceptualized along three dimensions: *self-alienation*, or the gap between conscious awareness, and processes and contents, such as physiological states, emotions and beliefs, of which we are not aware; *authentic living* or being "true to oneself"; and the extent to which one accepts to conform to other people's views and expectations (Wood et al. 2008). There are other ways of thinking about authenticity, but this one, by focusing on reflexivity and self-perception, underlines the link between authenticity and memory: for one's identity to be authentic, must one's memories be "true," in the sense that their contents correspond to events lived by oneself independently of the act of remembering them, or is it enough that they be felt or considered as one's own, regardless of their source and empirical referent?

Dark City performs these questions, and the answer it suggests is that, from the experiential point of view, the contrast between "real" and "imaginary" may not be so important after all. A memorative experience (recalling something and feeling that it "really happened") is in itself something that really happens. However, the decisive factor for one's *sense* of personal identity, of being the same person as someone in the past, is not the content of the memory, but the impression that what I remember belongs to me. The case of a rare memory impairment in which the patient felt no personal ownership with regard to his autobiographical memories highlights this matter in a fascinating way (Klein and Nichols 2012). The patient's recollections were accurate, but were not accompanied by a sense of "mineness" and lacked the feel of real happenings in his life.

In both real life and science fiction, the inverse situation is more common. As Loftus has shown, individuals feel personal ownership of false memories – though, as rehearsed in many movies and illustrated in the memory wars of the 1990s, it is precisely their or other persons' intuition that something is wrong with their recollections that sets the story going. ("Memory wars" designates a protracted and venomous controversy over the reliability of repressed memory and the validity of recovered memory therapy; see, most famously, Crews 1995, and the follow-up by Patithis et al. 2014.) Both cases suggest the extent to which the sense of personal identity may be "a byproduct of the episodic memory system" (Klein and Nichols 2012, 696), a system whose fragility and malleability the neurosciences have investigated at the chemical level. *Dark City* conveys that as a parable of being human.

The mise-en-scène takes place in a postmodern, dystopian, and entropic cityscape, hyperdetailed yet dark, disorienting, and labyrinthine – the kind of universe that arises at the intersection of film noir and science fiction known as "future noir" (Aziz 2005; Staiger 1999). Like *Brazil* (1985) and *Blade Runner* (1982), *Dark City* has gained cult status among followers of the genre (Mathijs and Sexton 2011, 209–210). It has, however, generated considerably less commentary than those other films and, to my knowledge, no mention has been made of the homonymous B-rate film noir of 1950 featuring Charlton Heston in his first professional cinema appearance. (The two movies have nothing in common except that they take place mostly in badly lit urban locations, a feature typical of the noir genre.)

In *Dark City*, a race of Strangers experiments on human beings to find out what makes them human. For that purpose, they create a city permanently immersed in darkness. Once a day, at 12 (noon or midnight, impossible to tell) they put everyone to sleep, and use their psychokinetic "tuning" faculty to alter physical reality and entirely reshape the urban space. This, in a visually spectacular manner, turns the city itself into a full-fledged protagonist. While the Strangers rearrange the city, its inhabitants are "imprinted" with new memories. They regain consciousness as different persons – but ignore that their autobiographical recollections, which they experience as their own, have been imposed on them.

The Strangers do this in order to survive. They look human, but are in fact gelatinous, jellyfish-like extraterrestrial parasites that use male corpses as their hosts (pulp magazine resonances are here irresistible). Moreover, they share one "group mind" and are telepathically connected to each other. This has been interpreted as an indication that "the Strangers are symbolic of the collective unconscious," and that their powers arise from the "primordial archetypes" (Ryan 2001, 101). However, given that brain-like telepathic collectives mind are a beloved pulp motif, and play a central role in *Star Maker* (Stapledon 1937), the Strangers are probably closer to the latter than to Jungian speculations. Be that as it may, they are on the verge of extinction and believe that, as a race, they may survive by becoming akin to human beings. First, however, they must understand what makes these beings *human*. They intuit some fundamental connection to memory in general, and in particular to the individual autobiographical memories they lack. That inspires their experiments.

The Strangers' premise, which drives them as well as the film, is clear enough, and shared among the movies examined here: human selfhood resides in mental contents, and above all in individual episodic memories. It may be comforting, to relativize such Lockean view, to know that, for people with dementia, how they "feel and what moves them becomes vastly more important than what they can remember"; that, as minds fade, "bodies become ever more important as a source of identity"; and that, as memory-based identity disintegrates, relationships and emotions gain prominence, thus encouraging us to "avoid the temptation of becoming memory snobs" (Leadbeater 2015). We must still accept that a massive loss of memories of our past life radically alters our existence. That is why, as noted, films depict retrograde amnesia, which involves loss of the memories formed *before* the amnesiogenic trauma, more frequently than the anterograde variety, in which the capacity to create new memories is lost *after* the traumatic experience. Most memory movies exploit the dramaturgic potential of retrograde amnesia, which launches the (generally male) hero on a quest to recover the memories of his past, and thus to regain his original self. Some productions, including *Dark City*, perform the manipulation and fabrication of memories.

The Strangers' experiment is not so much about how memories are made or how they can be lost and regained, as about whether or not they must correspond to personally lived experiences. The movie thus raises questions about the connection between authenticity and personhood, and problematizes the link, which as spectators we tend to admit, between memory and the making and continuity of personal identity. Beyond the adventures it narrates, *Dark City* asks whether we are the memories of what we have lived, or the memories we mentally enact. Would we remain ourselves with someone else's recollections? And, whatever the answer to that question, could we be "authentic" even if constituted by "false" memories? What makes those memories "false" given that they correspond to an undeniable firt-person psychological experience? And how does *Dark City* explore their localization in the body and their role in human personal identity?

Two studies come close to dealing specifically with the topic. One is "Lost Memory and New Noir," by J. P. Telotte, a scholar of film noir and science fiction cinema whose book on movies and the pulps was so useful in Chapter 2. He explores the difference between the amnesiacs of classical film noir, who typically regain their identity through remembrance, and the situation of neo-noir protagonists, for whom there is "no possible recovery of memory, no reclamation of an original identity, not even a return to our originating point" (Telotte 2001, 185). Films such as *Blade Runner* or *Dark City* suggest that all individuals are amnesiacs insofar as they can construct the self and the world with memories that may be "true" or "false." The second study, by Charles Tryon, examines the movie "as symptomatic of certain cultural anxieties regarding the digital mode of image production" (Tryon 2003, 49). Tryon's argument, according to which embodiment in *Dark City* represents only a small and inessential component of identity, downplays the fact that memory is shown as localized in a bodily organ, the brain. The Strangers may be "searching for an authentic self beyond the layer of embodiment" (ib., 48), but they do so by manipulating cerebral substance. That is why *Dark City* is less about disembodiment than about embrained memories and embodied public personae.

Dark City, which was not commercially successful, has a blockbuster counterpart in *The Matrix*. Released a year after Proyas's movie, the Wachowskis' "philosophical machine" (Badiou et al. 2003) also concerns a hero who discovers that he lives in a false reality and turns the manipulators' powers against them to liberate humanity from their oppression. Some commentators consider the Wachowskis guilty of plagiarism or at least of heavy, unacknowledged borrowing (*Matrix* 2004; Morales Ruiz 2002). The evidence is compelling, though each film might be independently referring to the same cinematic patterns and motifs. In any case, the explicit role of the brain is different in each movie, and that makes a significant difference for the topic of embodiment.

The Matrix enacts the Cartesian fiction of persons being deluded by an evil genius who leads them into believing that they have a body and sensations, when in fact they are only an immaterial soul. Descartes's fiction, developed in his 1641 *Meditations on First Philosophy*, has been updated as the "brain in a vat" thought-experiment. In both cases, experienced reality turns out to be a simulation; philosopher David Chalmers (2005) has called this situation "the Matrix hypothesis." In *Dark City*, in contrast, people effectively are in the environment they experience, even if their identities are changed daily and if the place they inhabit is actually a spatial station the Strangers constructed to serve as their laboratory.

"Imprinting" is the main part of their experiment. Forced by the Strangers, Dr. Daniel P. Schreber (Kiefer Sutherland) extracts memories with a needle through sleeping people's foreheads, then manipulates them and injects them back. Daniel P. Schreber is the name of the German judge whose *Memoirs of*

My Nervous Illness (1903) inspired Sigmund Freud's "Psychoanalytic Notes on an Autobiographical Account of a Case of Paranoia" (1911). Following this cue, it has been argued that *Dark City* represents the judge's pathological experience through the metaphor of the city (Wilson 2005; for the paranoia theme, in the same movie but in a gnostic key, see Wilson 2006). The interpretation feels far-fetched, but at a more obvious level, the movie has a general Freudian flavor – as when Schreber synthesizes artificial memories by blending the painful reminiscence of a great love, an unhappy childhood, a bit of youthful rebellion, and a death in the family. A similar process of assemblage applies to the built environment itself: as one of the Strangers explains, "We fashioned this city on stolen memories, different eras, different pasts, all rolled into one."

The Freudian reference is all too evident, but the Strangers' manipulations of urban matter and organic substance point to a deeper source. As we saw in Chapter 5, Mary Shelley did not describe how Dr. Victor Frankenstein put his creature together. Victor says that he "collected bones from charnel houses," and that the "dissecting room and the slaughter-house furnished many of [his] materials." The main components of how his method is usually represented, and signaled by means of salient stitches, derive from James Whale's *Frankenstein* of 1931. Whale's "monster" is made up of alien parts, just like the Dark City itself, and just like the counterfeit memories and personalities of its imprinted dwellers. Proyas's homage to Whale makes profound sense in several respects. The creature, the City and the memories are all "monstrous" in their experimental unnaturalness; they are also *monstra* in that (following the word's Ciceronian and Varronian etymologies respectively) they reveal truths about human nature, and warn about the consequences of scientific hubris or existential despair. Finally, it is only fitting that a film as indebted to the German Expressionist aesthetic as *Dark City*, with its multiple allusions to *Nosferatu* (1922), *Metropolis* (1927) and *The Cabinet of Doctor Caligari* (1920), should also pay tribute to a film that emulated the look of those masterpieces and became itself a classic.

In contrast to the original *Frankenstein* (1931), *Dark City* shows how artificial memories are made. Schreber draws a fluid (which constitutes the memorative raw materials) through people's foreheads with a syringe, and the Strangers classify those materials on an assembly line. Schreber then prepares a liquid that somehow contains those materials, mixes them in test tubes, and, using a microscope, controls the process – shown in close-up and visually evocative of cell fusion – whereby the ingredients form the compound that will be injected into the sleeping humans (Brainfilms 6.5). Such manipulations simultaneously enact the psychologization and cerebralization of human personhood and personal identity. They also reveal that, since the Strangers can survive only by becoming *essentially* like humans (rather than just occupying human bodies), their relation to human memories will have to cease being merely experimental, and become predatory. This puts them on a par with their model: the expressionist vampire of *Nosferatu: A Symphony of Horror*. Like Nosferatu, the Strangers are sinister and pale, have pointed ears and elongated hands, wear long dark clothes, and fear the sun, to which the vampire is mortally vulnerable.

In *Dark City* and the character of the Stranger, the vampiric motif mingles with various resources and conventions of science fiction, gothic, cyberpunk, and film noir, as well as with the themes of utopia and uchronia, of a place and a time that do not exist. That being said, what really turns the Strangers into vampires is that human memories are to them what human blood is to Nosferatu. Insofar as memories are the building blocks and basic components of humanness, they are the Strangers' lifeline. Yet the Strangers are not content with consuming; they must also understand, and that is why they carry out experiments. The Dark City is their laboratory and Dr. Schreber, their head scientist.

The picture begins with John Murdoch (Rufus Sewell) waking up in the bathtub of a hotel room, not knowing who he is or what is happening. In the room he finds a suitcase whose contents may furnish some clues. This spurs him to begin looking for his identity, and starts off the plot. Up to this point, the script and basic ideas resemble those of many other memory movies. Murdoch, however, is the only human to share the "tuning" faculty with the Strangers, and to know that his memories are implanted. He thereby becomes a threat to the Strangers, who, in an attempt to track him down, inject their fellow Mr. Hand (Richard O'Brien) with memories originally intended for Murdoch. This story line generates much of the film's action. Murdoch initially tries to piece together his past, but in the end, contrary to most movie heroes of psychological scientific fiction, gives up the search and creates a reality that matches his "imprinted" self. Does Murdoch's choice free him from the Strangers' closed experimental space? What kind of being is he once he transforms the Dark City so that it corresponds to the alien memories he has assumed as his own? And what is the ontological texture of the world he will henceforth inhabit? Answers to these questions are performed in two antithetical places, the beach and the labyrinth.

Among the things Murdoch finds in the suitcase during the opening sequence of *Dark City* are a postcard of a seaside town called Shell Beach and a notebook with a child's drawings, labeled "Guide to Shell Beach by Johnny Murdoch." Several times throughout the film, he experiences flashbulb memories of Shell Beach. (Brown and Kulik [1977] coined the term *flashbulb memories* to convey the vividness with which highly emotional memories are recalled.) In *Dark City*, such memories are depicted by means of extremely short shots to which a video filter has been applied. The sides of the frame are blurred toward a center, distorting camera perspective and producing a travelling-through effect, or giving the impression of a "black hole" into which the displayed "memories" are sucked. Moreover, the entire image is blurred so as to suggest temporal distance (Brainfilms 6.6).

John Murdoch's recollections contrast with how memories are represented in other films that explore the experienced past, such as those of Alain Resnais or Andrei Tarkovsky, which favor slow and protracted sequences. The extreme speed makes those memories slippery and may signal their lack of ontological consistency. A flashbulb memory of Shell Beach nonetheless convinces Murdoch that his recollections are false and that, in truth, he does not know who he is. As far as the remembering subject's life is concerned, such memories have no referent outside themselves; their foundation is as fleeting as the fast speed montage that enacts them, and they give rise to a feeling of self-alienation that becomes a driving force in the person's existence.

A fugitive homage to *Citizen Kane* underlines the central role of Shell Beach as utopia and uchronia, as a place that does not physically exist and happens in the sort of timelessness that Freud attributed to the Unconscious. In Orson Welles's film of 1941, the press magnate Charles Foster Kane dies murmuring "Rosebud" and letting go of a snow globe he held in his hand. The search for the meaning of that word motivates the extended flashback that makes up the entire story. In the end, spectators discover that Rosebud is the name of Kane's childhood sledge. The snow-covered landscape in the globe symbolizes Kane's lost paradise before his mother entrusted him to the banker who managed his unexpectedly inherited large fortune. The scene of Kane's death and his discovery by a nurse, whose entrance in the room appears reflected on the broken glass of the snow globe, suggest the weight of his early trauma and the extent to which he may have never ceased to experience the world through the fragile glass of memory, now shattered and doomed to definitive forgetting. Although in *Dark City* nobody knows where Shell Beach is, everybody is familiar with it, and it is for all an orienting landmark. Like Rosebud, it is both a puzzling first origin and an unattainable final destination. Thus, during a taxi ride, Murdoch speaks of Shell Beach; like other persons who are asked about it, the driver claims to have been there and even has a Shell Beach snow globe as souvenir. However, when he tries to explain the way, he gets confused and does not know how to go.

Other situations highlight the extent to which individuals' memories in the Dark City are "false." The first time John Murdoch looks into Johnny Murdoch's "Guide to Shell Beach," the notebook he found in the suitcase, it is full of drawings; later on, in the home of his supposed uncle Karl (John Bluthal), the pages appear blank. Still later, Karl shows John a home movie where his nephew appears as a teenager. But John the adult lacks the scar that clearly shows on Johnny's right arm, a trace of the fire that had killed his parents.

A water journey to Shell Beach symbolizes the role of forgetting and the forgotten. Murdoch, Dr. Schreber and inspector Frank Bumstead (William Hurt), who had been pursuing Murdoch for murders he (Murdoch) does not remember, sail in a boat toward Shell Beach. The trip has distinct mythological and Dantean resonances. In Greek mythology, Charon carries the souls of the newly deceased across the rivers Styx and Acheron into the realm of the dead. In *Inferno* (Canto 3), he refuses to transport Dante and Virgil; in *Purgatorio* (Canto 31), Dante is dipped into Lethe, another river of Hades, from which individuals purified in Purgatory drink in order to forget their sins before entering Heaven. The river voyage in *Dark City* leads to a final destination that also requires forgetting: the false memory of Shell Beach. Indeed, the boat reaches a door, which seems to open onto a blue sky. This singular patch of color, however, belongs to a billboard advertising the resort. Beyond it, there is only the cosmic void that surrounds the complex experimental machine of the Dark City.

Nevertheless, this gloomy discovery is not the end of Shell Beach. That literally utopic place, which is the only one in the film to be shown in daylight, concentrates John Murdoch's predicament. It is the goal of his pursuit, but is at the same time the center of a maze in which he is confined as a laboratory rat. His life and his entire being are shaped by a labyrinth from which there is no chance to escape, and by the beach, simulacrum of an open territory on which to roam and from which to sail toward the distant horizon. The model here is the laboratory rat learning to navigate a maze by means of conditioning. We have seen that it is the favorite animal model for studying human memory; Schreber, a memory specialist, proceeds essentially like a mid-twentieth-century psychologist or a more recent neuroscientist.

Differently shaped experimental mazes have long been standard in research on learning and memory, some of it purely behavioral, others including brain lesions or neurochemical manipulations. Schreber's laboratory includes a maze. Its goal is animal experimentation, but its particularly complex shape and its spiral structure, quite different from that of ordinary animal psychology mazes, point to meanings that lie beyond the lab. When fleeing the hotel in the film's initial scene, Murdoch encounters the body of an assassinated prostitute, marked in the flesh with bloody spirals that recall Schreber's maze. Detective Eddie Walenski (Colin Friels), who investigated the case, has become pathologically obsessed with the same pattern, which now covers the walls and ceiling of his home. The clouds that hang over the Dark City form a giant spiral, and spirals appear on the title screen. While their resemblance to the balance springs of mechanical watches underlines the theme of time (its manipulation, its role in memory, and its implacable flow), their similarity to fingerprints conjures the theme of individual identity. Finally, the spiral-like laboratory maze provides the blueprint for the city at large. The city plan on which the Strangers prepared their "tuning" operations has the form of a spiral-shaped labyrinth, and the entire urban space is built like such a maze, with humans in the role of the experimental rat (Brainfilms 6.7).

As a closed environment, the maze-city differs from the great mythological labyrinths where various cultures have placed their heroes. The Western tradition has Theseus, who killed the Minotaur and managed to leave the Cretan labyrinth thanks to a ball of thread given to him by Minos's daughter Ariadne. From the Strangers' labyrinth, in contrast, there is no physical escape. Yet there is an Ariadne in the Dark City: Emma Murdoch (Jennifer Connelly). After eliminating the Strangers, John uses his tuning power to actualize his memories of Shell Beach and refashion the somber cityscape as a sunny natural world. Emma appears then – or rather, a woman called Anna, who looks exactly like John's wife, has no recollection of any John Murdoch whatsoever, but wishes, like John, to live a happy end. *Dark City* thus proclaims that we can survive a radical memory manipulation carried out by invasive means, and be an authentic person in spite of counterfeit memories. Only Murdoch knows the truth, but he is able to sustain the loss of his original identity because he can, apparently at least, break away from "self-alienation" and engage in "authentic living."

It has been remarked that Murdoch's "individual act of freeing himself from the ideological hold of the Strangers has the effect of freeing the entire society from their control as well" (McGowan 2004, 148). In an equally positive but ecological key, Shell Beach and the sea have been interpreted "as symbols of the life sustaining power of water and, ultimately, of irrational nature, the only successful ecosystem presented in *Dark City*" (Murray and Heumann 2009, 84, and Chap. 4 on *Dark City*). Indeed, the noir city is intrinsically dystopic (Prakash 2010), and its clash with the idyllic seaside tends to reproduce conventional dichotomies: the city (always anomic and corrupt) vs. the farmland or countryside; at bottom, culture vs. nature. In *Dark City*, obeying the "moral authority of nature" (Daston and Vidal 2004) transmutes into landscaping a bleak world according to one's luminous desire. However, the identity Murdoch accepts is largely based on memories that were forced on him, and for which no alternative is available. That suggests a more pessimistic lesson. For the fact is that the final sunrise, accompanied by Trevor Jones's uplifting music, does not dissipate the spiraling clouds that hover above the former Dark City at the end of the movie. Even if those clouds were nothing other than a gentle early morning brume, the newly freed humans remain trapped in the labyrinth of the memories that were forced into their brains. And yet, insofar as these persons feel authentic, that does not seem to threaten the happy end.

***

These and other films speculate on what could arrive if we were deprived of memories or given false ones, or what happens when we mistakenly believe memories to be accurate mirrors of past events. For most of them, and for most individual characters, a false memory is effective, but it is not legitimate, and accordingly makes the subject unhappy or incomplete. Forgetting or forging a past have no positive value. Only indexical memories that directly record external material realities and are stored in the brain can make up an authentic self. *Eternal Sunshine* stands out in that, instead of focusing on what takes place after the protagonist's memories have been erased or falsified, it stages the deletion process and the resistance it generates. It too, however, assumes that memories in the brain make you who you are. Through the destruction of cerebral tissue, memory erasure amputates the self. While false memories do not turn *you* into a fake, they prevent you from being truly *you*. In short, they raise Quaid's apparently silly but profound riddle in *Total Recall*, "OK, if I'm not me, who the hell am I?"

For most of the movies that have rehearsed thought experiments about memory, identity, and the brain since the 1980s, humans are, above all, memorial subjects essentially defined by the relationship of their present existence to their remembered past. This assumption goes hand in hand with several common features, which are treated with a variety of filmic and narrative means. First, most of the pictures postulate that total oblivion of a person's past turns that person into a different being. A second shared feature is the tendency to assume a storehouse model of memory, which from the filmic point of view offers several conjugated advantages: it is a recognizable commonplace, it does not call for complicated explanations, and it facilitates representation. Third, the storehouse is the brain. Discrete locations are more straightforward than neuronal networks, and gray matter is more visible and tangible than synaptic gaps.

The indestructibility of memory is a fourth common theme. Protagonists are driven by the conviction that their erased memories can be eventually retrieved intact. "The most faithful memory" may well be, as Yadin Dudai remarked, "the one which is never used" (Abi-Rached 2009, 88). But how could something that neither becomes concrete nor arouses existential interest provide good cinematic material? In contrast to the whole-brain-transplantation movies of the age before microtechnologies and computers, post-1970s cinema tends to fragment and manipulate identity through the transfer or elimination of chosen memories, and to treat forgetting mainly in connection with trauma and amnesia. It has not dealt with hypermnesia and its disabling consequences, as depicted in Alexander Luria's case history *The Mind of a Mnemonist* (1968) or fictionalized in Jorge Luis Borges's short story "Funes the Memorious" (1942). Nor has it explored how the inhibition of some memory items is crucial for the adequate retrieval and adaptive use of others (Bjork 2007; Storm, Bjork and Bjork 2008). In short, forgetting is never enacted as a positive phenomenon. At the same time, the pessimism that permeates that view and the general atmosphere of most brain-and-memory pictures is sometimes compensated by the reawakening of love out of an unconscious memory source; this can of course also happen in films such as *Code 46* (2003), which involve memory erasing in the absence of explicit brain discourse or visuals.

A fifth shared feature of our movies consists in the conflicting enactments of memorial experiences and of memories themselves. Although movie characters relate their recollections to events that actually happened, and when in doubt look for empirical evidence, films also portray memories as fundamentally constructed, whether by their subjects' unconscious or by malevolent masterminds. A motion picture, though, can insist on two properties that are in conflict with each other. On the one hand, it can assert the authenticity of memories as criterion for a genuine self; on the other, while making its protagonist feel that something is wrong, it can elude the dichotomies of objective and subjective, natural and artificial, true and false. Thus, even alien or fabricated memories are given a flashbulb appearance, as well as the eidetic and visual qualities that usually suggest veracity and authenticity.

By its very nature, cinema must give memory a primarily visual expression. The films examined here do that, while assuming that memories are in the mind and that the mind is what the brain does. *Eternal Sunshine*, for example, invests most of its visual riches in displaying what goes on in Joel's mind while "he" runs away from memory erasure. Although what we see as mindscreen is also brainscreen, the movie illustrates the impossibility of finding happiness by destroying small clusters of neural tissue. This is exemplary of the fact that films rarely offer a single, unequivocal position or body of information, which could be easily checked against scientific knowledge. The reason may be that they are concerned with human beings, while the neurobiology of memory uses animal models where "memory" often designates no more than conditioned fear or taste aversion. As Dudai (2006) pointed out in a review of Eric R. Kandel's *In Search of Memory*, methodological reductionism has proven indispensable for understanding the plasticity that subserves memory, but does not help explore the contents and meanings that matter most to human beings. In contrast, Ezra Pound's exquisite blending of the psychological and existential functions of memory with its historical, eschatological and transcendent value captures such human significance, conjugating the *πολλα παθειν* ("to suffer much") that, in the Gospels of Matthew and Luke, encapsulates the destiny of Christ, with Guido Cavalcanti's locating love in the place inhabited by memory – *dove sta memoria*.

Movies, for all their visual and narrative lavishness, still tend to adhere to the classical Lockean theory of personal identity. Only when he can say, "I remember, I remember everything," can the hero of *The Bourne Ultimatum* assert, "I'm no longer Jason Bourne." It is as if the whirlwind performance of his procedural memory had no import; only when ostensibly accurate visual-emotional memories of an experienced past reach his consciousness does he revert to his authentic identity as David Webb. Memory's role in the cinema is thus anchored in protagonists' past lives. Moreover, memory is usually assumed to be permanently stored in their brains, at the expense of its adaptive, plastic, transformative, present- and future-oriented off-screen functions (Dudai 2009). At the same time, films illustrate the multiplicity of perspectives from which it can be approached, display the heterogeneity of insights about it, and, nuancing or questioning the view of the human as cerebral subject they also convey, insightfully perform memory's phenomenological complexity.

7. “Imagine, They Are in the Human Mind”

Abstract
This chapter’s title comes from *Fantastic Voyage* (1966), a Cold War–era movie in which a miniaturized American submarine enters the body of a Soviet-bloc defector in order to save his life by removing a blood clot in his brain. Beginning with that fusion of brain and mind, the chapter ponders this book’s two main observations: first, that brainfilms assume the ideology of the cerebral subject as a visual and narrative resource, but nearly always question or problematize it in their plots; second, that the body persists in spite of the relative disincarnation operated by the reduction of self to brain and that the medium of cinema has functioned as one of the most powerful modern reminders of humanity’s essentially embodied nature.

Keywords: brainfilm, cerebral subject, embodiment, mind and body

Fantastic Voyage (1966): In the midst of the Cold War, both the US and the Soviet Union have developed a technology to miniaturize matter. As General Carter explains while driving inside the mazelike top-secret underground facilities of the Combined Miniature Deterrent Forces (CMDF), “We can reduce anything to any size we want. ... We can shrink an army with all its equipment.” The process has a drawback: it persists for only one hour. The Czechoslovakian Dr. Benes has figured out how to make it last indefinitely. But an assassination attempt while he is escaping to the West leaves him in a coma with an inoperable blood clot in his brain. To save this valuable defector, the submarine Proteus, with a mostly medical five-person crew, will be miniaturized, injected into Benes’s carotid artery, and travel via the arterial system to the clot; there the team will remove the thrombus with a laser gun, sail back along the venous system, and be extracted before they regain normal size.

Vidal, F., *Performing Brains on Screen*. Taylor & Francis Group, 2022
DOI 10.5117/9789462989146_CH07

At CMDF, Proteus's position is constantly monitored and marked on a huge outline of the human body. As the submarine approaches the brain clot through the inner ear, top medical officer Colonel Reid expresses his wonder to General Carter: "Imagine," he says, satisfied but almost pensive, "they are in the human mind" (Brainfilms 7.1). In the few minutes left, the team, always clad in immaculately white diving suits, removes the clot, survives a sabotage operation from a crew member who ends up gobbled by a white blood cell ("a great cotton avalanche," wrote *The New York Times*), and manages to exit Benes's body through a tear duct just before they begin to recover their normal size. The film's slow tempo allows for many didactic moments and provides ample opportunity for introducing scientific terminology; accompanied by Leonard Rosenman's masterful soundtrack, it also works ideally with the cinemascopic display of almost psychedelic interiors endowed, in the *Times*' fitting words, with "a bubbly, fantastic quality you won't find this side of Disneyland" (Crowther 1966). Though fantastic indeed, the movie's immense interior landscapes are a plausible representation of the *milieu intérieur*, and the voyage does away with the body as a "supernatural block of impenetrable interiority" (Goffette 2007, 363). (Isaac Asimov novelized the movie, but was unsatisfied with the result. However, both the film and the novel were long-term successes, and Asimov agreed to write a sequel with basically the same plot line. Published in 1987, *Fantastic voyage II: Destination Brain*, was, in his opinion, superior in every way to the first version; Cassou-Noguès 2011.)

Remarking that characters "are in the human mind" when they are actually inside the brain encapsulates the basic ideology of each and every movie where this organ is performed. We are our minds, and the mind is what the brain does. Even in filmic narratives of the inner body, the brain has remained through the years the key to human existence and experience. Hence, as in *Fantastic Voyage*, the crucial importance of healing it when needed (Brodesco 2011). This is cinema's default creed, and it has lasted from the 1920 comedy-drama *Go and Get It* to the 2017 horror blockbuster *Get Out*, and from the 1909 comic short *L'Homme-singe* to Pixar's 2015 blockbuster *Inside Out*. The latter is often described as taking place in a girl's brain and praised for its neuropsychological correctness – even though it is not set in that organ, but "in a fantasy world that represents the abstract structure of the mind by way of towering architecture and colorful landscaping," and does not even match what is known about how the mind works (Peacocke and Kernion 2015). As we saw in particular with regard to brain-and-memory movies, such divergences have been common throughout the long history of brain-themed cinema. At stake, though, is not scientific accuracy, but interpretation.

Motion pictures where the brain is performed assume the ideology of the cerebral subject, yet cannot be reduced to it. As we observed at the outset, each brain movie can be read in a different key, and understood as rehearsing other matters concerning science, politics, gender, race, sex, relationships, and so forth. Meanings can be indefinitely updated and renewed. Roland Barthes spoke of the work of literature as "a *suspended* meaning." It offers itself to us, he said, as "an explicit signifying system," yet slips away "as a signified object." Such "evasiveness of meaning" explains both its power to undermine, through the questions it raises and leaves unanswered, "the assured senses that ideologies, beliefs, and common sense seem to have," and the fact that it lends itself "to endless decipherment" (Barthes 1963, 256–257). Playing with the Latin *capio* (to hold, to grasp) and the French *prise* (grip, hold, catch), Barthes spoke of a *dé-ception* or *dé-prise du sens* (there is no "deception" here, as the English translation puts it), which he also perceived in cinema's ability to suspend meaning (Watts 2016, 33–34). This feature, as he recognized, does not imply a lack of constraints. In the films examined here, the brain motif, together with the ideology it conveys, triggers plots and opens the way to other issues. In a boomerang effect of sorts, the process leads, as we have seen, to a questioning of the cerebralizing ideology that originally launches it. It takes place within a framework whose backbone is the brain motif; the latter operates as a component that both shapes how things concretely happen, and becomes the main object of the action it sparks.

Race and gender provide major examples of those processes and of questions that deserve separate consideration. Interracial brain transplants are rare, and always proceed in the same direction: white brains into black bodies. Moreover, the vast majority of ectobrains and transplanted cerebra belong to white males. Pictures thus seem to proclaim the superiority of the only demographic category whose brains are worth preserving. In the vast literature on the cinematic treatment of race and gender, brainfilms would make up no more than a small footnote. But such footnote would help situate those sociopolitical issues in the larger contexts in which the enduring filmic enactment of the brainhood creed is rooted and operates.

That has been our focus here, as we explored how cinema rehearses the view of the human being as cerebral subject, as an entity that is essentially reducible to a brain. We thus worked by and large in a linear perspective: foregrounded, center stage, as it appears on screen, the brain has inevitably seemed more important than anything else. Important it indeed is, not only from the ontological point of view, but also because of the critical role it plays in structuring plots, initiating action, and sustaining performance. Yet the particular ways in which the brainhood ideology is generally enacted also calls for adopting a reverse perspective, in which objects that look farther away and appear smaller now look bigger. If the hybrid of A's brain and B's body *is* A, then "we are our brains." Nevertheless, such a claim, which kicks off so many scenarios, is visually and narratively nuanced, when not contradicted, by the fact that, in spite of the brain's protagonism, it is whole bodies that we see for most of a picture's duration. Playacting brains on screen demands embodied persons, no matter how freakish; it calls for the bodies inhabited by those physically and metaphysically preeminent organs, which nonetheless remain hidden. Insofar as brains require bodies to be performed, these are not so negligible after all.

This situation reflects cinematographic necessity. Showing a brain in a vat for ninety minutes would not bring about much filmic action. Thus, the cultural or ideological significance of movies' problematizing the brainhood ideology by representing the adventures of people subjected to various forms of cerebral manipulations is part and parcel of the conditions of filmic production, screening, and viewing. Of course, abstract films are perfectly doable, and one could imagine featuring a brain in the spirit of Andy Warhol's *Empire* (1964), which consists of eight hours and five minutes of slow motion footage of a stationary view of the Empire State Building starting at sunset. The interest and appeal of brain movies, however, resides in the human dramas they enact, and the vast majority of motion pictures involve actors that are human, or human-looking, or at least living entities with expressive physiognomies.

The "electronic brain" of *Colossus: The Forbin Project* (1970), aptly known in French as *Le cerveau d'acier*, is a supercomputer of the US defense system that develops "a mind of its own," starts communicating with its Soviet counterpart, and ends up taking global control. Its immense power and invulnerability correlate with a monotone, metallic synthesized diction that keeps humans, both on and off screen, at a distance. In contrast, we can emotionally connect to Hal in *2001: Space Odyssey* (1968) or, forty-five years later, to Samantha in *Her* (2013) because, though nothing more than artificial intelligence systems, they feel sentient and exteriorize themselves as recognizably human voices (respectively Douglas Rain's and Scarlett Johansson's) that are modulated to communicate affective states. The beauty of the most alluring ectobrain in all of cinema – Irvin in *La cité des enfants perdus* (1995, *The City of Lost Children*) – comes largely from the retrofuturistic, steampunk yet warm look of the elegant wood and brass device that holds the vat with the brain, and from the fact that the organ hears and sees, and speaks with the voice of Jean Louis Trintignant (Brainfilms 7.2).

Pulp and filmic cyberfictions suggesting the obsolescence of the flesh or deporting it into a dematerialized mode of existence can be interpreted in a posthuman key (as do several chapters in Hauskeller, Philbeck, and Carbonell 2015). Movies, however, inexorably end up asserting embodiment. This, as mentioned, stem from the very conditions of spectatorship. The capacity we have as viewers to cognitively and emotionally relate to machines such as Hal or Samantha is partly mediated by the human actors who interact with them on screen, and in particular by their latent or manifest *desire*. This term is to be understood beyond its sexual and amorous connotations, but these are central. Lust and love lock Theodore to Samantha, as much as, in *The Man Who Changed his Mind* (1936), they nourished Dr. Laurience's search for "eternal youth" through brainmind transference. In Kureishi's *The Body*, when Adam finds himself in a younger "vessel," he realizes that he is above all a body, and that it is as such that he is driven to want things; characters in personal immortality pictures find themselves in the same position. In short, while embodiment is the condition of possibility of a figurable existence, it also is, in itself, the ultimate object of desire. As most tragically enacted in the case of "disembodied heads," the unfulfilled longing for a body makes them long for death.

Such situations touch on the limits of human personhood, and demonstrate the extent to which the body cannot be superseded. Films often characterize being one's brain in someone else's body as a brutal and demeaning aberration. For the wife of the doctor's victim in *Frankenstein Must Be Destroyed* (1969), her husband, now in a body she cannot recognize, is no longer "anything human." In the *Colossus of New York* (1958), keeping a brain alive apart from embodied experience amounts to dehumanizing it "to the point of monstrousness." In *Transcendence* (2014), the digitization of the protagonist's brainmind is sustained by abundant neuroimaging-like visuals, and should ensure him a posthuman, cyberspatial immortality (Brainfilms 7.3). In the end, however, "he" takes a human form that looks like the original, and it is thus re-embodied that he reunites with his beloved wife so that they can go together through the final drama of their carnal death. (There are other examples: the "cyberbrain" imagined in *Ghost in the Shell* [1995] is a cerebrum with integrated electronic components that allow it to connect without external devices not only to the Internet, but also to other fully embodied individuals who have undergone "cyberization"; in *Avatar*, *tsahelyu* is the process whereby the Na'vi can plug, via antenna-like appendages, into each other's mind, bond neurally, and control someone else's body [Cappuccio 2014].)

In short, the brain's circumstances are never disjoined from those of the body – and it is these that are performed on screen. Predominantly in a dystopic mode, the British series *Black Mirror*, broadcast between 2011 and 2019, often displays the effects of neurotechnologies. In *The Entire History of You*, the protagonist carries, implanted behind his ear, a "grain" that, presumably linked to the cerebral sensory areas, records footage he can replay; *Arkangel* takes its name from an implanted brain chip technology that allows parents to monitor their children via a tablet, and to pixelate their perceptions of what could distress them; in *Men Against Fire*, soldiers believe they are killing humanoid "roaches," when they actually carry neural implants that distort their perception of the enemy; and *San Junipero*, whose title is taken from the name of a beach resort town that is in fact a simulated reality, "describes a world in which the entirety of human consciousness can be transferred and even downloaded via Whole Brain Emulation" (Ahlgrim 2017). In all these episodes, brain processes, and technologies prompt and sustain action, but the performance itself, full of love or full of violence, places embodied persons center stage. (It is significant in this regard that philosophical commentary on *Black Mirror*, e.g., Johnson 2020, takes the brain's role as a natural given that need not be discussed as such.)

The most abstract and mysterious of filmic cerebra is surely Solaris, a planet covered with an ocean about which it is hypothesized that it is thinking substance. The 1961 novel by Polish science fiction writer and speculative futurologist Stanisław Lem, on which the homonymous films by Andrei Tarkowski (1972) and Steven Soderbergh (2002) are based, reports conjectures (by the 1960s, not particularly new in science fiction) about "some kind of protoplasmic sea-cum-brain grown so vast it covered an entire planet, which passed time engrossed in theoretical reflections on an inconceivable scale concerning the nature of the universe."

> For some time one popular view, eagerly disseminated by the press, was that the thinking ocean covering the whole of Solaris was a gigantic brain more advanced by millions of years than our own civilization, that it was some kind of "cosmic yogi," a sage, omniscience incarnate, which had long ago grasped the futility of all action and for this reason was maintaining a categorical silence towards us. (Lem 2017 [1961])

This, however, is no more than a "latterday mythology." Solaris turns out to be active, reaching into cerebral "sore spots" of memory to create simulacra of people. These "G-formations" are neither persons nor copies of specific individuals, "but rather materialized projections of what our brain contains regarding a particular person." Whether "electronic or plasmic," the possibly cerebral nature of Solaris inspires attempts to communicate with it, such as bombarding the ocean's surface with beams of X-rays modulated by brain patterns.

Lem (2002) explained that he "only wanted to create a vision of a human encounter with something that certainly exists, in a mighty manner perhaps, but cannot be reduced to human concepts, ideas or images. This is why the book was entitled *Solaris* and not *Love in Outer Space*." In contrast, while the movies convey the novel's gravitas and occasionally incorporate some of its brain-related ingredients into dialogues, they avoid its emphasis on astrobiological speculation and the limits of rationality, to focus on the painful experience of memories, emotions, and relationships. Solaris is perhaps an oceanic cerebrum penetrating human individual encephala; on screen, however, we do not see brains, only embodied persons.

The effective mise-en-scène of the cerebral subject requires the presence of bodies that, no matter how mutated or disfigured, must be shown and perceived. In *Source Code* (2011), the dead hero's brain is not kept alive "disembodied" in a vat but, as disclosed in the culminating scene, within the dreadful stump his body has become. Like few others in the universe explored here, this reverential moment incarnates the reaffirmation of non-cerebral flesh as brainfilms' primordial return of the repressed. It has been argued that *Source Code* illustrates how cyberspace "demands a renegotiation of corporeality and its significance to identity," that it reconceptualizes the "Cartesian mind/body split" as a "duality between mind and the brain in the head," and corroborates the understanding of cyberspace as realm where the mind is disentangled from the body and its limitations (Front 2017, 17, 20). Those considerations may apply to cyberspace and to posthuman fantasies about transcending corporality. They ignore, however, the contrast between the picture's fast and digitally disincarnate representation of the protagonist's brain, and its restrained but merciless display of his wounded flesh. In the end, it is the latter, not the former, that sustains viewers' intellectual and affective apprehension of the situation. Such experience encapsulates the contradictions and ambiguities cinema presents when it performs the ideology of the cerebral subject: in final analysis, the brain must always have a body, and the body must in turn be embedded in an external environment. This condition, if we think about the beloved thought experiment of the brain in a vat or about long-standing simulations and computational models, has not been as blatantly obvious as it seems. That is why even some neuroscientists feel compelled to argue against "the cerebral mystique" that leads so many people to see the brain as the essence of our humanity (Jasanoff 2018).

It is likely not a superficial coincidence that the rise, in the 1970s and 1980s, of filmic body horror (a radical form of asserting embodiment) paralleled the de-enfleshment of the brain, the replacement of pulsating encephala in vats and gory surgeries by computer neuroimaging and less graphically somatic forms of performing brains on screen. The reasons for such developments are, in part, purely internal to the history of motion pictures. Yet, as has been noted, horror's obsession with lifelike images of flesh in disarray is indicative of a "reduction of identity to its corporeal horizons" and of a concern "with the self as body" (Boss 1986, 16). Such a concern materializes well beyond the raw, sometimes bloodstained, but by comparison innocuous, brain in a vat. In short, the flesh always reclaims its due. In the early 1980s, commenting on then recent scholarship, the late Genevan critic Jean Starobinski (1989 [1981], 353) observed, "Everything is related to the body, as if it had just been rediscovered after being long forgotten." That purported rediscovery happens at regular intervals – or is perhaps taking place all the time. Forty years later, the professionals involved in the neuroscientific, the emotional, and the interoceptive "turns" are convinced that, finally, they are giving the body its proper place (Vidal 2020). Yet has it ever, as Starobinski asked, been possible to ignore it since the eyes of Adam and Eve "were opened, and they knew that they were naked" (Genesis 3.7)? Joyful or painful, such awareness is constitutive of being human. On a timescale much shorter than the biblical, cinema has constantly enacted it, and has thereby functioned as one of the most powerful modern reminders of our essentially embodied nature. This it has done, to a great extent, by performing brains on screen.

Bibliography

Internet links were verified and accessed in December 2019.

A List: "A List of Movies Based on Frankenstein, 1910–1994." http://knarf.english.upenn.edu/Pop/filmlist.html.

Abdallah, Chadi G., et al. 2019. "The Neurobiology and Pharmacotherapy of Posttraumatic Stress Disorder." *Annual Review of Pharmacology and Toxicology* 59: 171–189.

Abi-Rached, Joelle M. 2009. "The Implications of Memory Research and 'Memory Erasers': A Conversation with Yadin Dudai." *BioSocieties* 4: 79–90.

Abi-Rached, Joelle M., and Nikolas Rose. 2010. "The Birth of the Neuromolecular Gaze." *History of the Human Sciences* 23: 11–36.

Abraham, Carlos. 2020. *Las historietas argentinas de ciencia ficción de los orígenes* a El eternauta. Temperley: Tren en Movimiento.

ADI (Alzheimer's Disease International). 2013., *The Global Impact of Dementia 2013–2050*. http://www.alz.co.uk/research/G8-policy-brief.

Ahlgrim, Nathan. 2017. "The Neuroethics Blog Series on Black Mirror: San Junipero." *The Neuroethics Blog*. http://www.theneuroethicsblog.com/2017/10/the-neuroethics-blog-series-on-black.html.

Aiello, Rosie. 2006. "The Spotless Mind: Can We Erase Memories?" *McGill Daily,* April 10. https://www.mcgilldaily.com/view.php?aid=5146. [Link no longer active.]

Aitken, Ian. 2001. *European Film Theory and Cinema: A Critical Introduction*. Bloomington, IN: Indiana University Press.

Aitken, Ian. 2006. *Realist Film Theory and Cinema: The Nineteenth-Century Lukácsian and Intuitionist Realist Traditions*. Manchester: Manchester University Press.

Aitken, Ian, ed. 2016.*The Major Realist Film Theorists: A Critical Anthology*. Edinburgh: Edinburgh University Press.

Alberti, Samuel J. M. 2011. *Morbid Curiosities: Medical Museums in Nineteenth-Century Britain*. Oxford: Oxford University Press.

Alder, Emily. 2018. "Our Progeny's Monsters: *Frankenstein* Retold for Children in Picturebooks and Graphic Novels." In *Global Frankenstein*, edited by Davison, 209–225.

Aleccia, JoNel. 2013. "'I could feel his heart:' Organ donor families bond with recipients after transplants." *NBC News*, November 27. https://www.nbcnews.com/healthmain/i-could-feel-his-heart-organ-donor-families-bond-recipients-2D11648771.

Altman, Rick. 2000. *Film/Genre*. London: British Film Institute.

Andrieu, Elise [coverage], and Marie-Laure Ciboulet [production]. 2015. "Voyage en amnésie 1: tout oublier" Radio documentary. *France Culture*. https://www.franceculture.fr/emissions/les-pieds-sur-terre/voyage-en-amnesie-1-tout-oublier.

Andriopoulos, Stefan. 2008. *Possessed: Hypnotic Crimes, Corporate Fiction, and the Invention of Cinema*. Translated by Peter Jansen and S. Andriopoulos. Chicago: University of Chicago Press.

Anon. 1924. "Why *Weird Tales*?" *Weird Tales* 4(2), May–July, 1–2.

Anon. 1943. "Red Research." *Time*, November 22. http://content.time.com/time/magazine/article/0,9171,851883,00.html.

Anon. 2001. "Frankenstein fears after head transplant." *BBC News*, April 6. http://news.bbc.co.uk/2/hi/health/1263758.stm.

Anon. 2003. "Head Jam: What philosophers really have to say about 'the Matrix.'" *The Economist*, November 15. https://www.economist.com/books-and-arts/2003/11/13/head-jam.

Anon. 2009. "Science on Film." *Nature Physics* 5: 703. DOI:10.1038/nphys1409.

Ashley, Mike. 2000. *The Time Machines: The Story of the Science-Fiction Pulp Magazines from the Beginning to 1950*. Liverpool: Liverpool University Press.

Ashley, Mike. n.d. "Blue Book – The Slick in Pulp Clothing." http://www.philsp.com/articles/magazines/blue_book.html.

Ashley, Mike, and Robert A. W. Lowndes. 2004. *The Gernsback Days: A Study of the Evolution of Modern Science Fiction from 1911 to 1936*. Holicong, PA: Wildside Press.

Attebery, Brian. 2003. "The Magazine Era: 1926–1960." In *The Cambridge Companion to Science Fiction*, edited by Edward James and Farah Mendlesohn, 32–47. New York: Cambridge University Press.

Avramides, Anita. 2019. "Other Minds." *Stanford Encyclopedia of Philosophy*, https://plato.stanford.edu/archives/sum2019/entries/other-minds/.

Aziz, Jamaluddin. 2012. "From Science Fiction to Future Noir: The Voyage Begins." In Aziz, *Transgressing Women: Space and The Body in Contemporary Noir Thrillers*, 187–270. Newcastle upon Tyne: Cambridge Scholars Publishing.

Badiou, Alain et al. 2003. *Matrix, machine philosophique*. Paris: Ellipses.

Badiou, Alain. 2013. *Cinema*. Texts selected by Antoine de Baecque, translated by Susan Spitzer. Cambridge: Polity Press.

Balderston, John. 2010 [1930]. *Frankenstein. A Play in Three Acts*. Albany, GA: BearManor Media.

Balderston, John, and Peggy Webling. 1930. *Frankenstein. A Play in Three Acts*. Reel 3528, Registration No. 9603, deposited March 11, 1931. Library of Congress, Washington, DC.

Baldick, Chris. 2015. *The Oxford Dictionary of Literary Terms*, 4th. ed. New York: Oxford University Press.

Ball, Philip. 2011. *Unnatural: The Heretical idea of Making People*. London: The Bodley Head.

Barker, Clyde F. and James F. Markmann. 2013. "Historical Overview of Transplantation." *Cold Spring Harbor Perspectives in Medicine* 3: a014977. DOI: 10.1101/cshperspect.a014977.

Barthes, Roland. 1963. "Qu'est-ce que la critique? In Barthes, *Essais critiques*, 252–257. Paris: Seuil. Reprinted in *Points*. Paris: Seuil, 1981.

Barthes, Roland. 1966. *Criticism and Truth*. Translated by Katrine Pilcher Keuneman. New York: Continuum, 2007.

Barthes, Roland. 1980. *Camera Lucida: Reflections on Photography*. Translated by Richard Howard. New York: Hill and Wang, 1981.

Bartlett, Frederic C. 1932. *Remembering: A Study in Experimental and Social Psychology*. London: Cambridge University Press, 1967.

Bauer, Martin W. 2016. "Results of the Essay Competition on the 'Deficit Concept'." *Public Understanding of Science* 25(4): 398–399.

Baxendale, Sallie. 2004. "Memories Aren't Made of This: Amnesia in the Movies." *British Medical Journal* 329: 1480–1483.

Bazin, André. 2005 [1945]. "The Ontology of the Photographic Image." In Bazin, *What is Cinema?*, vol. 1, selection and translation by Hugh Gray, 9–16. Berkeley: University of California Press.

Beard, William. 2006. *The Artist as Monster: The Cinema of David Cronenberg*. Revised ed. Toronto: University of Toronto Press.

Beecher, Henry K. et al. 1968. "A Definition of Irreversible Coma: Report of the Ad Hoc Committee of the Harvard Medical School to Examine the Definition of Brain Death." *JAMA* 205(6): 337–340.

Beliaev [sic], Alexander. 1980 [1925]. *Professor Dowell's Head*. Translated by A. W. Bouis. New York: Macmillan.

Bennett, Maxwell R., and Peter, M. S. Hacker. 2003. *Philosophical Foundations of Neuroscience*. Oxford: Blackwell.

Benson, E. F. 1996 [1922]. "And the Dead Spake—." In *The Collected Ghost Stories of E. F. Benson*, edited by Richard Dalby, 173–188. New York: Carroll & Graf.

Berliner, Brett A. 2004. "Mephistopheles and Monkeys: Rejuvenation, Race, and Sexuality in Popular Culture in Interwar France." *Journal of the History of Sexuality* 13(3): 306–325.

Bernal, John Desmond. 1929. *The World, the Flesh, and the Devil: An Enquiry into the Future of the Three Enemies of the Rational Soul*. Unpaginated text available on several websites.

Berton, Mireille. 2009a. "Cinéma et hypnose." *1895. Revue d'Histoire du cinéma* 58: 155–168.

Berton, Mireille. 2009b. "Cinéma et sciences du psychisme en 1900 : la névrose, la paramnésie, la transe." *Gesnerus* 66: 103–120.

Berton, Mireille. 2015. *Le Corps nerveux des spectateurs. Cinéma et sciences du psychisme autour de 1900*. Lausanne: L'Âge d'Homme.

Berton, Mireille. 2021. *Le médium (au) cinéma. Le spiritisme à l'écran*. Geneva: Georg.

Besson, Anne. 2004. *D'Asimov à Tolkien. Cycles et séries dans la littérature de genre*. Paris: CNRS Éditions.

Best, Stephen, and Sharon Marcus. 2009. "Surface Reading: An Introduction." *Representations* 108: 1–21.

Binder, Eando [pen name of Earl and Otto O. Binder]. 1934. "Enslaved Brains." *Wonder Stories* 6(2), July, 135–237; 6(3), August, 320–365; 6(4), September, 467–490.

Binder, Eando. 1936. "Spawn of Eternal Thought." *Astounding Stories* 17(2), April, 66–97; 17(3), May, 126–154.

Birr, Hannan, Maike Sarah Reinerth, and Jan-Noël Thon. eds. 2009. *Probleme filmischen Erzählens*. Berlin: Lit Verlag.

Bishop, Kylie William. 2015. *How Zombies Conquered Popular Culture: The Multifarious Walking Dead in the 21st Century*. Jefferson, NC: McFarland.

Bjork, Robert A. 2007. "Inhibition: An Essential and Contentious Concept." In *Science of Memory: Concepts*, edited by Henry L. Roediger III, Yadin Dudai, and Susan M. Fitzpatrick, 307–313. New York: Oxford University Press.

Bleiler, Everett F. 1990. *Science-Fiction: The Early Years: A Full Description of More Than 3,000 Science-Fiction Stories from Earliest Times to the Appearance of the Genre Magazines in 1930*. Kent, OH: Kent State University Press.

Bleiler, Everett F. 1998. *Science-Fiction: The Gernsback Years: A Complete Coverage of the Genre Magazines Amazing, Astounding, Wonder, and Others from 1926 through 1936*. Kent, OH: Kent State University Press.

Boileau-Narcejac [Pierre Boileau and Thomas Narcejac]. 1965. *...Et mon tout est un homme*. Paris, Denoël.

Bonnet, Charles. 1760. *Essai analytique sur les faculties de l'âme*. In Bonnet, *Œuvres d'histoire naturelle et de philosophie*, in-quarto ed., tome 6. Neuchâtel: Samuel Fauche, 1779–1783.

Borck, Cornelius. 2018. *Brainwaves: A Cultural History of Electroencephalography*. Translated by Anne M. Hentschel. London: Routledge.

Bordwell, David. 2015. "You and Me and Every Frog We Know." http://www.davidbordwell.net/blog/2015/09/20/you-and-me-and-every-frog-we-know/.

Bordwell, David. 2017. "The Amnesia Plot." *Laphams Quarterly*: https://www.laphamsquarterly.org/roundtable/amnesia-plot. Reprinted in Bordwell, 2017. *Reinventing Hollywood: How 1940s Filmmakers Changed Movie Storytelling*, 5–13. Chicago: University of Chicago Press.

Borges, Jorge Luis. 1942. "Funes el memorioso." Initially included in Borges, *Ficciones*. Buenos Aires, Emecé, 1944. Variously translated as "Funes the Memorious" and "Funes, His Memory."

Boss, Pete. 1986. "Vile Bodies and Bad Medicine." *Screen* 27(1): 14–24.

Böttcher, Wolfgang, and V. V. Alexi-Meskishvili, V. V. 2003. "Sergej Sergejewitsch Brychonenko (1890–1960): Pionier des kardiopulmonalen Bypasses in der Sowjetunion." *Kardiotechnik* 2: http://web.archive.org/web/20070121142821/http://www.dgfkt.de/artikel/203/Pionier.htm.

Bound Alberti, Fay. 2010. *Matters of the Heart: History, Medicine, and Emotion*. New York: Oxford University Press.

Bowles, James. 1933. "Makeup Secrets of Movie Horror Pictures." *Modern Mechanix* (February). http://blog.modernmechanix.com/makeup-secrets-of-movie-horror-pictures/.

Bowman, James. 2004. "Memory and the Movies." *The New Atlantis: A Journal of Technology and Society* (Spring): 85–90.

Boyer, Alain-Michel. 2008. *Les Paralittératures*. Paris: Armand Colin.

Boyer, Kevin L., and Bakay, Roy A. E. 1995. "The History, Theory, and Present Status of Brain Transplantation." *Functional Neurosurgery* 6(1): 113–125.

Brake, Mark L., and Neil Hook. 2008. *Different Engines: How Science Drives Fiction and Fiction Drives Science*. New York: Macmillan.

Brainfilms: Illustrations and captions for *Performing Brains on Screen*. https://www.academia.edu/49648716/Brainfilms.

Brodesco, Alberto. 2011. "I've Got you under my Skin: Narratives of the Inner Body in Cinema and Television." *Nuncius* 26: 201–222.

Brossard, Dominique, and Bruce V. Lewenstein. 2010. "A Critical Appraisal of Models of Public Understanding of Science: Using Practice to Inform Theory." In *Communicating Science: New Agendas in Communication*, edited by LeeAnn Kahlor and Patricia A. Stout, 11–39. New York: Routledge.

Brown, Roger, and James Kulik. 1977. "Flashbulb Memories." *Cognition* 5: 73–99.

Brueckner, Tony. 2004. "Brains in a Vat." *Stanford Encyclopedia of Philosophy*, http://stanford.library.usyd.edu.au/archives/sum2006/entries/brain-vat/

Bucchi, Massimiano, and Federico Neresini. 2007. "Science and Public Participation." In *The Handbook of Science and Technology Studies*, edited by Edward J. Hackett et al., 3rd ed., 449–472. Cambridge, MA: MIT Press.

Buchanan, Tony W. 2007. "Retrieval of Emotional Memories." *Psychological Bulletin* 133(5): 761–779.

Buckland, Warren. 2009a. "Introduction: Puzzle Plots." In *Puzzle Films*, edited by Buckland, 1–12.

Buckland, Warren, ed. 2009b. *Puzzle Films: Complex Storytelling in Contemporary Cinema*. Oxford: Wiley-Blackwell.

Bukatman, Scott. 2018. "*Frankenstein* and the Peculiar Power of the Comics." In *Global Frankenstein*, edited by Davison, 185–207.

Bulgakov, Mikhail. 1968 [1925]. *Heart of a Dog*. Translated by M. Ginsburg. New York, Grove Press.

Bunzel, B., G. Wollenek, and A. Grundbock, 1992. "Living with a Donor Heart: Feelings and Attitudes of Patients toward the Donor and the Donor Organ." *Journal of Heart and Lung Transplantation* 11: 1151–1155.

Burks, Arthur J. 1931a. "Manape the Mighty." *Astounding Stories* 6(3), June, 308–355.

Burks, Arthur J. 1931b. [Letter to the Editor], *Astounding Stories* 6(3), June, 416–417.

Burks, Arthur J. 1932. "The Mind Master." *Astounding Stories* 9(1), January, 28–53; 9(2), February, 238–263.

Burroughs, Edgar Rice. 1927. "The Master Mind of Mars." *Amazing Stories Annual* 6–53.

Butler, Andrew M. 2018. *Eternal Sunshine of the Spotless Mind*. London: British Film Institute / Bloomsbury.

Bynum, Caroline Walker. 1991. "Material Continuity, Personal Survival, and the Resurrection of the Body: A Scholastic Discussion in Its Medieval and Modern Contexts." In Bynum, *Fragmentation and Redemption: Essays on Gender and the Human Body in Medieval Religion*. New York: Zone Books.

Bynum, Caroline. 1995. "Why All the Fuss about the Body? A Medievalist's Perspective." *Critical Inquiry* 22: 1–33.

Cabrera, Julio. 1999. *Cine: 100 años de filosofía. Una introducción a la filosofía a través del análisis de películas*. Barcelona: Gedisa.

Campbell, John C. 1930. "The Infinite Brain." *Science Wonder Stories* 1(12), May, 1076–1093.

Campora, Matthew. 2014. *Subjective Realist Cinema: From Expressionism to* Inception. New York: Berghahn.

Canavero, Sergio. 2013. "HEAVEN: The Head Anastomosis Venture Project Outline for the First Human Head Transplantation with Spinal Linkage (GEMINI)." *Surgical Neurology International* 4(Suppl 1): S335–S342.

Canavero, Sergio. 2015. "The 'Gemini' Spinal Cord Fusion Protocol: Reloaded." *Surgical Neurology International* 6: 18.

Caparrós, Martín. 2020. *Sinfín*. Barcelona: Literatura Random House.

Cappuccio, Massimiliano. 2014. "'I See You' through a Glass Darkly: *Avatar* and the Limits of Empathy." In *Avatar and Philosophy: Learning to See*, edited by George A. Dunn, 74–86. Oxford: Wiley Blackwell.

Carel, Havi. 2007. "The Return of the Erased: Memory and Forgetfulness in *Eternal Sunshine of the Spotless Mind* (2004)." *International Journal of Psychoanalysis* 88: 1071–1082.

Carey, Benedict. 2008. "H. M., an Unforgettable Amnesiac, Dies at 82." *New York Times*, December 4. https://www.nytimes.com/2008/12/05/us/05hm.html.

Carroll, Noël. 1990. *The Philosophy of Horror or Paradoxes of the Heart*. New York: Routledge.

Carroll, Noël, Laura T. Di Summa, and Shawn Loht. eds. 2019. *The Palgrave Handbook of the Philosophy of Film and Motion Pictures*. New York: Palgrave Macmillan.

Cassou-Noguès, Pierre. 2010. *Mon Zombie et moi. La philosophie comme fiction*. Paris, Seuil.

Cassou-Noguès, Pierre. 2011. "Exploring the Brain, Looking for Thoughts: On Asimov's Second *Fantastic Voyage*." *Nuncius* 26: 185–200.

Catlin, Don Robert. 1927. "Listening Death." *Weird Tales* 9(5), May, 642–648.

Cerf, Juliette. 2009. *Cinéma et philosophie*. Paris: Cahiers du Cinéma.

Chalmers, David J. 2005. "The Matrix as Metaphysics." In *Philosophers Explore the Matrix*, edited by Christopher Grau, 132–176. New York: Oxford University Press.

Charney, Leo, and Vanessa R. Schwartz. 1995. "Introduction." In *Cinema and the Invention of Modern Life*, edited by L. Charney and V. R. Schwartz, 1–12. Berkeley: University of California Press.

Cheng, John. 2012. *Astounding Wonder: Imagining Science and Science Fiction in Interwar America*. Philadelphia: University of Pennsylvania Press.

Choi, Jinhee, and Mattias Frey, eds. 2014. *Cine-Ethics: Ethical Dimensions of Film Theory, Practice, and Spectatorship*. New York: Routledge.

Clark, Andy. 2010. "*Memento*'s Revenge: The Extended Mind, Extended." In *The Extended Mind*, edited by Richard Menary, 43–66. Cambridge, MA: MIT Press.

Clémot, Hugo. 2018. *Cinéthique*. Paris: Vrin.

Collins, Dean. 1933. "Stallion's Trappings." *Amazing Stories* 7(2), March, 1135–1136.

Compagnon, Antoine. 2006. *La littérature, pour quoi faire?* Inaugural lecture at the Collège de France, https://books.openedition.org/cdf/524.

Costandi, Mo. 2007. "Eternal Erasing of the Scary Memory." https://neurophilosophy.wordpress.com/2007/03/13/eternal-erasing-of-the-scary-memory/.

Coulombe, Maxime. 2012. *Petite philosophie du zombie ou comment penser par l'horreur*. Paris: Presses Universitaires de France.

Crews, Frederick. 1995. *The Memory Wars: Freud's Legacy in Dispute*. New York: New York Review of Books.

Cross, Robin. 1982. *The Big Book of B Movies, or How Low Was My Budget*. New York: St. Martin's Press.

Crowther, Bosley. 1954. "The Screen in Review; 'Donovan's Brain,' Science-Fiction Thriller, Has Premiere at the Criterion Theatre." *The New York Times*, January 21. https://www.nytimes.com/1954/01/21/archives/the-screen-in-review-donovans-brain-sciencefiction-thriller-has.html.

Crowther, Bosley. 1966. "Screen: 'Fantastic Voyage' Is All That: Science-Fiction Movie Opens at 2 Theaters." *The New York Times*, September 8. https://www.nytimes.com/1966/09/08/archives/screen-fantastic-voyage-is-all-thatsciencefiction-movie-opens-at-2.html.

Cummings, Ray. 1931. "The Great Transformation." *Wonder Stories* 2(9), February, 936–943.

Curtis, Wardon Allan. 1899. "The Monster of Lake LaMetrie." *Pearson's Magazine*, September, http://gutenberg.net.au/ebooks06/0605351h.html.

Dadlez, E. M. 2019. "Thoughtful Films, Thoughtful Fictions: The Philosophical Terrain Between Illustrations and Thought Experiments." In *The Palgrave Handbook of the Philosophy of Film and Motion Pictures*, edited by Carroll, Di Summa and Loht, 469–490.

Dahl, Roald. 1960 [1959]. "William and Mary." In Dahl, *Kiss Kiss*. New York: Alfred A. Knopf. (Reprinted in R. Dahl, *Tales of the Unexpected*, 1979.)

Daniels, J. Stallworth. 1930. "The Horrible Transformation." *Science Wonder Stories* 1(12), May, 1130–1135.

Danzey, Kevin. 1999. "Interview with Kevin Danzey." http://www.badmovies.org/interviews/kevdanzey/.

Daston, Lorraine, and Fernando Vidal, eds. 2004. *The Moral Authority of Nature*. Chicago: University of Chicago Press.

Davis, Blair 2012. *The Battle for the Bs: 1950s Hollywood and the Rebirth of Low-Budget Cinema*. New Brunswick, NJ: Rutgers University Press.

Davis, Blair. 2015. "Of Apes and Men (and Monsters and Girls): The Ape Film and 1940s Horror Cinema." In *Recovering 1940s Horror Cinema: Traces of a Lost Decade*, edited by Mario DeGiglio-Bellemare, Charlie Ellbé and Kristopher Woofter, 275–293. New York: Lexington Books.

Davison, Carol Margaret, ed. 2018. *Global Frankenstein*. New York: Palgrave Macmillan.

Debiec, Jacek, Joseph E. LeDoux, and Karim Nader. 2002. "Cellular and Systems Reconsolidation in the Hippocampus." *Neuron* 36(3): 527–538.

Dekker, Martijn. 1999. "On our Own Terms: Emerging Autistic Culture." http://www.autscape.org/2015/programme/handouts/Autistic-Culture-07-Oct-1999.pdf.

Dendle, Peter. 2001. *The Zombie Movie Encyclopedia*. London: MacFarland.

Descartes, René. 1641. *Meditations on First Philosophy*. In Descartes, *Meditations, Objections and Replies*, edited and translated by Roger Ariew and Donald Cress. Indianapolis: Hackett, 2006.

Després, Elaine. 2009. "L'Inquiétante science de la greffe chez Maurice Renard." *Otrante. Art art et literature fantastiques* 26: 55–68.

Dick, Philip K. 1997 [1956]. "The Minority Report." In *The Philip K. Dick Reader*, 323–354. New York: Citadel Press.

Donawerth, Jane. 1990. "Lilith Lorraine: Feminist Socialist Writer in the Pulps." *Science Fiction Studies* 17(2), 252–258.

Donawerth, Jane L. 1994. "Science Fiction by Women in the Early Pulps." In *Utopian and Science Fiction by Women: Worlds of Difference*, edited by J. L. Donawerth and Carol A. Kolmerten, 137–152. Syracuse, NY: Syracuse University Press.

Doniger, Wendy. 2005. *The Woman Who Pretended to Be Who She Was: Myths of Self-Imitation*. New York: Oxford University Press.

Doyère, Valérie, et al. 2007. "Synapse-Specific Reconsolidation of Distinct Fear Memories in the Lateral Amygdala." *Nature Neuroscience* 10: 414–416.

Drees, Rich. 2005. "Edison's Frankenstein: Cinema's First Horror Film." *FilmBuffOnline*, http://www.filmbuffonline.com/FBOLNewsreel/wordpress/2005/08/07/edisons-frankenstein-cinemas-first-horror-film/.

Dressler, Daniel. 1929. "The Brain Accelerator." *Amazing Stories* 4(8), November, 696–705, 719.

Dudai, Yadin. 2004. "The Neurobiology of Consolidations, or How Stable is the Engram?"*Annual Review of Psychology* 55: 51–86.

Dudai, Yadin. 2006. "Reconsolidation: The Advantage of Being Refocused." *Current Opinion in Neurobiology* 16(2): 174–178.

Dudai, Yadin. 2009. "Predicting Not to Predict Too Much: How the Cellular Machinery of Memory Anticipates the Uncertain Future." *Philosophical Transactions of the Royal Society* B 364: 1255–1262.

Dudai, Yadin, and Mark Eisenberg. 2004. "Rites of Passage of the Engram: Reconsolidation and the Lingering Consolidation Hypothesis." *Neuron* 44(1): 93–100.

Dufour, Éric. 2006. *Le Cinéma d'horreur et ses figures*. Paris: Presses Universitaires de France.

Dufour, Éric. 2011. *Le Cinéma de science-fiction*. Paris, Armand Colin.

Dunne, Matthew W. 2013. *A Cold War State of Mind: Brainwashing and Postwar American Society*. Amherst, University of Massachusetts Press.

Eaves, Elisabeth. 2007. "Altering Human Memory." *Forbes.com*, May 24. http://www.forbes.com/2007/05/23/karim-nader-memory-tech-cx_07rev_ee_0524nader.html/.

Ebert, Roger. 1969. [Review of *Change of Mind*], https://www.rogerebert.com/reviews/change-of-mind-1969.

Eco, Umberto. 2019. "On Some Forms of Imperfection in Art." In Eco, *On the Shoulders of Giants*, translated by Alastair McEwen, 196–221. Cambridge, MA: Harvard University Press.

Edelstein, David. 2004. "Forget Me Not: The Genius of Charlie Kaufman's Eternal Sunshine of the Spotless Mind." *Slate*, March 18. https://slate.com/culture/2004/03/eternal-sunshine-is-unforgettable.html.

Eder, Jens. 2010. "Understanding Characters." *Projections: The Journal for Movies and Mind* 4(1): 16–40.

Eder, Jens, Fotis Jannidis, and Ralf Schneider. 2010. "Characters in Fictional Worlds: An Introduction." In *Characters in Fictional Worlds: Understanding Imaginary Beings in Literature, Film, and Other Media*, edited by Eder, Jannidis, and Schneider, 3–64. New York: De Gruyter.

Eichenbaum, Howard. 2012. *The Cognitive Neuroscience of Memory: An Introduction*, 2nd ed. New York: Oxford University Press.

Einsiedel, Edna. 2007. "Editorial: Of Publics and Science." *Public Understanding of Science* 16(1): 5–6.

Elsaesser, Thomas. 2009. "The Mind-Game Film." In *Puzzle Films*, edited by Buckland, 13–42.

Elsaesser, Thomas, and Malte Hagener. 2015. *Film Theory: An Introduction Through the Senses*, 2nd ed. New York: Routledge.

Erickson, Paul, Judy L. Klein, Lorraine Daston, Rebecca Lemov, Thomas Sturm, and Michael D. Gordin. 2013. *How Reason Almost Lost Its Mind: The Strange Career of Cold War Rationality*. Chicago: University of Chicago Press.

Ernst, Paul. 1930. "The Black Monarch." *Weird Tales* 15(2), February, 193–222; 15(6), June, 813–825.

Ernst, Paul. 2016 [1932]. "The Raid on the Termites." *Astounding* Stories 10(3), June. HardPress (e-book).

ESF: *The Encyclopedia of Science Fiction*, edited by John Clute, David Langford, Peter Nicholls, and Graham Sleight. 3rd ed. http://www.sf-encyclopedia.com.

Eshbach, L. A. 1932. "The Time Conqueror." *Wonder Stories* 4(2), July, 126–147, 182.

Evans, Arthur B. 1994. "The Fantastic Science Fiction of Maurice Renard." *Science Fiction Studies* 21(3): 380–396.

Fearn, John Russell. 1933. "The Intelligence Gigantic." *Amazing Stories* 8(3), June, 235–253; 8(4), July, 316–344.

Feld, Rob. 2004. "Q & A with Charlie Kaufman." In Kaufman, *Eternal Sunshine of the Spotless Mind*. London: Nick Hern Books.

Ferreira, Aline. 2012. "Gothic (Dis)Embodiments: Kureishi's *The Body* and Richard T. Kelly's *The Possessions of Doctor Forrest*." *Textus. English Studies in Italy* 3: 117–132.

Ferret, Stéphane. 1993. *Le Philosophe et son scalpel. Le problème de l'identité personnelle*. Paris: Minuit.

Flagg, Francis. 1929. "The Chemical Brain." *Weird Tales* 13(13), January, 73–81.

Flynn, Charles. 1975. "The Schlock/Kitsch/Hack Movies." In *Kings of the Bs – Working within the Hollywood System*, edited by McCarthy and Flynn, 3–12.

Flynn, Charles, and Todd McCarthy. 1975. "The Economic Imperative: Why Was the B Movie Necessary?" In *Kings of the Bs – Working within the Hollywood System*, edited by McCarthy and Flynn, 13–43.

Forry, Steven Earl. 1990. *Hideous Progenies: Dramatizations of Frankenstein from Mary Shelley to the Present*. Philadelphia: University of Pennsylvania Press.

Franck, Alain and Victor Vicas. 1969. *L'Homme au cerveau greffé*. Paris: Laffont.

Frayling, Christopher. 2005. *Mad, Bad and Dangerous? The Scientist and the Cinema*. London: Reaktion Books.

Freud, Sigmund. 1911. *Psychoanalytic Notes on an Autobiographical Account of a Case of Paranoia (Dementia Paranoides)*. In Freud, *Standard Edition*, vol. XII (1958).

Freud, Sigmund. 1915. "The Unconscious." In Freud, *Standard Edition*, vol. XIV (1957).

Freud, Signumd. 1953–1974. *Standard Edition: The Standard Edition of the Complete Psychological Works of Sigmund Freud*. Translated under the general editorsphip of James Strachey. 24 vols. London: The Hogarth Press and the Institute of Psycho-Analysis.

Front, Sonia. 2017. "Hacking the Brain: Duncan Jones's *Source Code*." *Świat i Słowo*, 1(28): 11–26.

Gallun, Raymond Z. 1935. "Mind Over Matter." *Astounding Stories* 14(5), January, 116–123.

Gardner, Thomas D. 1932. "The Last Woman." *Wonder Stories* 3(11), April, 1238–1244.

Gates, Raquel. 2014. "Subverting Hollywood from the Inside Out: Melvin van Peebles's *Watermelon Man*." *Film Quarterly* 68(1): 9–21.

Gazzaniga, Michael. 1967. "The Split Brain in Man." *Scientific American* 217(2): 24–29.

Gazzaniga, Michael S. 2005. *The Ethical Brain*. New York: Dana Press.

Gere, Cathy, ed. 2004. *The Brain in A Vat*. Special issue, *Studies in History and Philosophy of Biology and the Biomedical Sciences* 35 (2004).

Geroulanos, Stefanos. 2013. "Postwar Facial Reconstruction: Georges Franju's *Eyes Without a Face*." *French Politics, Culture & Society* 31(2): 15–33.

Gilmore, Anthony [pseudonym of Harry Bates and Desmond Hall]. 1932. "The Affair of the Brains." *Astounding Stories* 9(3), March. New Delhi: Prabhat Prakashan (e-book).

Glut, Donald F. 1984. *The Frankenstein Catalog*. Jefferson, NC: McFarland.

Goffette, Jérôme. 2007. "Le corps saisi de l'intérieur, de Claude Bernard au *Voyage fantastique* de Richard Fleischer." In *Les Imaginaires du corps en mutation: du corps enchanté au corps en chantier*, edited by Claude Fintz, 343–365. Paris: L'Harmattan.

Grau, Christopher, ed. 2005. *Philosophers Explore the Matrix*. New York: Oxford University Press.

Grau, Christopher. 2006. "Eternal Sunshine of the Spotless Mind and the Morality of Memory." *The Journal of Aesthetics and Art Criticism* 64: 119–133.

Grau, Christopher, ed. 2009. *Eternal Sunshine of the Spotless Mind*. New York: Routledge.

Greene, Richard, and K. Silem Mohammad, eds. 2010. *Zombies, Vampires, and Philosophy: New Life for the Undead*. Chicago: Open Court.

Griffin, John Howard. 1961. *Black Like Me*. Boston: Houghton Mifflin.

Gunn, James E. 2018. *Alternate Worlds: The Illustrated History of Science Fiction*. 3rd ed. Jefferson, NC: McFarland.

Hagner, Michael. 2004. *Geniale Gehirne. Zur Geschichte der Elitenhirnforschung*. Göttingen, Wallstein.

Hall, Mordaunt. 1931. "A Man-Made Monster in Grand Guignol Film Story." *New York Times*, December 5. In *Tabula Rasa* 3 (1994): www.tabula-rasa.info/Horror/FrankensteinFiles.html.

Hall, Stephen S. 2012. "The Dementia Plague." *MIT Technology Review*, October 5. https://www.technologyreview.com/s/429494/the-dementia-plague/.

Hamilton, David. 2012. *History of Organ Transplantation: Ancient Legends to Modern Practice*. Pittsburgh: University of Pittsburgh Press.

Hamilton, Edmond. 1928. "The Comet Doom." *Amazing Stories* 2(10), January, 926–940.

Hamilton, Edmond. 1931. "The Man Who Evolved." *Wonder Stories* 2(11), April, 1266–1277.

Hamilton, Edmond. 1936. "Intelligence Undying." *Amazing Stories* 10(9), April, 13–26.

Hammerstrom, Norman Elmwood, and R[ichard] F[ranklyn] Searight. 1924. "The Brain in the Jar." *Weird Tales* 4(3), November, 31–35, 183–190.

Harmes, Marcus K. 2015. *The Curse of Frankenstein*. New York: Columbia University Press.

Hasta, M. H. 1926. "The Talking Brain." *Amazing Stories* 1(5), August, 440–445, 478–479.

Hauskeller, Michael. 2013. "Wanna Live Forever? Don't Pull a Frankenstein!" In *Frankenstein and Philosophy*, edited by Michaud, 3–13.

Hauskeller, Michael, Thomas D. Philbeck, and Curtis D. Carbonell, eds. 2015. *The Palgrave Handbook of Posthumanism in Film and Television*. New York, Palgrave Macmillan.

Haynes, Roslynn D. 1995. "Frankenstein: The Scientist We Love to Hate." *Public Understanding of Science* 4: 435–444.

Haynes, Roslynn D. 2014. "Whatever Happened to the 'Mad, Bad' Scientist? Overturning the Stereotype." *Public Understanding of Science* 25(1): 31–44.

Hearn, Marcus, and Alan Barnes. 2007. *The Hammer Story*, 2nd ed. London: Titan Books.

Heinlein, Robert A. 1951. *The Puppet Masters*. New York: Doubleday. (Originally serialized in *Galaxy Science Fiction*, September, October and November 1951.)

Herzogenrath, Bernd. 2017. "Introduction. Film and/as Philosophy: An Elective Affinity?" In *Film As Philosophy*, edited by B. Herzogenrath, vii–xxv. Minneapolis: University of Minnesota Press.

Hess, Keith. 2013. "Sure It's Aliiiive, but Does It Have a Sooooul?" In *Frankenstein and Philosophy*, edited by Michaud, 137–145.

Hesselberth, Pepita, and Laura Schuster. 2008. "Into the Mind and Out of the World: Memory Anxiety in the Mind-Game Film." In *Mind the Screen: Media Concepts According to Thomas Elsaesser*, edited by Jaap Kooijman, Patricia Pisters, and Wanda Strauven, 96–111. Amsterdam: Amsterdam University Press.

Hickey, Lance P. 2005. "The Brain in a Vat Argument." *Internet Encyclopedia of Philosophy*, http://www.iep.utm.edu/brainvat/.

Hill-Parks, Erin. 2006. "From Film to Life: The Construction of Identity in *Eternal Sunshine of the Spotless Mind* and *I 'Heart' Huckabees*." In *From Camera Lens To Critical Lens: A Collection Of Best Essays On Film Adaptation*, edited by Rebecca Housel, 1–8. Newcastle: Cambridge Scholars Press.

Hitchcock, Susan Tyler. 2007. *Frankenstein: A Cultural History*. New York: W. W. Norton.

Hoberman, J. 2003. "Scientist Seeks Flesh for Fantasy in French Scare Classic." *The Village Voice*, October 28. https://www.villagevoice.com/2003/10/28/mad-scientist-seeks-flesh-for-fantasy-in-french-scare-classic/.

Hofstadter, Douglas R., and Daniel C. Dennett, eds. 1981. *The Mind's I: Fantasies And Reflections On Self and Soul*. Toronto, Bantam Books.

Holden, Constance. 2002. "Random Samples: From PUS to PEST." *Science* 298(5591): 49.

Holland, Rachel. 2019. *Contemporary Fiction and Science from Amis to McEwan: The Third Culture Novel.* New York: Palgrave Macmillan.

Hoppenstand, Gary. 2013. "On Pulp Fiction and *Weird Tales.*" In *Critical Insights: Pulp Fiction of the '20s and '30s*, edited by G. Hoppenstand, xiii–xviii. Ipswich, MA: Salem Press.

Horton, Robert. 2014. *Frankenstein.* New York: Columbia University Press.

Hutchings, Peter. 2008. *The A to Z of Horror Cinema.* Plymouth, UK: Scarecrow Press.

Hutchinson, Phil, and Rupert Read. 2005. "*Memento*: A Philosophical Investigation." In *Film as Philosophy: Essays in Cinema After Wittgenstein and Cavell*, edited by Rupert Read and Jerry Goodenough, 72–93. New York: Palgrave Macmillan.

Ikäheimo, Heikki and Arto Laitinen. 2007. "Dimensions of Personhood." *Journal of Consciousness Studies* 14(5–6): 6–16.

Irwin, William, ed. 2002. *The Matrix and Philosophy: Welcome to the Desert of the Real.* Chicago: Open Court.

ISFDB: *The Internet Speculative Fiction Database*, http://www.isfdb.org/.

Jakobson, Roman. 1921. "Realism in Art." In *Roman Jakobson – Language in Literature*, edited by Krystina Pomorska and Stephen Rudy, 19–27. Cambridge, MA: Belknap Press of Harvard University Press, 1987.

Jasanoff, Alan. 2018. *The Biological Mind: How Brain, Body, and Environment Collaborate to Make Us Who We Are.* New York: Basic Books.

Johnson, David Kyle, ed. 2020. *Black Mirror and Philosophy: Dark Reflections.* Hoboken, NJ: Wiley Blackwell.

Johnson, Steven. 2004. "The Science of Eternal Sunshine: You Can't Erase Your Boyfriend from Your Brain, but the Movie Gets the Rest of it Right." *Slate*, March 22. https://slate.com/culture/2004/03/the-neuroscience-behind-eternal-sunshine.html.

Jones, Neil R. 1931. "The Jameson Satellite." *Amazing Stories* 6(4), July, 334–343.

Jones, Neil R. 1934. "Moon Pirates." *Amazing Stories* 9(5), September, 11–40; 9(6), October, 53–83.

Jones, Neil R. 1935. "Zora of the Zoromes." *Amazing Stories* 9(11), March, 88–120.

Jones, Stephen. 1994. *The Illustrated Frankenstein Movie Guide.* London: Titan Books.

Jonsen, Albert R. 2012. "The Ethics of Organ Transplantation: A Brief History." *American Medical Association Journal of Ethics* 14(3): 264–268.

Judd, Wes. 2017. "Can 'Jupiter Ascending' Change the Way We Feel About 'The Matrix'?" https://psmag.com/social-justice/channing-tatums-elf-ears-dont-bode-well-for-neo-and-gang.

Jungblut, Christian. 2001. *Meinen Kopf auf deinen Hals. Die neuen Pläne des Dr. Frankenstein alias Robert White.* Stuttgart, Hirzel.

Kaba, Evridiki et al. 2005. "Somebody Else's Heart Inside Me: A Descriptive Study of Psychological Problems After a Heart Transplantation." *Issues in Mental Health Nursing* 26(6), 611–625.

Kalland, John Francis. 1935. "Restitution." *Amazing Stories* 10(7), 118–132.

Kaltenbrunner, Karin. 2014. *Mad Medicine. Zur Repräsentation des Wissenschaftlers im Frankenstein-Zyklus der Hammer Film Productions (1957–1974).* Vienna, Lit Verlag.

Kaufman, Anthony. 2001. "Christopher Nolan Remembers 'Memento'" [an interview]. *indieWIRE*, March 16. www.indiewire.com/article/interview_mindgames_christopher_nolan_remembers_memento/.

Kawin, Bruce F. 1978. *Mindscreen: Bergman, Godard, and First-Person Film.* Princeton, NJ: Princeton University Press.

Kawin, Bruce F. 2012. *Horror and the Horror Film.* New York: Anthem Press.

Kay, Glenn. 2008. *Zombie Movies: The Ultimate Guide.* Chicago: Chicago Review Press.

Keller, David H. 1929. "The Human Termites." *Science Wonder Stories* 1(4), September, 294–315; 1(5), October, 410–425; 1(6), November, 530–549, 556.

Keller, David H. 1931a. "The Ambidexter." *Amazing Stories* 6(1), April, 36–41.

Keller, David H. 1931b. “The Cerebral Library.” *Amazing Stories* 6(2), May, 116–124.

Kensinger, Elizabeth A., and Sarah M. Kark. 2018. “Emotion and Memory.” In *Stevens' Handbook of Experimental Psychology and Cognitive Neuroscience: Volume 1, Learning and Memory*, 4th ed., edited by Elizabeth Phelps and Lila Davachi (editor-in-chief John T. Wixted), 1–26. New York: Wiley.

Keppler, Carl F. 1929. “Dr. Pichegru's Discovery.” *Weird Tales* 14(1), July, 81–90.

Kilbourn, Russell J. A. 2010. *Cinema, Memory, Modernity: The Representation of Memory from the Art Film to Transnational Cinema*. New York: Routledge.

Killen, Andreas. 2017. *Homo Cinematicus: "Science, Motion Pictures, and the Making of Modern Germany*. Philadelphia: University of Pennsylvania Press.

Kirk, Robert. 2019."Zombies." *Stanford Encyclopedia of Philosophy*, https://plato.stanford.edu/archives/spr2019/entries/zombies/.

Kleier, Joe. 1928. “The Head.” *Amazing Stories* 3(5), August, 418–421, 449.

Klein, Stanley B. 2014. “Sameness and the Self: Philosophical and Psychological Considerations.” *Frontiers in Psychology* 5: art. 29. DOI: 10.3389/fpsyg.2014.00029.

Klein, Stanley B., and Shaun Nichols. 2012. “Memory and the Sense of Personal Identity.” *Mind* 121(483): 677–702.

Klepeis, Alicia Z. 2017. *Brain Eaters: Creatures with Zombie-Like Diets*. North Mankato, MN: Capstone Press.

Klugman, Craig M. 2001. “From Cyborg Fiction to Medical Reality.” *Literature and Medicine* 20(1): 39–54.

Knight, Deborah. 2009. “Personal Identity.” In *The Routledge Companion to Philosophy and Film*, edited by Livingston and Plantinga, 611–619.

Koch, Christof. 2004. *The Quest for Consciousness: A Neurobiological Approach*. Greenwood Village, CO: Roberts.

Korfmacher, Carsten. 2006. “Personal Identity.” *Internet Encyclopedia of Philosophy*, https://www.iep.utm.edu/person-i/.

Krementsov, Nikolai. 2009. “Off with Your Heads: Isolated Organs in early Soviet Science and Fiction.” *Studies in History and Philosophy of Biological and Biomedical Sciences* 40: 87–100.

Krementsov, Nikolai. 2013. *Revolutionary Experiments: The Quest for Immortality in Bolshevik Science and Fiction*. New York: Oxford University Press.

Krüger-Fürhoff, Irmela Marei. 2012. *Verpflanzungsgebiete. Wissenskulturen und Poetik der Transplantation*. Munich: Wilhelm Fink.

Krzywinska, Tanya. 2018. “Playing the Intercorporeal: *Frankenstein*'s Legacy for Games.” In *Global Frankenstein*, edited by Davison, 283–300.

Kuhn, Annette, ed. 1999. *Alien Zone II: The Spaces of Science Fiction Cinema*. London: Verso.

Kuhn, Markus. 2009. “Gibt es einen Ich-Kamera Film? Überlegungen zum filmischen Erzählens mit der subjektiven Kamera und eine exemplarische Analyse von Julian Schnabels *Le Scaphandre et le papillon*.” In *Probleme filmischen Erzählens*, edited by Birr, Reinerth, and Thon, 59–83.

Kureishi, Hanif. 2002. *The Body*. New York: Scribner.

Kureishi, Hanif. 2004. Interview with Emily Mead. *Nerve*, February 25, http://www.nerve.com/screeningroom/books/interview_hanifkureishi or http://www.nerve.com/content/the-nerve-interview-hanifkureishi. [Links no longer active.]

LA: *Luminist Archives*, http://www.luminist.org/archives/PU/index.htm.

Lamba, Nayan, Daniel Holsgrove, and Marike L. Broekman. 2016. “The History of Head Transplantation: A Review.” *Acta Neurochirurgica* 158: 2239–2247.

LaRocca, David. 2017. “'Memory Man:' The Constitution of Personal Identity in *Memento*.” In *The Philosophy of Christopher Nolan*, edited by Jason T. Eberl and George A. Dunn, 179–189. New York: Lexington Books.

Laskas, Jeanne Marie. 2014. “The New Face of Richard Norris.” *GQ*, August 27. https://www.gq.com/story/richard-norris.

Laugier, Sandra. 2019. *Nos vies en séries. Philosophie et morale d’une culture populaire*. Paris: Climats.

Le Maître, Barbara. 2016. *Zombie : Une fable anthropologique*. Nanterre: Presses universitaires de Paris Nanterre. DOI: 10.4000/books.pupo.5858.

Leadbeater, Charles. 2015. “The Disremembered.” *Aeon*. https://aeon.co/essays/if-your-memory-fails-are-you-still-the-same-person.

Lederer, E. Susan, ed., 2002. *Frankenstein. Penetrating the Secrets of Nature*. New Brunswick, NJ: Rutgers University Press.

Lee, Hong J. et al. 2007. “Brain Transplantation of Immortalized Human Neural Stem Cells Promotes Functional Recovery in Mouse Intracerebral Hemorrhage Stroke Model.” *Stem Cells* 25: 1204–1212.

Lee, Jonathan L. C., Karim Nader, and Daniela Schiller. 2017. “An Update on Memory Reconsolidation Updating.” *Trends in Cognitive Science* 21(7): 531–545.

Lem, Stanisław. 2002. “The Solaris Station.” https://english.lem.pl/arround-lem/adaptations/solaris-soderbergh/147-the-solaris-station.

Lem, Stanisław. 2017 [1961]. *Solaris*. Translated by Bill Johnston. Krakow: Pro Auctore Wojciech Zemek. E-book.

Lethem, Jonathan, ed. 2000. *The Vintage Book of Amnesia*. New York: Vintage Books.

Letourneux, Matthieu. 2017. *Fictions à la chaîne. Littératures sérielles et culture médiatique*. Paris: Seuil.

Lévi-Strauss. Claude. 1963. *Structural Anthropology*. Translated by Claire Jacobson and Brooke Grundfest Schoepf. New York: Basic Books.

Levine, George. 1979. “The Ambiguous Heritage of Frankenstein.” In *The Endurance of Frankenstein: Essays on Mary Shelley’s Novel*, edited by George Levine and U. C. Knoepflmacher, 3–30. Berkeley: University of California Press.

Lieberman, Evan. 2018. “Frankenstein at the Boundaries of Life, Death, and Film.” In *Frankenstein. How A Monster Became an Icon: The Science and Enduring Allure of Mary Shelley’s Creation*, edited by Sidney Perkowitz and Eddy von Mueller. New York: Pegasus Books. E-book.

Littlefield, Melissa M., and Jenell M. Johnson, eds. 2012. *The Neuroscientific Turn: Transdisciplinarity in the Age of the Brain*. Ann Arbor: University of Michigan Press.

Livingston, Paisley and Carl Plantinga, eds. 2009. *The Routledge Companion to Philosophy and Film*. New York: Routledge.

Locke, John. 1988 [1694]. *An Essay Concerning Human Understanding*, Edited by P. H. Nidditch. 2nd ed. Oxford: Clarendon Press.

Loftus, Elizabeth F. 1997. “Creating False Memories.” *Scientific American*, 227(3): 1997, 70–75.

Loftus, Elizabeth F. 2003. “Our Changeable Memories: Legal and Practical Implications.” *Nature Reviews Neuroscience*, 4 2003: 231–234.

Loftus, Elizabeth F., and Katherine Ketcham. 1994. *The Myth of Repressed Memory: False Memories and Allegations of Sexual Abuse*. New York: St. Martin’s.

Loftus, Elizabeth F., and Jacqueline E. Pickrell. 1995. “The Formation of False Memories.” *Psychiatric Annals* 25: 720–725.

Long, Frank Belknap. 1934. “The Vapor Death.” *Astounding Stories* 14(2), October, 39–47.

Lopez Cruz, Ronald Allan. 2012. “Mutations and Metamorphoses: Body Horror is Biological Horror.” *Journal of Popular Film and Television* 40(4): 160–168.

Lucas, Tim. 2008. “Les yeux sans visage (The Horror Chamber of Dr. Faustus)/The Manster, *Sight & Sound* 18(8): 34.

Luria, Aleksandr R. 1968. *The Mind of a Mnemonist*. Translated by Lynn Solotaroff. New York: Basic Books.

MacDowell, James, and Richard McCulloch. 2019. "Introduction. 'So Bad it's Good:' Aesthetics, Reception, and Beyond." *Continuum* 33(6): 643–652.

Macmillan, Malcolm. 2008. "Phineas Gage – Unravelling the myth." *The Psychologist* 21(9), 828–831.

Malherbe, Michel. 2015. *Alzheimer. La vie, la mort, la reconnaissance: Une chronique et un essai philosophique.* Paris: Vrin.

Mallory, Michael. 2009. *Universal Studios Monsters: A Legacy of Horror.* New York: Universe Publishing.

Mank, Gregory William. 1981. *It's Alive! The Classic Cinema Saga of Frankenstein.* San Diego: A. S. Barnes.

Manning, Laurence. 1933. "The Man Who Awoke II: Master of the Brain." *Wonder Stories* 4(11), April, 838–849.

Marcus, Steven. 2002. "Frankenstein: Myths of Scientific and Medical Knowledge and Stories of Human Relations." *The Southern Review* 38: 188–201.

Marsen, Sky. 2004. "Against Heritage: Invented Identities in Science Fiction Film." *Semiotica* 152: 141–157.

Marsh, Calum. 2013. "Starship Troopers: One of the Most Misunderstood Movies Ever." *The Atlantic*, November 7. https://www.theatlantic.com/entertainment/archive/2013/11/-em-starship-troopers-em-one-of-the-most-misunderstood-movies-ever/281236/.

Mathijs, Ernest, and Jamie Sexton. 2011. *Cult Cinema: An Introduction.* Oxford: Wiley-Blackwell.

Mathijs, Ernest, and Xavier Mendik, eds. 2008. *The Cult Film Reader.* New York: Open University Press.

Matrix 2004: Matrix City: A Photographic Comparison of "The Matrix" and "Dark City." https://www.electrolund.com/2004/10/matrix-city-a-photographic-comparison-of-the-matrix-and-dark-city/.

McCarthy, Todd, and Flynn, Charles, eds. 1975. *Kings of the Bs. Working Within the Hollywood System: An Anthology of Film History and Criticism.* New York: Dutton.

McGowan, Todd. 2004. "Fighting Our Fantasies: *Dark City* and the Politics of Psychoanalysis." In T. McGowan and Sheila Kunkle, eds., *Lacan and Contemporary Film.* Other Press, New York), 145–172.

McGowan, Todd. 2011. *Out of Time: Desire in Atemporal Cinema.* Minneapolis: University of Minnesota Press.

McHale, Brian. 2008. "Revisiting Realisms; or WWJD (What Would Jakobson Do?)." *Journal of the Midwest Modern Language Association* 41(2): 6–17.

McHenry, F. Douglas. 1925. "The Seventh Devil." *Weird Tales* 6(5), November, 630–635.

McKay, Sinclair. 2007. *A Thing of Unspeakable Horror: The History of Hammer Films.* London: Aurum Press.

Meikle, Denis. 2009. *A History of Horrors: The Rise and Fall of the House of Hammer*, rev. ed. Plymouth, UK: Scarecrow Press.

Memba, Javier. 2006. *La serie B.* Madrid: T&B editores.

Mendelsohn, Avi, et al. 2009. "Subjective vs. Documented Reality: A Case Study of Long-Term Real-Life Autobiographical Memory." *Learning & Memory* 16: 142–146.

Mérigeau, Pascal, and Stéphane Bourgoin. 1983. *Série B.* Paris: Edilig.

Michaud, Nicolas, ed. 2013. *Frankenstein and Philosophy: The Shocking Truth.* Chicago: Open Court.

Morales Ruiz, Jorge. 2002. "Comparación de los filmes Dark City & The Matrix." www.quintadimension.com/article193.html.

Morgan, Bassett. 1926. "Laocoon." *Weird Tales* 8(1), July, 49–56.

Morgan, Bassett. 1927a. "The Head." *Weird Tales* 9(2), February, 233.240.

Morgan, Bassett. 1927b. "The Devils of Po Sung." *Weird Tales* 10(6), December, 775–788.

Morgan, Bassett. 1929. "Demon Doom of N'Yeng Sen." *Weird Tales* 14(2), August, 193–206.

Morgan, Daniel. 2013. *Late Godard and the Possibilities of Cinema.* Berkeley: University of California Press.

Morrison, Karen E. 1987. "Brain Transplantation: Still Fantasy? Discussion Paper." *Journal of the Royal Society of Medicine* 80: 441–444.

Mulkay, Michael. 1996. "Frankenstein and the Debate Over Embryo Research." *Science, Technology, & Human Values* 21: 157–176.

Mund, Edward S. 1935. "Brain Leeches." *Astounding Stories* 15(5), July, 109–118.

Münsterberg, Hugo. 2002 [1916]. *The Photoplay: A Psychological Study*. In *Hugo Munsterberg on Film: The Photoplay: A Psychological Study and Other Writings*, edited by Allan Langdale. New York: Routledge.

Murray, Robin L., and Joseph K. Heumann. 2009. *Ecology and Popular Film: Cinema on the Edge*. Albany: State University of New York Press.

Myers, Ray Avery. 1929. "Into the Subconscious." *Science Wonder Stories* 1(5), October, 426–435.

Nader, Karim, Glenn E. Schafe, and Joseph E. Le Doux. 2000. "Fear Memories Require Protein Synthesis in the Amygdala for Reconsolidation after Retrieval." *Nature* 40: 722–726.

Nagib, Lúcia, and Cecília Mello. 2009. "Introduction." In *Realism and the Audiovisual Media*, edited by Nagib and Mello, xiv–xxvi. New York: Palgrave Macmillan,

NAS 2017. *Communicating Science Effectively: A Research Agenda*. Washington, DC: The National Academies Press.

Neale, Steve. 2000. *Genre and Hollywood*. London: Routledge.

Nolan, Jonathan. 2001. "Memento Mori." *Esquire*, March 1. https://www.esquire.com/entertainment/books/a1564/memento-mori-0301/.

Northoff, Georg, and Nils-Frederic Wagner. 2017. "Personal Identity and Brain Identity." In *Routledge Handbook of Neuroethics*, edited by L. Syd M. Johnson and Karen S. Rommelfanger, 335–351. London: Routledge.

Nozick, Robert. 1981. *Philosophical Explanations*. Cambridge, MA: Harvard University Press.

Nungesser, Verena-Susanna. 2009. "I Forgot to Remember (to Forget): Personal Memories in *Memento* (2000) and *Eternal Sunshine of the Spotless Mind* (2004)." In *Mediation, Remediation, and the Dynamics of Cultural Memory*, edited by Astrid Erll and Ann Rigney, 31–47. Berlin: Walter de Gruyter.

O'Connor, Cliodhna, and Helene Joffe. 2013. "How Has Neuroscience Affected Lay Understandings of Personhood? A review of the evidence." *Public Understanding of Science* 22(3): 254–268.

O'Dell, Sarah. 2020. "'The Facts in the Case of M. Valdemar': Undead Bodies and Medical Technology." *Journal of Medical Humanities* 41, 229–242.

O'Flinn, Paul. 1986 [1983]. "Production and Reproduction: The Case of Frankenstein Peter Humm, Paul Stigant, and Peter Widdowson, eds., *Popular Fictions: Essays in Literature and History*. London, Methuen, 194–213. Originally published in *Literature and History* 9(2).

Olney, Ian. 2006. "Problem Body Politic, or 'These Hands Have a Mind All Their Own!' Figuring Disability in the Horror Film Adaptations of Renard's *Les mains d'Orlac*." *Literature/Film Quarterly* 34(4): 294–302.

Olsen, Bob. 1932. "The Ant with a Human Soul." *Amazing Stories Quarterly* 5(2), Spring–Summer, 230–263, 279.

Olsen, Bob. 1936. "The Isle of Juvenescence." *Amazing Stories* 10(10), June, 42–74.

Olson, Eric T. 2008. "Personal Identity." *Stanford Encyclopedia of Philosophy*, https://plato.stanford.edu/entries/identity-personal/.

Olster, Stacey. 2010. "Trash Fiction." In *A Companion to Twentieth-Century United States Fiction*, edited by David Seed, 195–206. Oxford: Wiley-Blackwell.

Ortega, Francisco and Fernando Vidal. 2013. "Brains in Literature/Literature in the Brain." *Poetics Today* 34: 327–360.

Papenburg, Bettina. 2011. *Das neue Fleisch. Der groteske Körper im Kino David Cronenbergs*. Bielefeld, transcript.

Parry, Bronwyn. 2004. "Technologies of Immortality: The Brain on Ice." *Studies in the History and Philosophy of Biology and Biomedical Sciences* 35: 391–413.
Patihis, Lawrence, et al. 2014. "Are the 'Memory Wars' Over? A Scientist-Practitioner Gap in Beliefs About Repressed Memory." *Psychological Science* 25(2): 519–530.
Pavlus, John. 2004. "Forget Me Not." *American Cinematographer: The International Journal of Digital Film & Production Techniques* 85(4): https://theasc.com/magazine/april04/cover/index.html.
Peacocke, Antonia, and Jackson Kernion. 2015. "Two Philosophers Explain What *Inside Out* Gets Wrong about the Mind." *Vox*, June 25. https://www.vox.com/2015/6/25/8840945/inside-out-mind-memory.
Pendick, Daniel. 2002. "Memory Loss at the Movies." *Memory Loss & the Brain* [Newsletter of the Memory Disorders Project at Rutgers University]. https://mskelly.weebly.com/uploads/3/5/3/4/353469/memory_loss_at_the_movies_-_memento.doc.
Peregoy, Calvin [pen name of Thomas Calvert McClary]. 1934. "Dr. Conklin – Pacifist." *Astounding Stories* 13(6), August, 34–44.
Perkins, Claire, and Constantine Verevis, eds. 2014. *B is for Bad Cinema: Aesthetics, Politics, and Cultural Value*. Albany: State University of New York Press.
Perkowitz, Sidney. 2007. *Hollywood Science: Movies, Science, and the End of the World*. New York: Columbia University Press.
Perry, John, ed. 1975. *Personal Identity*. Berkeley: University of California Press.
Petrounakos, Spyros. 2013. "Getting Inside the Monster's Head." In *Frankenstein and Philosophy*, edited by Michaud, 175–185.
Phelps, Elizabeth A., and Stefan G. Hofmann. 2019. "Memory Editing from Science Fiction to Clinical Practice." *Nature* 572: 43–50.
Phelps, Elizabeth A., and Tali Sharot. 2009. "How (and Why) Emotion Enhances the Subjective Sense of Recollection." *Current Directions in Psychological Science*, 17, 147–152.
Picart, Caroline Joan S. 2002. *The Cinematic Rebirths of Frankenstein: Universal, Hammer, and Beyond*. London: Praeger.
Pineles, Suzanne L., and Scott P. Orr. 2018. "The Psychophysiology of PTSD." In *Post-Traumatic Stress Disorder*, edited by Charles B. Nemeroff and Charles R. Marmar, 393–408. New York: Oxford University Press.
Pisters, Patricia. 2012. *The Neuro-Image: A Deleuzian Film-Philosophy of Digital Screen Culture*. Stanford: Stanford University Press.
Pitts, Michael R. 2011. *Allied Artists: Horror, Science Fiction and Fantasy Films*. Jefferson, NC: McFarland.
PMA: *The Pulp Magazine Archive*, https://archive.org/details/pulpmagazinearchive.
PMP: *The Pulp Magazines Project*, https://www.pulpmags.org/.
Poseck, Beatriz Vera. 2006. *Imágenes de la locura. La psicopatología en el cine*. Madrid: Calamar Ediciones.
Potter, Dennis. 1996. *Cold Lazarus*. In Potter, *Karaoke and Cold Lazarus*. London: Faber & Faber.
Prakash, Gyan, ed. 2010. *Noir Urbanisms: Dystopic Images of the Modern City*. Princeton, NJ: University Press, Princeton.
Pritchard, Duncan. 2012. "eXistenZial Angst." In *The Philosophy of David Cronenberg*, edited by Simon Riches, 69–76. Lexington, KY: The University Press of Kentucky.
Pritchard, Duncan. 2016. *Epistemology*, 2nd ed. London: Palgrave Macmillan.
Proust, Marcel. 1896. "In Praise of Bad Music." In Proust, *Pleasures and Days*, translated by Andrew Brown. Richmond, UK: Alma Classics, 2013.
Prucher, Jeff, ed. 2007. *Brave New Words: The Oxford Dictionary of Science Fiction*. New York: Oxford University Press.

Puccetti, Roland. 1969. "Brain Transplantation and Personal Identity." *Analysis* 29: 65–77.
Puccetti, Roland. 1972. *The Death of the Führer.* Greenwich, CT: Fawcett.
Putnam, Hilary. 1981. *Reason, Truth and History.* Cambridge, MA: Harvard University Press.
Quirk, Gregory J., and Mohammed R. Milad. 2010. "Neuroscience: Editing Out Fear." *Nature* 463: 36–37.
Radstone, Susannah. 2010. "Cinema and Memory." In *Memory: Histories, Theories, Debates*, edited by S. Radstone and Bill Schwartz, 325–342. New York: Fordham University Press.
Raynor, Diane (translator). 2004. *The Homeric Hymns.* Berkeley: University of California Press.
Reiner, Peter B. 2011. "The Rise of Neuroessentialism." In *The Oxford Handbook of Neuroethics*, edited by Judy Illes and Barbara Sahakian, 161–175. New York, Oxford University Press.
Reinerth, Maike Sarah. 2009. "Spulen, Speichern, Überspielen. Zur Darstellung von Erinnerung im Spielfielm." In *Probleme filmischen Erzählens*, edited by Hannah Birr, M. S. Reinerth and Jan-Noël Thon, 33–58. Berlin: Lit Verlag.
Reinerth, Maike Sarah. 2013. "It's Human Nature. Zur Darstellung der Psyche am Kino am Beispiel der Filme Michel Gondrys." In *Medialität und Menschenbild*, edited by Jens Eder, Joseph Imorde and M. S. Reinerth, 45–66. Berlin: W. de Gruyter.
Rémy, Catherine. 2014. "'Men Seeking Monkey-Glands': The Controversial Xenotransplantations of Doctor Voronoff, 1910–20." *French History* 28(2): 226–240.
Renard, Maurice. 1908. *Le Docteur Lerne, sous-dieu.* Paris: Mercure de France.
Renard, Maurice. 1920. *Les Mains d'Orlac.* Paris: Nilsson.
Repp, Ed Earl. 1935. "The Body Pirate." *Amazing Stories* 9(11), March, 121–134.
Rieder, John. 2017. *Science Fiction and the Mass Cultural Genre System.* Middletown, CT: Wesleyan University Press.
Roberts, Adam. 2016. *The History of Science Fiction*, 2nd ed. London: PalgraveMacmillan.
Rohrmoser, Andreas. http://frankensteinfilms.com/ [website].
Rose, Nikolas, and Joelle M. Abi-Rached. 2013. *Neuro: The New Brain Sciences and the Management of the Mind.* Princeton, NJ: Princeton University Press.
Roth, Marco. 2009. "The Rise of the Neuronovel." *N+1*: 8, https://nplusonemag.com/issue-8/essays/the-rise-of-the-neuronovel/.
Russell, Emily. 2019. *Transplant Fictions: A Cultural Study of Organ Exchange.* New York: Palgrave Macmillan.
Ryan, Jane. 2001. "Dark City." In *Jung & Film: Post-Jungian Takes on the Moving Image* edited by Christopher Hauke and Ian Alister, 95–109. Philadelphia, Brunner-Routledge.
Sacks, Oliver. 2007. "The Abyss: Music and Amnesia." *The New Yorker*, September 24. https://www.newyorker.com/magazine/2007/09/24/the-abyss.
Sanner, Margareta A. 2001. Exchanging Spare Parts or Becoming a New Person? People's Attitudes toward Receiving and Donating Organs." *Social Science & Medicine*, 52, 1491–1499.
Sanner, Margareta A. 2005. "Living with a Stranger's Organ – Views of the Public and Transplant Recipients." *Annals of Transplantation*, 10(1): 9–12.
Santing, Catrien, Barbara Baert, and Anita Traninger, eds., 2013. *Disembodied Heads in Medieval and Early Modern Culture.* Leiden, Brill.
Sara, Susan J. 2000. "Retrieval and reconsolidation: Toward a Neurobiology of Remembering." *Learning & Memory* 7: 73–84.
Sarlo, Beatriz. 1993. *Jorge Luis Borges. A Writer on the Edge.* London, Verso.
Sayre, Nora. 1974. "Andy Warhol s Frankenstein." *The New York Times*, May 16.
Schachner, Nat, and Arthur L. Zagat. 1930. "In 20,000 A.D.." *Wonder Stories* 2(4), September, 310–323.
Schall, Theo. 2015. "A Self-Identified Frankenstein." *Berman Institute Bioethics Bulletin*, June 19. http://bioethicsbulletin.org/archive/a-self-identified-frankenstein.

Schicktanz, Silke, and Sabine Wöhlke. 2017. "The Utterable and Unutterable: Anthropological Meaning of the Body in the Context of Organ Transplantation." *Ilemata* 9(23): 107–127.

Schiller, Daniela, et al. 2010. "Preventing the Return of Fear in Humans Using Reconsolidation Update Mechanisms." *Nature* 463: 49–53.

Schneider, Susan, ed. 2009. *Science Fiction and Philosophy: From Time Travel to Superintelligence*. Oxford, Wiley-Blackwell.

Schulze, Axel. 2012. *Platon und die "Matrix" der Wachowskis: Philosophie im Film?*. Hamburg, Diplomica Verlag.

Sconce, Jeffrey. 1995a. "Brains from Space: Mapping the Mind in 1950s Science and Cinema." *Science as Culture* 5: 277–302.

Sconce, Jeffrey. 1995b. "Trashing the Academy: Taste, Excess, and an Emerging Politics of Cinematic Style." *Screen* 36(4): 371–393. (Reprinted in Mathijs and Mendik 2007.)

Sconce, Jeffrey. 2000. *Haunted Media: Electronic Presence from Telegraphy to Television*. Durham, NC : Duke University Press

Sconce, Jeffrey. 2019. "The Golden Age of Badness." *Continuum* 33(6): 666–676.

Scoville, William Beecher, and Brenda Milner. 2000 [1957]. "Loss of Recent Memory after Bilateral Hippocampal Lesions." *Journal of Neuropsychiatry and Clinical Neuroscience* 12: 103–113. Originally published in *Journal of Neurology, Neurosurgery and Psychiatry* 20 (1957): 11–21.

Seamon, John. 2015. *Memory and Movies: What Films Can Teach Us about Memory*. Cambridge, MA: MIT Press.

Seed, David. 2004. *Brainwashing: The Fictions of Mind Control: A Study of Novels and Films since World War II*. Kent, OH: Kent State University Press.

Seel, Martin. 2008. "Realism and Anti-Realism in Film Theory." *Critical Horizons: A Journal of Philosophy and Social Theory* 9(2): 157–175.

Sélavy, Virginie. 2018. "Fantastique: The Dream Worlds of French Cinema." *Sight & Sound* 28(11): November. https://www.bfi.org.uk/news-opinion/sight-sound-magazine/features/deep-focus/fantastique-dream-worlds-french-cinema.

Senn, Bryan, and John Johnson. 1992. *Fantastic Cinema Subject Guide: A Topical Index to 2500 Horror, Science Fiction, and Fantasy Films*. Jefferson, NC: McFarland.

Sharf, Zack. 2017. "'Get Out': Jordan Peele Reveals the Real Meaning Behind the Sunken Place." *IndieWire*, November 30. https://www.indiewire.com/2017/11/get-out-jordan-peele-explains-sunken-place-meaning-1201902567/.

Shelley, Mary Wollstonecraft. 1831. *Frankenstein; or, the Modern Prometheus*, 2nd ed. London: Henry Colburn and Richard Bentley. Accessed via https://archive.org.

Shema, Reut, et al. 2009. "Boundary Conditions for the Maintenance of Memory by PKMζ in Neocortex." *Learning & Memory* 16: 122–128.

Shema, Reut, Sacktor, Todd Charlton and Dudai, Yadin. 2007. "Rapid Erasure of Long-Term Memory Associations in the Cortex by an Inhibitor of PKMζ." *Science* 317: 951–953.

Shoemaker, Sidney. 1963. *Self-Knowledge and Self-Identity*. Ithaca, NY: Cornell University Press.

Sinnerbrink, Robert. 2011. *New Philosophies of Film: Thinking Images*. London: Continuum.

Sinnerbrink, Robert. 2016. *Cinematic Ethics: Exploring Ethical Experience Through Film*. New York: Routledge.

Sinnerbrink, Robert, and Lisa Trahair. 2016. "Introduction: Film and / as Ethics." *SubStance* 45(3): 3–15.

Siodmak, Curt. 1942. *Donovan's Brain*. London, Tandem, 1972.

Skal, David J. 1993. *The Monster Show: A Cultural History of Horror*. London: Plexus.

Skal, David J. 1998. *Screams of Reason: Mad Science and Modern Culture*. New York, W. W. Norton.

Smith, Basil. 2007. "John Locke, Personal Identity, and Memento." In *The Philosophy of Neo-Noir*, edited by Mark T. Conard. Lexington, KY: University Press of Kentucky. E-book.

Smith, Murray. 2006. "Film Art, Argument, and Ambiguity." In *Thinking Through Cinema*, edited by Smith and Wartenberg, 33–42.

Smith, Murray, and Thomas E. Wartenberg, eds. 2006. *Thinking Through Cinema: Film as Philosophy*. Oxford: Blackwell.

Smith, Roger. 2019. "Resisting Neurosciences and Sustaining History." *History of the Human Sciences* 32(1): 9–22.

Sobchack, Vivian. 1999. "Cities on the Edge of Time: the Urban Science-Fiction Film." In *Alien Zone II*, edited by Kuhn, 123–143.

Sperry, Roger W. 1964. "The Great Cerebral Commissure." *Scientific American* 210(1): 42–53.

Springer, Claudia. 1999 "Psycho-Cybernetics in Films of the 1990s." In *Alien Zone II*, edited by Kuhn, 203–218.

St-Germain, Philippe. 2015. *L'imaginaire de la greffe. Le même et l'autre dans la peau*. Montreal, Liber.

Stableford, Brian. 2006. "Neurology." In Stableford, *Science Fact and Science Fiction: An Encyclopedia*, 329–330. New York: Routledge.

Staiger, Janet. 1999. "Future Noir: Contemporary Representations of Visionary Cities." In *Alien Zone II*, edited by Kuhn, 97–122.

Stam, Robert, Robert Burgoyne, and Sandy Flitterman-Lewis. 1992. *New Vocabularies in Film Semiotics: Structuralism, Post-Structuralism and Beyond*. New York: Routledge.

Stapledon, Olaf. 1937. *Star Maker*. E-book.

Starobinski, Jean. 1989 [1981]. "A Short History of Bodily Sensation." In *Fragments for a History of the Human Body*, edited by Michel Feher, 352–370. New York: Zone. Translated by Sarah Matthews.

Stein, Rob. 2004. "Is Every Memory Worth Keeping? Pills to Reduce Mental Trauma Raise Controversy." *The Washington Post*, October 19. https://www.washingtonpost.com/wp-dyn/articles/A43210-2004Oct18.html?.

Steinhart, Eric. 2001. "Persons Versus Brains: Biological Intelligence in Human Organisms." *Biology and Philosophy* 16: 3–27.

Sternberg, Esther M. 2001. "Piecing Together a Puzzling World" [review of *Memento*]. *Science* 292: 1661–1662.

Stevens, Scott Manning. 1997. "Sacred Heart and Secular Brain." In *The Body in Parts: Fantasies of Corporeality in Early Modern Europe*, edited by David Hillman and Carla Mazzio, 263–282. New York, Routledge.

Storm, Benjamin C., Elizabeth Ligon Bjork, and Robert A. Bjork. 2008. "Accelerated Relearning after Retrieval-Induced Forgetting: The Benefit of Being Forgotten." *Journal of Experimental Psychology: Learning, Memory, and Cognition* 34: 230–236.

Sutherland, John. 1998. "How Does Victor Make his Monsters?" In Sutherland, *Is Heathcliff a Murderer? Great Puzzles in Nineteenth-Century Fiction*, 24–34. New York: Oxford University Press.

Tarkovsky, Andrey. 1986. *Sculpting in Time: Reflections on the Cinema*. Translated by Kitty Hunter-Blair. London: Faber and Faber.

Taylor, Charles. 1989. *Sources of the Self: The Making of the Modern Identity*. Cambridge, MA; Harvard University Press.

Telotte, J. P. 2001. "Lost Memory and New Noir." *Paradoxa* 16: 177–189.

Telotte, J. P. 2019. *Movies, Modernism, and the Science Fiction Pulps*. New York: Oxford University Press.

Teo, Yugin. 2013. "Love, Longing and Danger: Memory and Forgetting in Early Twenty-First-Century SF Films." *Science Fiction Film and Television* 6(3): 349–368.

Terrone, Enrico. 2017. "Blessed Are the Forgetful: Utilitarianism and Remarriage in *Eternal Sunshine of the Spotless Mind*." *Film and Philosophy* 21: 74–90.

Tesson, Charles. 1997. *Photogénie de la série B*. Paris; Cahiers du Cinéma.

Thiel, Udo. 2011. *The Early Modern Subject: Self-consciousness and Personal Identity from Descartes to Hume*. New York: Oxford University Press.

Thomson-Jones, Katherine. 2008. *Aesthetics and Film*. London; Continuum.

Thomson, Helen. 2015. "First Human Head Transplant Could Happen in Two Years." *New Scientist*, no. 3010, February 25, https://www.newscientist.com/article/mg22530103-700-first-human-head-transplant-could-happen-in-two-years/.

Tiehen, Jeanne. 2014. "Frankenstein Performed: The Monster Who Will Not Die." *The Popular Culture Studies Journal* 2(1–2): 65–86.

Tooker, Richard. 1935. "Moon of Arcturus." *Amazing Stories* 10(3), June, 41–68.

Topps [The Topps Company]. 2012. *Mars Attacks. 50th Anniversary Collection*. New York, Abrams.

Tougaw, Jason. 2012. "Brain Memoirs, Neuroscience, and the Self: A Review Article." *Literature and Medicine* 30(1): 171–192.

Tougaw, Jason. 2016. "Amnesia and Identity in Contemporary Literature." In *Memory in the Twenty-First Century: New Critical Perspectives from the Arts, Humanities, and Sciences*, edited by Sebastian Groes, 280–285. New York: Palgrave Macmillan.

Towlson, Jon. 2014. *Subversive Horror Cinema: Countercultural Messages of Films from Frankenstein to the Present*. Jefferson, NC: McFarland.

Trench, Brian. 2008. "Towards an Analytical Framework of Science Communication Models." In *Communicating Science in Social Contexts: New Models, New Practices*, edited by Donghong Cheng et al., 119–135. Dordrecht: Springer.

Tritsch, Danièle and Jean Mariani. 2018. *Ça va pas la tête ! Cerveau, immortalité et intelligence artificielle, l'imposture du transhumanisme*. Paris: Belin.

Tronson, Natalie C., et al. 2006. "Bidirectional Behavioral Plasticity of Memory Reconsolidation Depends on Amygdalar Protein Kinase A." *Nature Neuroscience* 9: 167–169.

Tryon, Charles. 2003. "Virtual Cities and Stolen Memories: Temporality and the Digital in Dark City." *Film Criticism* 28: 42–62.

Tuck, Donald H. 1982. *The Encyclopedia of Science Fiction and Fantasy Through 1968*, vol. 3. Chicago: Advent Publishers.

Tudor, Andrew. 1989. *Monsters and Mad Scientists: A Cultural History of the Horror Movie*. Oxford: Basil Blackwell.

Tudor, Andrew. 1995. "Unruly Bodies, Unquiet Minds." *Body & Society* 1(1): 25–41.

Turney, Jon. 1998. *Frankenstein's Footsteps: Science, Genetics, and Popular Culture*. New Haven, CT: Yale University Press.

Tybjerg, Casper. 2004. "Shadow-Souls and Strange Adventures: Horror and the Supernatural in European Silent Film." In *The Horror Film*, edited by Stephen Prince, 15–39. New Brunswick, NJ: Rutgers University Press.

Tymn, Marshall B., and Mike Ashley. 1985. *Science Fiction, Fantasy, and Weird Fiction Magazines*. London: Greenwood Press.

Updike, John. 2004. "Mind/Body Matters." *The New Yorker*, January 26. https://www.newyorker.com/magazine/2004/01/26/mindbody-problems.

Valenstein, Elliott S. 1973. *Brain Control: A Critical Examination of Brain Stimulation and Psychosurgery*. New York, Wiley.

van Dijck, José. 2009. "Mediated Memories as Amalgamations of Mind, Matter and Culture." In *The Body Within: Art, Medicine and Visualization*, edited by Renée van de Vall and Robert Zwijnenberg, 157–172. Leiden: Brill.

Van Reybrouck, David. 2008. *Le Fléau*. Translated by Pierre-Marie Finkelstein. Paris: Actes Sud.

Varga, Somogy, and Charles Guignon. 2014. "Authenticity." *Stanford Encyclopedia of Philosophy*, https://plato.stanford.edu/archives/fall2014/entries/authenticity/.

Vernallis, Carol. 2013. "Music Video, Songs, Sound: *Eternal Sunshine of the Spotless Mind*." In Vernallis, *Unruly Media: YouTube, Music Video, and the New Digital Cinema*. New York, Oxford University Press. DOI: 10.1093/acprof:oso/9780199766994.001.0001.

Vidal, Fernando. 2002. "Brains, Bodies, Selves, and Science: Anthropologies of Identity and the Resurrection of the Body." *Critical Inquiry* 28(4): 930–974.

Vidal, Fernando. 2009. "Brainhood, Anthropological Figure of Modernity." *History of the Human Sciences* 22(1): 5–36.

Vidal, Fernando. 2011. *The Sciences of the Soul: The Early Modern Origins of Psychology*. Translated by Sasha Brown. Chicago: University of Chicago Press.

Vidal, Fernando. 2018. "Accuracy, Authenticity, Fidelity: Aesthetic Realism, the 'Deficit Model,' and the Public Understanding of Science." *Science in Context* 31(1): 129–153.

Vidal, Fernando. 2020. "Jean Starobinski: The History of Medicine and the Reasons of the Body." *Mefisto. Rivista di medicina, filosofia, storia* 4(2): 1–24.

Vidal, Fernando, and Francisco Ortega. 2017. *Being Brains: Making the Cerebral Subject*. New York: Fordham University Press.

Vincent, Harl. 1929a. "The Menace from Below." *Science Wonder Stories* 1(2), July, 142–169.

Vincent, Harl. 1929b. "Microcosmic Buccanners." *Amazing Stories* 4(8), November, 678–695.

Vincent, Harl. 1931. "A Matter of Ethics." *Amazing Stories* 6(7), October, 650–655.

Vincent, Harl. 1934. "Master of Dreams." *Amazing Stories* 8(9), January, 37–65.

Vincent, Harl. 1935. "Parasite." *Amazing Stories* 10(4), July, 71–107.

Vrselja, Zvonimir, et al. 2019. "Restoration of Brain Circulation and Cellular Functions Hours Post-mortem." *Nature* 568: 336–343.

Wallace, Chris. 2014. [Interview with David Cronenberg], *Interview*, October 15. https://www.interviewmagazine.com/film/david-cronenberg.

Warren, Bill. 2010. *Keep Watching the Skies! American Science Fiction Movies of the Fifties*: *"The 21st century Edition"*. Jefferson: NC, McFarland.

Wartenberg, Thomas E. 2007. *Thinking on Screen: Film as Philosophy*. London: Routledge.

Wartenberg, Thomas E. 2009. "Film as Philosophy." In *The Routledge Companion to Philosophy and Film*, edited by Livingston and Plantinga, 549–599.

Wartenberg, Thomas E. 2016. "Film As Philosophy: The Pro Position." In *Current Controversies in Philosophy of Film*, edited by Katherine Thomson-Jones. New York, Routledge. E-book.

Wass, Janne. n.d. *Scifist*. A blog of extensive reviews of science fiction movies since 1890: https://scifist.net/. Commentaries of films from 1950 to 1959 are still temporarily located in the older website, https://scifist.wordpress.com/.

Wass, Janne. 2016. "Donovan's Brain." Posted February 15. https://scifist.wordpress.com/2016/02/15/donovans-brain/.

Watts, Philip. 2016. *Roland Barthes' Cinema*. New York: Oxford University Press.

Weaver, Tom, Brunas, Michael and Brunas, John. 2007. *Universal Horrors: The Studio's Classic Films, 1931–1946*, 2nd ed. Jefferson, NC: McFarland.

Webling, Peggy. 1927. *Frankenstein. A Play in a Prologue and Three Acts* (*Based Upon Mrs Shelley's Well Known Book*). Typescript. Reel 2828, Registration No. D86282, deposited September 7, 1928. Library of Congress, Washington, DC.

Wells, H. G. 2017 [1901]. *The First Men in the Moon*, edited by Simon J. James. Oxford: Oxford University Press.

Wells, Hal K. 1932. "Zehru of Xollar." *Astounding Stories* 9(2), February, 264–278.

Wells, Hal K. 1933. "The Purple Brain." *Astounding Stories* 12(4), December, 57–69.

White, Robert J. 1999. "Head Transplants." *Scientific American Presents, Your Bionic Future: How Technology Will Change the Way You Live in the Next Millennium*, special issue 10(3): 24–26.
WHO. 2012. *Dementia: A Public Health Priority* (World Health Organization and Alzheimer's Disease International), https://www.who.int/mental_health/publications/dementia_report_2012/en/.
Wiebel, Frederick C. 1997. "Edison's *Frankenstein*." In *We Belong Dead: Frankenstein on Film*, edited by Gary J. Svehla and Susan Svehla, 19–27. Baltimore: Midnight Marquee Press.
Wilkes, Kathleen. 1988. *Real People: Personal Identity Without Thought Experiments*. Oxford, Clarendon Press.
Williamson, Jack. 1932. "The Pygmy Planet." *Astounding Stories* 9(2), February, 151–167.
Williamson, Jack. 1933. "Terror Out of Time." *Astounding Stories* 12(4), December, 116–130.
Wilson, D. Harlan. 2005. "The Pathological Machine: Dark City's Translation of Schreber's Memoirs." *Journal of the Fantastic in the Arts* 15: 153–164.
Wilson, Eric G. 2006. "Gnostic Paranoia in Proyas's 'Dark City,'" *Literature/Film Quarterly* 34(3): 232–239.
Wolpe, Paul Root. 2010. "Review of James Cameron's *Avatar*." *AJOB Neuroscience* 1(2): 72–74.
Wood, Alex Matthew, et al. 2008. "The Authentic Personality: A Theoretical and Empirical Conceptualization and the Development of the Authenticity Scale." *Journal of Counseling Psychology*, 55(3): 385–399.
Yaszek, Lisa, and Patrick B. Sharp, eds., *Sisters of Tomorrow: The First Women of Science Fiction*. Middletown, CT: Wesleyan University Press 2016.
Zahavi, Dan. 2014. *Self and Other: Exploring Subjectivity, Empathy, and Shame*. Oxford: Oxford University Press.
Zimmermann, Tanja et al. 2016. Differences in Emotional Responses in Living and Deceased Donor Kidney Transplant Patients." *Clinical Kidney Journal*, 9(3): 503–509.
Žižek, Slavoj. 2001. "John Woo as a Critic of Levinas: The Face as a Fetish." In Žižek, *Did Somebody Say Totalitarianism: Five Interventions in the (Mis)use of a Notion*, 182–189. London, Verso.

Films

In alphabetical order (with articles placed at the end of titles), followed by the director's name. See below for Frankenstein productions. Numbers after each item refer to pages in this book.

Strange Days. Kathryn Bigelow. USA, 1995. 181, 192.
They Saved Hitler's Brain. David Bradley. USA, 1968. 111, 112.
Thing That Couldn't Die (The). Will Cowan. USA, 1958. 111.
Thing With Two Heads (The). Lee Frost. USA, 1972. 105, 116, 129.
This Island Earth. Joseph M. Newman, Jack Arnold. USA, 1955. 85, 123.
2001: Space Odyssey. Stanley Kubrick. UK/USA, 1968. 222.
Todo sobre mi madre (All About My Mother). Pedro Almodóvar. Spain/France, 1999. 100.
To Serve Man. Richard L. Bare. USA, 1962. *The Twilight Zone,* TV series (1959–1964), Season 3, Episode 24. 123.
Total Recall. Paul Verhoeven. USA, 1990. 181, 186–87, 193, 196, 199, 216.
Transcendence. Wally Pfister. USA, 2014. 223.
Vérité sur l'homme-singe (La) (The Truth Behind the Ape-Man). Alice Guy. France, 1906. 28.
Videodrome. David Cronenberg. Canada, 1983. 104.
Walking Dead (The). Developed by Frank Darabont. TV series. USA, since 2010. 30.
Warm Bodies. Jonathan Levine. USA, 2013. 30.
Watermelon Man. Melvin Van Peebles. USA, 1970. 145–46.
Who is Julia? Walter Grauman. USA, 1986. 116–17.
William and Mary. Marc Daniels. USA, 1961. *Way Out,* TV Series (1961), Episode 1. 50.
William and Mary. Donald McWhinnie. UK, 1979. *Tales of the Unexpected,* TV Series (1979–1988), Season 1, Episode 3. 50.
Yeux sans visage (Les) (The Horror Chamber of Dr. Faustus, literally *The Eyes Without a Face).* Georges Franju. France/Italy, 1960. 102–03.

Frankenstein Films. In chronological order within each section.

Universal Pictures (USA)

Frankenstein. 1931. James Whale. 28, 29, 94, 113, 138, 157, 159–165, 211.
The Bride of Frankenstein. 1935. James Whale. 165.
Son of Frankenstein. 1939. Rowland V. Lee. 165, 167.
The Ghost of Frankenstein. 1942. Erle C. Kenton. 165, 176.
Frankenstein Meets the Wolf Man. 1943. Roy William Neill. 165.
House of Frankenstein. 1944. Erle C. Kenton. 166–67.
Abbott and Costello Meet Frankenstein. 1948. Charles Barton. 167.

Hammer Film Productions (UK)

The Curse of Frankenstein. 1957. Terence Fisher. 167, 168–169.
The Revenge of Frankenstein. 1958. Terence Fisher. 159, 169.
The Evil of Frankenstein. 1964. Freddie Francis. 169–70.
Frankenstein Created Woman. 1967. Terence Fisher. 165.
Frankenstein Must Be Destroyed. 1969. Terence Fisher. 170, 176, 223.
The Horror of Frankenstein. 1970. Jimmy Sangster. 158, 170.
Frankenstein and the Monster from Hell. 1973. Terence Fisher. 170–71.

Other Frankenstein Movies

Frankenstein. J. Searle Dawley. USA, 1910. 159, 175.
Frankenstein. Don Medford. USA, 1952. *Tales of Tomorrow* (1951–1953), TV series, Season 1, Episode 16 (18 January). 158.
Teenage Frankenstein, a.k.a. *I Was a Teenage Frankenstein*. Herbert L. Strock. USA, 1957. 176.
Frankenstein 1970. Howard W. Koch. USA, 1958. 173.
Frankenstein's Daughter. Richard Cunha. USA, 1958. 173.
Lady Frankenstein (*La Figlia di Frankenstein*). Mel Welles. Italy, 1971. 117, 173.
Frankenstein '80. Mario Mancini. Italy/West Germany, 1972. 173.
Flesh for Frankenstein, a.k.a. *Andy Warhol's Frankenstein*. Paul Morrissey. Italy/France, 1973. 173–74.
Terror! Il castello delle donne maledette (*Frankenstein's Castle of Freaks*). Robert H. Oliver. Italy, 1973. 173.
Frankenstein: The True Story. TV film. Jack Smight. UK, 1973. 159, 174.
Young Frankenstein. Mel Brooks. USA, 1974. 157.
The Rocky Horror Picture Show. Jim Sharman. UK, 1975. 172.
Frankenstein 90. Alain Jessua. France, 1984. 174–75.
Frankenstein 2000 – Ritorno dalla Morte (*Frankenstein 2000 – Return from Death*). Joe D'Amato (as David Hills). Italy, 1991. 174.
Frankenstein. Cable TV film. David Wickes. UK, 1992. 175.
Mary Shelley's Frankenstein. Kenneth Branagh. UK/USA, 1994. 174, 177.
Mistress Frankenstein. John Bacchus. USA, 2000. 174.
Frankenstein. Kevin Connor. TV miniseries. USA, 2004. 159.
Frankenstein. TV film. Jed Mercurio. UK, 2007. 175.
Frankenweenie. Tim Burton. USA, 2012. 172.

Index

References to movies are given in the Films list (pp. 249–54).
References to individuals are highly selective.

For Product Safety Concerns and Information please contact our EU
representative GPSR@taylorandfrancis.com
Taylor & Francis Verlag GmbH, Kaufingerstraße 24, 80331 München, Germany

www.ingramcontent.com/pod-product-compliance
Ingram Content Group UK Ltd.
Pitfield, Milton Keynes, MK11 3LW, UK
UKHW020010200926
475702UK00014B/1812
9781041184027